This book is du

Nutrition and Health

Adrianne Bendich, PhD, FASN, FACN, Series Editor

For further volumes:
http://www.springer.com/series/7659

Mandy L. Corrigan · Arlene A. Escuro
Donald F. Kirby

Editors

Handbook of Clinical
Nutrition and Stroke

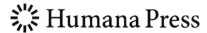 Humana Press

Editors
Mandy L. Corrigan, MPH, RD, LD, CNSC
Nutrition Support Team
Cleveland Clinic
Cleveland, OH, USA

Arlene A. Escuro, MS, RD, LD, CNSC
Nutrition Therapy
Cleveland Clinic
Cleveland, OH, USA

Donald F. Kirby, MD, FACP, FACN, FACG,
  AGAF, CNSC, CPNS
Center for Human Nutrition
Department of Gastroenterology
Cleveland Clinic
Cleveland, OH, USA

ISBN 978-1-62703-379-4   ISBN 978-1-62703-380-0 (eBook)
DOI 10.1007/978-1-62703-380-0
Springer New York Heidelberg Dordrecht London

Library of Congress Control Number: 2013932865

Printed on acid-free paper

Humana Press is a brand of Springer
Springer is part of Springer Science+Business Media (www.springer.com)

*To my husband, Adam, thank you for all your
support and unconditional love.
To my son Max with all my love.*
                                    –Mandy L. Corrigan

*To my husband, Ed, thank you for your
patience, support, and love.*
                                    –Arlene A. Escuro

*Dedicated to my wonderful family,
Debra, Ran, and Sydney.*
                                    –Donald F. Kirby

Foreword

Stroke is the fourth leading cause of death in America and the second-leading cause of death worldwide. It occurs more often in women than men, with African Americans having almost twice the risk of first-ever stroke compared with Caucasians. Stroke is a leading cause of adult disability. Aside from the short-term and long-term disability to the individual, the estimated direct and indirect financial costs of stroke to society are staggering. Unless there are changes in diet and lifestyle, it is likely that there will be increases in the occurrence of stroke due to the prevalence of nutritional and lifestyle risk factors associated with urbanization and the Western-style diet.

Despite the prevalence and seriousness of the disease, little attention has been given to the nutritional aspects of stroke, until now. The Handbook of Clinical Nutrition and Stoke is edited by Mandy L. Corrigan, M.P.H., R.D., L.D., C.N.S.C., Arlene A. Escuro, M.S., R.D., L.D., C.N.S.C. and Donald F. Kirby, M.D., F.A.C.P., F.A.C.N., F.A.C.G., A.G.A.F., C.N.S.C., C.P.N.S. from Cleveland Clinic. They are well known for their work in nutrition. This book is a comprehensive reference on nutrition for the multidisciplinary team caring for stroke patients. It includes a total of 19 chapters covering a range of topics relevant to stroke and nutrition. The first section of the book provides an overview of stroke including epidemiology, types of stroke, risk factors, and global trends. A review of malnutrition in stroke is also included in this section and introduces the reader to the concept of the development of malnutrition following stroke.

There are certain risk factors such as age, family history, gender, and race which are beyond our control. Yet, up to 80 % of strokes are preventable. With appropriate lifestyle and medical changes, the risk for stroke can be reduced. Part 2 of the book covers prevention and includes recommendations for lifestyle changes in the face of diabetes, hypertension, dyslipidemia, and obesity, all of which are amenable to diet, exercise, and medical interventions.

Although stroke occurs most often in adults, it can occur any time throughout the lifespan. Part 2 addresses the specific nutrition issues of stroke in pediatrics and adolescence up through adulthood. This is an important section as nutritional management of the pediatric stroke patient requires knowledge of age-specific nutritional requirements, as well as normal and disease-specific growth and development considerations. For the adult population, the etiology of stroke is diversified and correctly identifying underlying causes for stroke is essential for determination of effective treatment.

Part 3 expands on the treatment and management of these patients from the acute care setting though rehabilitation. The authors address the entire scope of nutrition interventions from the use of parenteral nutrition, enteral tube feeding placement, enteral formulas, unique nutrient requirements, oral dysphagia diets, and transitional feedings toward a goal of achievement of nutritional autonomy.

Complex issues surrounding rehabilitation, ethics, and community resources are addressed in the final chapters of this book. The text will be a valuable practical reference for all practitioners caring for patients with stroke. It fills a void in books that provide practical, comprehensive information on this complex patient population.

Greenville, NC, USA

Laura E. Matarese, PhD, RD, LDN,
FADA, FASPEN, CNSC
Associate Professor
Department of Internal Medicine
Division of Gastroenterology
Hepatology and Nutrition
Brody School of Medicine and
Department of Nutrition Science
East Carolina University
Greenville, NC, USA

Preface

This Handbook of Clinical Nutrition and Stroke is intended to serve as a comprehensive reference on nutrition for the multidisciplinary team caring for stroke patients. Our aim is for this handbook to provide practical information to clinicians working with the stroke population as well as the most up to date, evidence-based information currently available. Until this book was published, there was a gap in publications that provide comprehensive information on this population and specifically the area of nutrition support.

The book provides an introduction on the different types of stroke, associated risk factors, and uniquely feature global perspectives on stroke. In addition to discussing stroke risk factors, the treatment and management from the acute care setting though rehabilitation is outlined. We further capture the lifespan of patients affected by stroke (pediatric, younger adults, and older adults), and address prevention (from both nutritional and medical factors). Progression of the nutrition care plan is fully discussed from enteral tube feeding placement, enteral tube feedings, parenteral nutrition, unique nutrient requirements, oral dysphagia diets, and transitional feedings as patients regain their nutritional autonomy.

The authors were selected based on their areas of expertise with stroke patients. The dedication and expertise of the many contributing authors made this publication possible.

I would like to extend my sincere gratitude to Adrianne Bendich, Ph.D. and Humana Press for making the vision for this publication a reality.

Cleveland, OH, USA   Mandy L. Corrigan

Series Editor Page

The great success of the Nutrition and Health Series is the result of the consistent overriding mission of providing health professionals with texts that are essential because each includes: (1) a synthesis of the state of the science and relevant clinical applications, (2) timely, in-depth reviews by the leading researchers in their respective fields, (3) extensive, up-to-date fully annotated reference lists, (4) a detailed index, (5) relevant tables and figures, (6) identification of paradigm shifts and the consequences, (7) virtually no overt overlap of information between chapters, but targeted, inter-chapter referrals, (8) suggestions of areas for future research and (9) balanced, data-driven answers to patient as well as health professionals questions which are based upon the totality of evidence rather than the findings of any single study.

The Series volumes are not the outcome of a symposium. Rather, each editor has the potential to examine a chosen area with a broad perspective, both in subject matter as well as in the choice of chapter authors. The editor(s), whose training(s) is (are) both research and practice oriented, have the opportunity to develop a primary objective for their book, define the scope and focus, and then invite the leading authorities to be part of their initiative. The authors are encouraged to provide an overview of the field, discuss their own research and relate the research findings to potential human health consequences. Because each book is developed de novo, the chapters are coordinated so that the resulting volume imparts greater knowledge than the sum of the information contained in the individual chapters.

"Handbook of Clinical Nutrition and Stroke" edited by Mandy L. Corrigan, M.P.H., R.D., L.D., C.N.S.C., Arlene A. Escuro, M.S., R.D., L.D., C.N.S.C. and Donald F. Kirby, M.D., F.A.C.P., F.A.C.N., F.A.C.G., A.G.A.F., C.N.S.C., C.P.N.S. clearly exemplifies the goals of the Nutrition and Health Series. The major objective of this comprehensive text is to provide the multidisciplinary team of health professionals involved in the treatment of acute as well as the long-term care of stroke patients with up-to-date information on the nutritional aspects of care. This volume includes 19 informative review chapters that describe the current major dietary and health-related issues seen in the stroke patient and includes chapters that examine the complexities of stroke in the neonate and compare these to the effects of stroke through the other times of the life cycle. Stroke is a leading cause of significant disabilities that often impact the ability to eat and swallow food, and digest food optimally. Practicing health professionals, researchers, and academicians can rely on the chapters in this volume for objective data-driven overviews of nutritional concerns that affect the stroke patient whether the patient is a child, teen, young adult, or mature adult. This new comprehensive review of the science behind the nutritional strategies to undertake with the stroke patient is of great importance to the nutrition community as well as for health professionals who have to answer patient, client or family member questions about the newest clinical standards of practice and research on nutrition's role in maintaining the health and welfare of the stroke patient.

"Handbook of Clinical Nutrition and Stroke" begins with in-depth chapters that review the prevalence, types of strokes, risk factors, and long-term consequences of stroke. Transient ischemic attacks (TIA) are discussed as these can be precursors of stroke. Silent strokes or silent brain infarcts are included in discussions of diagnostic tests and clinically relevant findings. The first chapters, containing excellent tables and figures, provide overviews of the epidemiology of stroke that remind us that stroke is the leading cause of disability as well as the fourth leading cause of death in the US and is actually the second leading cause of death worldwide. The authors describe the three types and prevalence of strokes: 87 % are ischemic, 10 % are hemorrhagic strokes, and 3 % are subarachnoid hemorrhagic strokes. Major survey studies are reviewed including the REasons for Geographic and Racial Differences in Stroke (REGARDS) study and the INTERSTROKE study of global stroke rates. The studies documented five risk factors that accounted for more than 80 % of the global risk of all stroke: hypertension, current smoking, abdominal obesity, diet, and physical activity. An additional five factors increase the risk of stroke to 90 %: excessive alcohol consumption, dyslipidemia, cardiac causes, and psychosocial stress/depression. Thus, dietary factors that are modifiable may be able to reduce the risk of stroke by a considerable proportion.

In order to better understand the effects of stroke, the next chapter on the types of stroke includes a detailed description of the brain and its blood supply as well as the functions of different brain areas. Consequences of ischemic and hemorrhagic stroke are provided in detailed descriptions of brain functions that are affected by either the loss of blood or the exposure to blood following the hemorrhagic stroke. This chapter is especially valuable to health professionals who converse with patients and family members who request specific information about the brain areas affected and the clinical manifestations of the particular type of stroke. The importance of understanding the neuroanatomy and cerebral vascular anatomy of the brain are made clear in this well-illustrated chapter.

Critical risk factors for stroke are outlined in the next chapter that describes these in three categories: situational risk factors that are generally nonmodifiable, medical risk factors, and lifestyle risk factors that are both potentially modifiable and include dietary intake and nutritional considerations. Age is one of the most important nonmodifiable situational risk factors. For every 10 years after the age of 55 years, the stroke rate doubles. More than half of all strokes occur in people over age 75 and more than 80 % of strokes occur in ages over age 65. Other nonmodifiable factors include, but are not limited to the sex of the patient, family history, genetic predisposition especially in young stroke victims, and being African American, Lifestyle risk factors that increase risk include lack of physical activity, obesity, diabetes, smoking, use of unlawful drugs, few fruits and vegetables in the daily diet, and higher than recommended alcohol consumption. Related to these increased risk factors are the medical risk factors that may be a consequence of the lifestyle choices of patients. Hypertension is the major medical risk factor associated with stroke. Atrial fibrillation is another serious risk factor. Treatments such as aspirin and anticoagulants have been shown to lower stroke risks in patients with these chronic cardiovascular conditions. Diabetes, dyslipidemia, depression, and sleep apnea are also discussed in this informative chapter.

The fourth chapter in the introductory section provides references to the newest standards of care for the stroke patient. The role of antiplatelet agents like aspirin, clopidogrel, and dipyridamole in primary stroke prevention are reviewed as are their uses in secondary prevention. Recombinant tissue plasminogen activator, which is currently the mainstay therapy for acute ischemic stroke, is described. In fact, if it is administered in the first 4.5 h after stroke onset, it may result in significant benefits to the patient. The chapter cites the recommendations of the American Heart Association that for large artery occlusion strokes, it recommends using intra-arterial fibrinolytic therapy in the first 3–6 h window after stroke. The recent advances in the interventional management of acute strokes and new ways to mechanically disrupt blood clots and/or retrieve them from the arteries are reviewed for the reader.

The second section contains five chapters that describe the major chronic diseases that significantly increase the risk of stroke. Also included are unique chapters that review the unexpected event of a stroke in children and adolescents and provides comparisons between stroke effects in younger compared to older adults. The first chapter describes the health effects of mainly Type 2 diabetes that are associated with increased stroke risk. Type 2 diabetes is defined by several diagnostic blood tests including higher than average serum levels of insulin, glucose, and hemoglobin A1C. About 8 % of the U.S. population is affected by diabetes. About 1/3 are undiagnosed. The risk of diabetes increases with age. About 27 % of adults who are 65 years or older have diabetes. Diabetes is a major cause of heart disease and stroke. The risk of stroke is 2–4 times higher among people with diabetes. Almost a quarter of the US adult population has pre-diabetes and this also increases the risk of stroke. Medical nutrition therapy is recommended for individuals with diabetes. Weight loss and dietary guidance in clinical studies has shown benefits of sustained improvements in hemoglobin A1C. A major goal is to achieve and maintain glucose levels in the normal range. Food intake (focusing on carbohydrate), medication, metabolic control (glycemia, lipids, and blood pressure), improvements in anthropometric measurements, and increased physical activity have all been shown to improve outcomes including lowering the risk of stroke.

Another critical risk factor for stroke is hypertension. Other risk factors are high total cholesterol and especially high concentrations of low density lipoproteins, and hyperhomocysteinemia. Hypertension, hyperlipidemia, and hyperhomocysteinemia are modifiable risk factors for stroke that can be beneficially affected by dietary interventions. The commonality between hypertension, hyperlipidemia, and hyperhomocysteinemia and risk of stroke is related to atherosclerosis as each of these conditions contributes to atherosclerosis. Atherosclerosis is the buildup of plaque along artery walls resulting in hardening and narrowing of arteries. Of relevance, the carotid arteries carry blood to the brain. Hardening or narrowing of carotid arteries can result in a rupture of the plaque that can result in stroke. This chapter reviews the important findings from the Dietary Approaches to Stop Hypertension (DASH) Eating Plan that is proven to lower blood pressure, restrict dietary fats that contribute to hyperlipidemia and incorporates micronutrients that are necessary to possibly prevent hyperhomocystinemia. Regular physical activity, along with diets such as the DASH diet, has been shown to prevent stroke.

Obesity is documented in over 1/3 of all US adults and in >20 % of those under 18 years. It is well accepted that obesity increases the risk of many chronic diseases including cardiovascular disease and diabetes, and this links obesity to increased risk of stroke. As research has progressed, it is clear that central adiposity (abdominal obesity) is associated with an increased risk of the obesity-related diseases and conditions including diabetes, hypertension, and dyslipidemia. Thus assessment of abdominal obesity by means of waist circumference and body mass index (BMI) should be used to describe the type of obesity seen in the patient. This important chapter, containing 11 excellent figures, links obesity to diabetes, hyperlipidemia, hypertension, metabolic syndrome and reviews the effects of bariatric surgery. The primary message from this chapter is the need for the development of effective obesity prevention programs as treatment of obesity through dietary means has not been shown to have long-term effects for the majority of obese patients.

Stroke in pediatric populations usually has different causes than stroke in adults. Most pediatric strokes have a genetic component. Atherosclerosis is a rare cause of pediatric stroke. Pediatric stroke, especially in neonates, is often associated with congenital heart disease, clotting disorders, metabolic disorders, mitochondrial disorders, sickle cell disease, and focal arteriopathy and most recently in older children and teens, is associated with obesity, diabetes, and metabolic syndrome. The treatment protocol for acute stroke is essentially the same for young and old patients, with a focus on administration of tissue plasminogen activator as a first-line treatment. Details concerning the etiology of pediatric ischemic strokes, treatment of the acute and chronic state and diagnostic methodologies are emphasized. In acute nutritional management of stroke, the main goal of medical nutrition therapy is to ensure optimal nutrition to promote healing and prepare the child for physical rehabilitation. Nutritional management in the chronic phase deals with long-term effects of stroke that may include swallowing problems, immobility, spasticity, limited physical activity, cognitive and behavior changes, limited weight-bearing in the lower extremities, pressure sores, constipation, and gastroesophageal reflux. Moreover, these sensitive and informative chapters describe nutritional management of the pediatric stroke patient that requires knowledge of childhood-specific nutritional requirements, as well as normal and disease-specific growth and development considerations.

The last section of the volume includes ten chapters that examine critical aspects of stroke care that involve nutrition support. The first chapter contains an overview of the recent trends in the medical management of stroke. Descriptions of the management of secondary damage that may be associated with the use of certain drugs during the acute stroke, delayed deterioration with vasospasm, blood glucose monitoring, avoidance of neurological "metabolic crisis," and modern nutrient and fluid delivery in stroke care are included in this comprehensive chapter. The next chapter indicates that currently there is no consensus definition of the term malnutrition and there are no agreed-upon indices. Thus, determining the prevalence of malnutrition following stroke is difficult since no nutritional assessment tools have been developed and validated for this population. Further, no existing, previously developed, disease-specific assessment tools have been validated for use in stroke. As a consequence, when a systematic review identified 18 studies in which the nutritional status of patients was assessed after inpatient admission for stroke, frequency of malnutrition ranged from 6 to 62 %. The chapter reviews the relevant studies that examine pre-stroke nutritional status and risk factors for poor recovery. Pre-morbid risk factors associated with the development of malnutrition following stroke include a history of smoking, advanced age, female sex, and residential care. The consequences of stroke can further increase a patient's risk for nutritional decline post stroke. Fatigue, depression and anxiety, and the inability to communicate food preferences due to aphasia also increase risk of malnutrition.

The chapter on electrolyte balance reminds us of the critical importance of sodium, potassium, chlorine, phosphorus, magnesium, calcium, bicarbonate, and glucose in the maintenance of health. Electrolyte disturbances in stroke patients are common. Many of the derangements may occur during the acute phase. Some electrolyte disturbances may increase the risk for stroke, stroke complications, and even mortality. This comprehensive chapter, that includes 11 informative tables, reviews topics including the roles of aldosterone, antidiuretic hormone, diabetes insipidus, cerebral salt wasting, and blood urea and includes discussions of diagnosis and management of electrolyte disturbances in the stroke patient.

Nutritional support is key to the recovery of the stroke patient. The chapter on the options for nutrition support emphasizes that enteral nutrition is the established, preferential route of nutrition support for this patient population, and should commence as early as feasible. Parenteral nutrition is limited to the patient with a non-functioning and/or inability to access the gastrointestinal tract. Nutrition assessment is reviewed and the components of the assessment are matched to the needs of the stroke patient and the timing of the assessment, from immediately following the event to weeks or longer after the stroke. The components of a comprehensive nutrition assessment that are described include evaluation of anthropometrics, biochemical markers, clinical examination, and the patient's recent diet history. As one example of the important clinically relevant information provided in the chapter, the authors indicate: "When limitations in mobility or paralysis are present, caloric requirements will be lower due to decreased activity. Early medical treatments in the acute care setting with barbiturates or induced hypothermia as a method to decrease intracranial pressure also decreases caloric requirements. Indirect calorimetry is ideal for assessment of nutritional needs in these clinical scenarios." Additional topics include timing of enteral and/or parenteral nutrition, formula selection, potential complications, and medication—nutrient interactions. The following chapter provides further detailed information concerning enteral nutrition options and timings for use including blind placement of nasoenteric and oroenteric feeding tubes, facilitated placement of nasoenteric feeding tubes, percutaneous gastrostomy and jejunostomy tubes, and surgical gastrostomy and jejunostomy tubes. This detailed, practice-oriented chapter provides valuable resources for the medical team that provides enteral nutrition to the stroke patient regardless of the degree of damage caused by the stroke event.

Difficulty in swallowing (dysphagia) has serious effects on the nutritional status of the stroke patient. The comprehensive chapter on dysphagia, with excellent figures, includes references to assessment tools and coordination of care with speech pathologists and other health providers who can best evaluate the patient. The chapter explains that swallowing, or deglutition, is the neuromuscular act involving sensory and motor components controlling the movement of food from the oral cavity through the pharynx and esophagus to the stomach. Dysphagia is difficulty in the act of swallowing due to weakness, impaired coordination or obstruction. The incidence of dysphagia following stroke is reported to be between 19 and 81 %. Usually, the larger the area of infarct, the more impaired the swallowing. Dysphagia is more prevalent when the stroke involves the brainstem. The chapter also includes an important description of the consequences if food or liquid enters the lungs and the potential for the development of pneumonia.

The final chapters of this comprehensive book examine the value of nursing care and the importance of facilities that will aid the patient in rehabilitation and hopefully back to their home. The chapter concerning nursing care discusses the process of moving the patient from the hospital to the next level of care or home. Specialized, comprehensive nursing care provided in designated stroke units is vital to improving and maintaining positive stroke outcomes. The chapter emphasizes the importance of the specialized nurse who may evaluate the patient before transport to a hospital, work as an integral part of an emergency team in an ambulance or in the emergency room at the hospital, in the intensive care unit, and/or at the bedside in the general care hospital room. The chapter reviews the national recommendations and protocols for assessment of acute critical care and the importance of prevention of secondary infections or injury. The nurse is often the primary contact for the patient and family during the transition from the hospital to the rehabilitation facility and advance practice nurses are important sources of best practice guidelines especially when they educate families about the National Stoke Center Certification programs that should be in place wherever the patient is provided care.

The chapter on stroke rehabilitation acknowledges that nutrition is an integral therapy to assist patients in maximizing their rehabilitation potential. Rehabilitation is particularly important as statistics show that nearly 25 % of people who experience and survive their first stroke have a significantly increased risk of having another stroke in 5 years. This comprehensive chapter reviews the importance of physical, occupational as well as speech therapy and the reestablishment of competence in the activities of daily living. A number of key stroke complications are described including spasticity, aphasia (both fluent and non fluent), dysphagia, pain, urinary tract infections, deep vein thrombosis, depression, and seizures.

The two last chapters describe ethical issues in the care of stroke patients and provide resources for the health provider as well as the patient and family members. Patients and their family members may be unaware that the majority of hospitals and healthcare facilities have dedicated staff members who specialize in bioethics. The Clinical Ethics staff member can provide important resources for patients, surrogates, and health care professionals facing difficult decisions after a patient or family member has experienced a stroke. The overriding ethical principle of respect for patient autonomy, wishes, and preferences is dependent upon the assessment of a stroke patient's decision-making capacity. It is of great importance for the medical staff to be able to identify goals of care and clinical management of the patient. The chapter reviews the continuum of decision making over the course of care. Decisions to forgo life-sustaining treatment, including artificial nutrition and hydration, should be based on patient wishes and preferences as well as guidance from the clinical staff. Of particular interest for the nutritionist are the areas of artificial or medical provision of nutrition and hydration to patients who are unable to eat and drink by mouth. As reviewed in this chapter on ethical issues, artificial nutrition and hydration (ANH) can be life-saving. As basic care, ANH can prevent sensations of hunger and thirst, help to maintain a patient's life, and prevent death by malnutrition or dehydration. Additionally, because of the symbolic, cultural and even religious associations with eating and drinking, not providing "food and water," even when it is "artificial" or "medical," may be viewed by some as starvation, neglectful, and inhumane. Included in this chapter is a discussion of the sensitive issue of recoverability after stroke, especially during the immediate and acute phase. The concept of the time-limited trial (TLT) of life-sustaining treatment is reviewed. The final chapter provides technical information useful for clinicians and health providers involved in the treatment of the nutritional needs of patients. Specific recommended nutritional instructions are provided for patients using certain drugs that can affect their nutritional status and/or ability to eat, digest, metabolize or eliminate digested food. Useful lists of Websites for organizations involved in stroke research and care of stroke patients are also included.

The logical sequence of the sections as well as the chapters within each section enhance the understanding of the latest information on the role of nutritional components and therapeutically administered nutrients and fluids in the care of the stroke patient during acute and chronic care. The volume contains unique chapters that are helpful for specialized clinicians, related health professionals including the dietician, nurse, pharmacist, physical therapist, behaviorist, psychologist, and others involved in the treatment of the many different consequences of stroke. Moreover, the volume highlights the importance of the medical condition of the patient prior to their stroke. This comprehensive volume has great value for academicians involved in the education of graduate students and postdoctoral fellows, medical students, and allied health professionals who plan to interact with patients, family members and/or clients who have suffered a stroke or are recovering from related nutritional disorders.

The volume contains over 70 detailed tables and figures that assist the reader in comprehending the complexities of brain and circulatory physiology as well as the details of many of the consequences of stroke on the ability to eat, digest, metabolize as well as eliminate food from the digestive tract. The overriding goal of this volume is to provide the health professional with balanced documentation and awareness of the newest research and therapeutic approaches including an appreciation of the complexity of the choices for enteral and parenteral feeding for the stroke patient. Hallmarks of the 19 chapters include key words and bulleted key points at the beginning of each chapter, complete definitions of terms with the abbreviations fully defined for the reader and consistent use of terms between chapters. There are over 850 up-to-date references; all chapters include a conclusion to highlight major findings. The volume also contains a highly annotated index.

This unique text provides practical, data-driven resources based upon the totality of the evidence to help the reader understand the basics, treatments, and preventive strategies that are available for the stroke patient and those who are at increased risk of stroke. Of equal importance, critical issues that involve patient concerns, such as ethical issues, standards of nursing care, resources including the Websites of national organizations, are included in well-referenced, informative chapters. The overarching goal of the editors is to provide fully referenced information on the nutritional choices for stroke patients to health professionals so they may have a balanced perspective on the value of various preventive and treatment options that are available today as well as in the foreseeable future.

In conclusion, "Handbook of Clinical Nutrition and Stroke" edited by Mandy L. Corrigan, M.P.H., R.D., L.D., C.N.S.C., Arlene A. Escuro, M.S., R.D., L.D., C.N.S.C. and Donald F. Kirby, M.D., F.A.C.P., F.A.C.N., F.A.C.G., A.G.A.F., C.N.S.C., C.P.N.S. provides health professionals in many areas of research and practice with the most up-to-date, well-referenced, and comprehensive volume on the current state of the science and clinical practice involving stroke patients and their care. This volume will serve the reader as the most authoritative resource in the field to date and is a very welcome addition to the Nutrition and Health Series.

Adrianne Bendich, Ph.D., F.A.C.N., F.A.S.N.
"Nutrition and Health" Series Editor

About the Series Editor

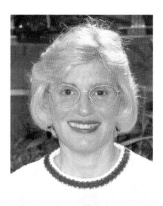

Dr. Adrianne Bendich has served as the "Nutrition and Health" Series Editor for over 15 years and has provided leadership and guidance to more than 100 editors who have developed the 50+ well respected and highly recommended volumes in the series.

In addition to "The Handbook of Clinical Nutrition and Stroke," edited by Mandy L. Corrigan, M.P.H., R.D., L.D., C.N.S.C., Arlene A. Escuro, M.S., R.D., L.D., C.N.S.C., and Donald F. Kirby, M.D., F.A.C.P., F.A.C.N., F.A.C.G., A.G.A.F., C.N.S.C., C.P.N.S., major new editions in 2012–2013 include the following:

1. *Nutrition in Infancy*, volumes one and two, edited by Dr. Ronald Ross Watson, Dr. George Grimble, Dr. Victor Preedy, and Dr. Sherma Zibadi, 2013.
2. *Carotenoids and Human Health*, edited by Sherry A. Tanumihardjo, 2013.
3. *Bioactive Dietary Factors and Plant Extracts in Dermatology*, edited by Dr. Ronald Ross Watson and Dr. Sherma Zibadi, 2013.
4. *Omega 6/3 Fatty Acids*, edited by Dr. Fabien De Meester, Dr. Ronald Ross Watson and Dr. Sherma Zibadi, 2013.

5. *Magnesium and Health*, edited by Dr. Ronald Ross Watson and Dr. Victor R. Preedy, 2012.
6. *Alcohol, Nutrition and Health Consequences*, edited by Dr. Ronald Ross Watson, Dr. Victor R. Preedy, and Dr. Sherma Zibadi, 2012.
7. *Nutritional Health, Strategies for Disease Prevention, Third Edition*, edited by Norman J. Temple, Ted Wilson, and David R. Jacobs, Jr., 2012.
8. *Chocolate in Health and Nutrition*, edited by Dr. Ronald Ross Watson, Dr. Victor R. Preedy, and Dr. Sherma Zibadi, 2012.
9. *Iron Physiology and Pathophysiology in Humans*, edited by Dr. Gregory J. Anderson and Dr. Gordon D. McLaren, 2012.

Earlier books included *Vitamin D, Second Edition* edited by Dr. Michael Holick; "Dietary Components and Immune Function" edited by Dr. Ronald Ross Watson, Dr. Sherma Zibadi and Dr. Victor R. Preedy; "Bioactive Compounds and Cancer" edited by Dr. John A. Milner and Dr. Donato F. Romagnolo; "Modern Dietary Fat Intakes in Disease Promotion" edited by Dr. Fabien DeMeester, Dr. Sherma Zibadi, and Dr. Ronald Ross Watson; "Iron Deficiency and Overload" edited by Dr. Shlomo Yehuda and Dr. David Mostofsky; "Nutrition Guide for Physicians" edited by Dr. Edward Wilson, Dr. George A. Bray, Dr. Norman Temple and Dr. Mary Struble; "Nutrition and Metabolism" edited by Dr. Christos Mantzoros and "Fluid and Electrolytes in Pediatrics" edited by Leonard Feld and Dr. Frederick Kaskel. Recent volumes include: "Handbook of Drug-Nutrient Interactions" edited by Dr. Joseph Boullata and Dr. Vincent Armenti; "Probiotics in Pediatric Medicine" edited by Dr. Sonia Michail and Dr. Philip Sherman; "Handbook of Nutrition and Pregnancy" edited by Dr. Carol Lammi-Keefe, Dr. Sarah Couch and Dr. Elliot Philipson; "Nutrition and Rheumatic Disease" edited by Dr. Laura Coleman; "Nutrition and Kidney Disease" edited by Dr. Laura Byham-Grey, Dr. Jerrilynn Burrowes and Dr. Glenn Chertow; "Nutrition and Health in Developing Countries" edited by Dr. Richard Semba and Dr. Martin Bloem; "Calcium in Human Health" edited by Dr. Robert Heaney and Dr. Connie Weaver and "Nutrition and Bone Health" edited by Dr. Michael Holick and Dr. Bess Dawson-Hughes.

Dr. Bendich was Director of Medical Affairs at GlaxoSmithKline (GSK) Consumer Healthcare and provided medical leadership for many well-known brands including TUMS and Os-Cal. Dr. Bendich had primary responsibility for GSK's support for the Women's Health Initiative (WHI) intervention study. Prior to joining GSK, Dr. Bendich was at Roche Vitamins Inc. and was involved with the groundbreaking clinical studies showing that folic acid-containing multivitamins significantly reduced major classes of birth defects. Dr. Bendich has coauthored over 100 major clinical research studies in the area of preventive nutrition. She is recognized as a leading authority on antioxidants, nutrition and immunity and pregnancy outcomes, vitamin safety and the cost-effectiveness of vitamin/mineral supplementation.

Dr. Bendich is President of Consultants in Consumer Healthcare LLC and is the editor of ten books including "Preventive Nutrition: The Comprehensive Guide For Health Professionals, Fourth Edition" coedited with Dr. Richard Deckelbaum (www.springer.com/series/7659). Dr. Bendich serves on the Editorial Boards of the

Journal of Nutrition in Gerontology and Geriatrics, and Antioxidants and has served as Associate Editor for "Nutrition" the International Journal; served on the Editorial Board of the Journal of Women's Health and Gender-Based Medicine and served on the Board of Directors of the American College of Nutrition.

Dr. Bendich received the Roche Research Award, is a *Tribute to Women and Industry* Awardee, and was a recipient of the Burroughs Wellcome Visiting Professorship in Basic Medical Sciences. Dr. Bendich was given the Council for Responsible Nutrition (CRN) Apple Award in recognition of her many contributions to the scientific understanding of dietary supplements. In 2012, she was recognized for her contributions to the field of clinical nutrition by the American Society for Nutrition and was elected a Fellow of ASN. Dr Bendich is Adjunct Professor at Rutgers University. She is listed in Who's Who in American Women.

About the Volume Editors Bios

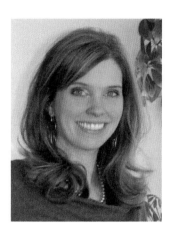

Mandy L. Corrigan is an advanced practice Nutrition Support Clinician in the Home Nutrition Support Team at Cleveland Clinic in Cleveland, Ohio. After becoming a registered dietitian, obtaining her master's degree in Public Health, and becoming a Board Certified Nutrition Support Clinician (CNSC) she continued specializing in clinical dietetics focusing on enteral and parenteral nutrition. She has held leadership positions at the national and state level including the Academy of Nutrition and Dietetics Dietitians in Nutrition Support (DNS) practice group, the American Burn Association, and the Ohio Society for Parenteral and Enteral Nutrition (O.S.P.E.N.). She serves as an editor for *Support Line*, a publication of DNS, and the *O.S.P.E.N. Access*.

Mandy has had many peer-reviewed publications including journal articles, case studies, and book chapters related to nutrition support and vascular access devices. She currently is specializing in the delivery and management of home parenteral nutrition to patients with intestinal failure. At present she is focusing her research efforts towards methods for prevention of life-threatening complications of parenteral nutrition, specifically catheter sepsis, at Cleveland Clinic, the center with the largest home parenteral nutrition program in the United States.

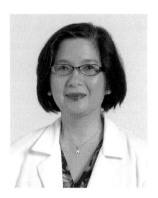

Arlene A. Escuro is an advanced practice registered dietitian in the Center for Human Nutrition, Section of Nutrition Therapy at the Cleveland Clinic. She has practiced in the field of clinical nutrition, with specialty practice in nutrition support, neurosciences, neurocritical care, colorectal surgery, and home enteral nutrition for over 20 years. She served as a nutrition specialist for the Cleveland Clinic Center for ALS and Related Disorders for 10 years. She is currently the inpatient home enteral nutrition coordinator, and she also provides nutrition therapy for colorectal surgery patients.

Arlene has several peer-reviewed articles, research abstracts, and professional presentations on the topic of nutrition support in stroke, amyotrophic lateral sclerosis, neurocritical care, and home tube feeding management. Her research study on *Enteral Nutrition in the Neurological Intensive Care Unit: Factors Impeding the Attainment of Tube Feeding Goals* was awarded Best Practice Poster by the American Society for Parenteral and Enteral Nutrition (ASPEN).

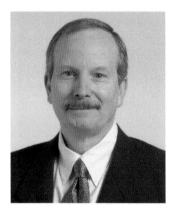

Donald F. Kirby is a gastroenterologist who specializes in Nutrition at the Cleveland Clinic in Cleveland, Ohio. He is Board Certified in Internal Medicine, Gastroenterology, and Nutrition Support. His practice encompasses from very malnourished patients, who may require intravenous nutrition, to those with morbid obesity. In addition, he is the Medical Director for the Intestinal Transplant Program and Program Director for the Nutrition Fellowship.

Contents

Part III   Medical Management of Stroke

Contributors

Stacey Claus, M.S.N., R.N., C.N.R.N., G.C.N.S-B.C. Nursing Education and Professional Practice Development, Cleveland Clinic, Cleveland, OH, USA

Mandy L. Corrigan, M.P.H., R.D., L.D., C.N.S.C. Cleveland Clinic, Nutrition Support Team, Cleveland, OH, USA

Janis Dale, H.B.Sc, R.D., C.D.E. Stroke and Neurological Rehabilitation Program, Neurotrauma Rehabilitation Program, St. Joseph's Health Care, Parkwood Hospital, London, ON, Canada

Omer J. Deen, M.D. Center for Human Nutrition, Digestive Disease Institute, The Cleveland Clinic, Cleveland, OH, USA

Michael De Georgia, M.D. Department of Neurology, University Hospitals Case Medical Center, Cleveland, OH, USA

Christina DeTallo, M.S., R.D., C.S.P., L.D. Pediatric Gastroenterology, Cleveland Clinic Children's Hospital, Cleveland, OH, USA

Andrea Vegh Dunn, R.D., L.D., C.D.E. Cleveland Clinic, Richard E. Jacobs Health Center, Avon, OH, USA

Melissa Ellis, M.S.N., A.C.N.P.-B.C. Neuro Intensive Care Unit, Cleveland Clinic, Cleveland, OH, USA

Arlene A. Escuro, M.S., R.D., L.D., C.N.S.C. Nutrition Therapy, Cleveland Clinic, Cleveland, OH, USA

Norine Foley, M.Sc., R.D. Aging, Rehabilitation and Geriatric Care Program, Lawson Health Research Institute, Parkwood Hospital, London, ON, Canada

Joao Gomes, M.D. Cerebrovascular Center, Cleveland Clinic, Cleveland, OH, USA

Brian J. Hedman, M.A., C.C.C.-S.L.P. Head and Neck Institute, Cleveland Clinic, Cleveland, OH, USA

Douglas Henry, M.D. Developmental and Rehabiliative Pediatrics, Cleveland Clinic Children's Hospital for Rehabilitation, Cleveland, OH, USA

Jennifer F.T. Jue, M.D. Department of Internal Medicine, Cleveland Clinic Foundation, Cleveland, OH, USA

Irene L. Katzan, M.D., M.S. Neurological Institute Center for Outcomes Research & Evaluation, Cleveland Clinic, Cleveland, OH, USA

Christine Kijak, H.B.Sc. Stroke and Neurological Rehabilitation Program, Amputee Rehabilitation Program, St. Joseph's Health Care, Parkwood Hospital, London, ON, Canada

Donald F. Kirby, M.D., F.A.C.P., F.A.C.N., F.A.C.G., A.G.A.F., C.N.S.C., C.P.N.S. Center for Human Nutrition, Department of Gastroenterology, Cleveland Clinic, Cleveland, OH, USA

Gursimran S. Kochhar, M.D. Department of Internal Medicine, Cleveland Clinic Foundation, Cleveland, OH, USA

Mei Lu, M.D., Ph.D. Cerebrovascular Center, Neurological Institute, Cleveland Clinic, Cleveland, OH, USA

Laura E. Matarese, Ph.D., R.D., L.D.N., F.A.D.A., F.A.S.P.E.N., C.N.S.C. Department of Internal Medicine, Division of Gastroenterology, Hepatology and Nutrition Brody School of Medicine and Department of Nutrition Science, East Carolina University, Greenville, NC, USA

J. Patrick McGowan, M.D. Consultative and Rehabilitation Unit, Physical Medicine and Rehabilitation, Virginia Commonwealth University, Richmond, VA, USA

Merideth Miller, R.D., C.S.P., L.D. Pediatric Gastroenterology, Cleveland Clinic Children's Hospital, Cleveland, OH, USA

Malissa Mulkey, M.S.N., R.N., C.C.R.N., C.C.N.S. Neuroscience Clinical Nurse Specialist, Department of Advanced Clinical Practice, Duke University Hospital, Durham, NC, USA

Craig Nielsen, M.D. Department of Internal Medicine, Cleveland Clinic Foundation, Cleveland, OH, USA

Kavita Nyalakonda, M.D. Cleveland Clinic, Richard E. Jacobs Health Center, Avon, OH, USA

Keely R. Parisian, M.D. Albany Gastroenterology Consultants, Albany, NY, USA

Katherine Patton, M.Ed., R.D., C.S.S.D., L.D. Center for Human Nutrition - Nutrition Therapy, Cleveland Clinic, Cleveland, OH, USA

J. Javier Provencio, M.D., F.C.C.M. Cerebrovascular Center and Neuroscience, Neurologic Institute, Cleveland Clinic, Cleveland Clinic Lerner College of Medicine, Cleveland, OH, USA

Bassel Raad, M.D. Department of Neurology, University Hospitals Case Medical Center, Cleveland, OH, USA

Sulieman Abdal Raheem, M.D. Center for Human Nutrition, Digestive Disease Institute, The Cleveland Clinic, Cleveland, OH, USA

Tina S. Resser, M.S.N., A.C.N.P.-B.C., C.N.R.N. Neurological Intensive Care Unit, Cleveland Clinic, Cleveland, OH, USA

Amy Calhoun Rosneck, M.A., C.C.C.-S.L.P. Head and Neck Institute, Cleveland Clinic, Cleveland, OH, USA

Martin L. Smith, S.T.D. Department of Bioethics, Cleveland Clinic, Cleveland, OH, USA

William S. Tierney, M.S. Cleveland Clinic Foundation, Cleveland Clinic Lerner College of Medicine, Cleveland Heights, OH, USA

Ari Marc Wachsman, M.D. Neurological Institute, The Cleveland Clinic, Cleveland, OH, USA

Part I
Introduction to Stroke

Chapter 1
Epidemiology of Stroke

Irene L. Katzan

Key Points

- Stroke is the fourth leading cause of death in the USA, and it is the *second* leading cause of death worldwide.
- Although there has been a decline in stroke incidence and mortality in the USA, this trend is not expected to last. With the aging of the population, the incidence and deaths from stroke are likely to skyrocket, and epidemiologists have warned of a stroke epidemic in the next 25 years.
- Stroke incidence and mortality will increase more quickly in low-income and middle-income countries because of the increases in the prevalence of risk factors for cardiovascular disease, including urbanization and Western-style dietary changes.

Keywords Epidemiology • Stroke • Mortality • Incidence • Intracerebral hemorrhage

Abbreviations

AF   Atrial Fibrillation
DALYs   Disability Adjusted Life Years
ICH   Intracerebral Hemorrhagic Stroke
SAH   Subarachnoid Hemorrhage
TIA   Transient Ischemic Attack

I.L. Katzan, M.D., M.S. (✉)
Neurological Institute Center for Outcomes Research & Evaluation, Cleveland Clinic,
9500 Euclid Avenue, S80, Cleveland, OH, USA
e-mail: katzani@ccf.org

M.L. Corrigan et al. (eds.), *Handbook of Clinical Nutrition and Stroke*,
Nutrition and Health, DOI 10.1007/978-1-62703-380-0_1,
© Springer Science+Business Media New York 2013

Overview of Stroke in the USA

Stroke is a major public health concern. The prevalence of stroke in the USA is roughly 3 % of the adult population. Each year, approximately 795,000 people experience a new or recurrent stroke. Most of these (610,000) are first-ever strokes. This translates to someone in the USA having a stroke every 40 s, on average [1]. Although stroke can occur at any age, the incidence increases with age: there is a doubling for each decade after age 55 [1].

Of all strokes, 87 % are ischemic, 10 % are intracerebral hemorrhagic strokes (ICH), and 3 % are subarachnoid hemorrhage strokes (SAH) [1]. Mexican Americans, Latin Americans, African Americans, Native Americans, Japanese people, and Chinese people have higher incidences of hemorrhagic stroke than do white Americans.

African Americans have a risk of first-ever stroke that is almost twice that of whites. The increased incidence is most prominent for young and middle-aged African Americans, who have a substantially higher risk of SAH and ICH than whites of the same age [2]. In 27,744 participants in the Reasons for Geographic and Racial Differences in Stroke (REGARDS) Study, which were followed over 4.4 years (2003–2010), the overall age and sex-adjusted black/white incidence rate ratio was 1.51, but it was lower for the very old and very young. For ages 45–54 years, it was 4.02, and for those ≥85 years of age, it was 0.86 [3].

Stroke ranks fourth among all causes of death, behind diseases of the heart, cancer, and chronic lower respiratory disease. In 2008, stroke accounted for ~1 of every 18 deaths in the USA. In comparison, coronary heart disease caused ~1 of every 6 deaths that year. On average, someone dies of a stroke every 4 min [4].

Several studies have shown a decrease in the age-adjusted annual incidence of first stroke among both men and women. One of the larger analyses is from the Framingham Heart Study. The age-adjusted incidence of first stroke per 1,000 person-years in this analysis declined in men from 7.7 during years 1950–1977, 6.2 during years 1978–1989, and down to 5.3 during 1990–2004. The decline in women was 6.2, 5.8, and 5.1 per 1,000 person-years, respectively. Although the incidence declined over time, the lifetime risk did not decline to the same degree, likely due to improved life expectancy.

In addition to the decline in incidence, there has been some decline in stroke mortality. From 1998 to 2008, the stroke death rate in the USA fell 34.8 %, and the actual number of stroke deaths declined 19.4 % [1]. This decline also occurred in heart disease; over the same time period, the rate of death from cardiovascular disease declined 30.6 %. The decline in mortality has been attributed to both a decreasing case fatality and a decrease in stroke incidence [1].

Although the incidence and mortality of overall stroke has decreased in the USA, a review of published studies and data from clinical trials found that hospital admissions for intracerebral hemorrhage have increased by 18 % in the past 10 years. This is likely due to an increase in age of population and the increasing use of anticoagulants, thrombolytics, and antiplatelet agents. In the Greater Cincinnati/Northern Kentucky Stroke Study, the annual incidence of anticoagulant-associated intracerebral hemorrhage per 100,000 people increased over time, from 0.8 (95 % CI 0.3–1.3) in

1988 to 1.9 (95 % CI 1.1–2.7) in 1993/1994 and 4.4 (95 % CI 3.2–5.5) in 1999 ($P < 0.001$ for trend). Among people ≥80 years of age, the rate of anticoagulant-associated intracerebral hemorrhage increased from 2.5 (95 % CI 0–7.4) in 1988 to 45.9 (95 % CI 25.6–66.2) in 1999 ($P < 0.001$ for trend). Over this period of time, incidence rates of cardioembolic ischemic stroke were similar, but warfarin use in the USA increased fourfold, suggesting a difference in preventive management strategies [1].

Worldwide Perspective

Although stroke is the fourth leading cause of death in the USA, it is the *second* leading cause of death worldwide. It is estimated that 87 % of stroke deaths occur in low- and middle-income countries. Stroke is also the fourth leading cause of lost productivity [5] and in disability-adjusted life years (DALYs) worldwide, behind only HIV/AIDS, unipolar depression and heart disease [6]. Disease burden is typically quantified in DALYs where 1 DALY is 1 year of "healthy" life lost. The burden of disease is defined as the gap between the current health of a population and an ideal situation in which everyone in the population lives to old age in full health [6]. Although incidence of stroke is higher in the elderly, because of the increased longevity of younger stroke survivors, two-thirds of the burden of stroke in the world occurs in people under age 70 years.

Worldwide estimates indicate that primary hemorrhages constitute a higher percentage of all strokes than in the USA, ranging from 10 to 25 %. Individuals of Asian, African, and Latin American origin tend to have a higher frequency of primary hemorrhage than persons of European origin [1].

Future Trends

Although there has been a decline in stroke incidence and mortality in the USA, this trend is not expected to last. With the aging of the population, the incidence and deaths from stroke are likely to skyrocket, and epidemiologists have warned of a stroke epidemic in the next 25 years [7–9]. Projections show that by 2030, an additional four million people in the USA will have had a stroke, a 24.9 % increase in prevalence from 2010 [10].

Using data from the National Center of Health Statistics and population projections from the US Census Bureau, Elkins and Johnston calculated an expected number of deaths in the USA from ischemic stroke in 30 years. They projected a 98 % increase over the 30-year period from 2002 to 2032. The total US population was projected to increase by only 27 % in the same period and much of this estimated increase in death was due to aging of the population and changes in the racial and ethnic composition of the USA [11].

It is possible that, although improvement in primary prevention efforts for stroke and heart disease will help, it may paradoxically complicate the problem to some extent. Patients treated with antithrombotics for stroke prevention may suffer a more severe hemorrhagic stroke, and patients who avoid cardiac death may survive and be at risk for the development of stroke, since the stroke risk increases with age [12].

The situation is even more dire when looking at projections worldwide. Stroke incidence and mortality will increase more quickly in low-income and middle-income countries because of the increases in the prevalence of risk factors for cardiovascular disease, including urbanization and Western-style dietary changes [6]. Without additional population-wide interventions, figures are predicted to increase to a 23 million first-ever strokes, 77 million stroke survivors, and 7.8 million deaths by 2030. This suggests that for any management strategies to have impact on world mortality, they must be implemented within low- and middle-income countries [6].

Risk Factors

Prevention is the most effective method of reducing the burden of stroke on society [6, 7]. The 2009 standardized case–control INTERSTROKE study provides important information on risk factors for stroke across the globe [13]. The study was the first large standardized case–control study of risk factors for stroke in which countries of low and middle income were included. The study evaluated attributable risk of stroke in 3,000 cases and 3,000 controls in 22 countries (Argentina, Australia, Brazil, Canada, Chile, China, Colombia, Croatia, Denmark, Ecuador, Germany, India, Iran, Malaysia, Mozambique, Nigeria, Peru, Philippines, Poland, South Africa, Sudan, and Uganda) and found the same risk factors in low- and middle-income countries as in high-income countries [13]. The study also found that five risk factors accounted for more than 80 % of the global risk of all stroke: hypertension, current smoking, abdominal obesity, diet, and physical activity [13]. An additional five risk factors increase the populational attributable risk of stroke to 90 %: excessive alcohol consumption, dyslipidemia (measured by ratio of apolipoproteins B to A1), cardiac causes (atrial fibrillation or flutter, previous myocardial infarction, rheumatic valvular heart disease, and prosthetic heart valve), and psychosocial stress/depression (see Table 1.1). Importantly, many of these risk factors are actionable. Some of the most significant ones are discussed below.

Hypertension

In INTERSTROKE, hypertension was associated with the highest estimated population-attributable fraction of 52 %, as has been seen in the past in prior epidemiology studies. Participants in INTERSTROKE with self-reported hypertension or blood pressure (BP) >160/90 mmHg were 2.8 times more likely to have a stroke than those without hypertension. Control of blood pressure is associated with a significant reduction in risk of stroke. A large meta-analysis of clinical trials found a 41 %

Table 1.1
Risk of stroke associated with risk factors in the INTERSTROKE study
(multivariate analyses)

Variable	Odds ratio (99 % CI)	Population-attributable risk
Hypertension (self-reported history of hypertension or BP >160/90 mmHg)	3.89 (3.33–4.54)	51.8 % (47.7–55.8)
Current smoker	2.09 (1.75–2.51)	18.9 % (15.3–23.1)
Waist-to-hip ratio		
Tertile 2 vs. tertile 1	1.42 (1.18–1.71)	26.5 % (18.8–36.0)[a]
Tertile 3 vs. tertile 1	1.65 (1.36–1.99)	
Diet risk score		
Tertile 2 vs. tertile 1	1.35 (1.12–1.61)	18.8 % (11.2–29.7)[a]
Tertile 3 vs. tertile 1	1.35 (1.11–1.64)	
Regular physical activity	0.69 (0.53–0.90)	28.5 % (14.5–48.5)
Diabetes mellitus	1.36 (1.10–1.68)	5.0 % (2.6–9.5)
Alcohol intake		
1–30 drinks per month	0.90 (0.72–1.11)	3.8 % (0.9–14.4)[a]
>30 drinks per month or binge drinker	1.51 (1.18–1.92)	
Psychosocial factors		
Psychosocial stress	1.30 (1.06–1.60)	4.6 % (2.1–9.6)
Depression	1.35 (1.10–1.66)	5.2 % (2.7–9.8)
Cardiac causes (atrial fibrillation or flutter, previous myocardial infarction, rheumatic valve disease, or prosthetic heart valve)	2.38 (1.77–3.20)	6.7 % (4.8–9.1)
Ratio of ApoB to ApoA1		
T2 vs. T1	1.13 (0.90–1.42)	24.9 % (15.7–37.1)[a]
T3 vs. T1	1.89 (1.49–2.40)	

T tertile, *Apo* apolipoprotein, *BP* blood pressure
[a]For variables expressed in tertiles, population-attributable risk was calculated from T2 plus T3 vs. T1. Population-attributable risk of alcohol calculated from any vs. none
Adapted from The Lancet, 360, O'Donnell MJ, Xavier D, Liu L, et al., "Risk factors for ischaemic and intracerebral haemorrhagic stroke in 22 countries (the interstroke study): A case-control study," 1903–1913, Copyright 2010, with permission from Elsevier

reduction in stroke for a BP reduction of 10 mmHg systolic or 5 mmHg diastolic regardless of BP before treatment [14]. The risk of stroke has a continuous association with blood pressure down to 115/75 mmHg [15]. Subjects with BP <120/80 mmHg have approximately half the lifetime risk of stroke of subjects with hypertension. Current guidelines for primary prevention of stroke recommend treatment of BP to a goal of 140/90 mmHg, and for patients with diabetes or renal disease, the BP goal is <130/80 mmHg [2].

Diabetes Mellitus

In 2008, approximately 8 % of the adult population in the USA, which comprise 18,300,000 people, had diagnosis of diabetes mellitus. An additional 3.1 % (7,100,000) had undiagnosed diabetes [1]. The prevalence of diabetes mellitus has been dramatically increasing over time, along with the increases in prevalence of overweight and obesity. Intensive glucose-lowering therapy (a glycolated hemoglobin [HbA$_{1c}$] level <7.0 %) has been shown to decrease the risk of microvascular complications and may or may not be beneficial for long-term reduction in the risk of cardiovascular disease [16]. Stroke risk can be reduced in patients with diabetes who receive risk factor modification in multiple areas. In the Steno-2 Study, 160 patients with type 2 diabetes and persistent microalbuminuria were assigned to receive either intensive therapy, including behavioral risk factor modification and a statin, antihypertensives, and an antiplatelet, or conventional therapy with a mean treatment period of 7.8 years. Patients were followed up for an average of 5.5 years. The risk of cardiovascular events was reduced by 60 % (HR, 0.41; 95 % CI, 0.25–0.67; $P < 0.001$) with intensive treatment vs. conventional therapy, and the number of strokes was reduced from 30 to 6 [17].

Obesity

The estimated prevalence of being overweight (having a body mass index (BMI) of 25–29.9 kg/m^2) and obesity (BMI $\geq$30 kg/m^2) in US adults $\geq$20 years of age is 67.3 % in 2008, representing 149,300,000 people. One-third of US adults are obese. Men and women of all race/ethnic groups in the population are affected by the epidemic of overweight and obesity [1] The relative risk of death from stroke is 1.39 (95 % CI 1.31–1.48) per increase of 5 kg/m^2 in BMI [18]. Although no clinical trials have evaluated the effects of weight loss on stroke risk, several trials have demonstrated a reduction in BP with weight reduction [2].

Cigarette Smoking

There is strong and pervasive evidence of the deleterious effects of smoking on stroke, cardiovascular disease in addition to cancer. In 2010, among Americans 18 years of age or older, 21.2 % of men and 17.5 % of women were cigarette smokers. Perhaps more disheartening, the rate is similar in adolescents: in 2009, 19.5 % of students in grades 9 through 12 reported current cigarette use [1]. The risk of stroke among smokers tends to peak at middle age and declines with advancing age [19].

Physical Activity

A meta-analysis of studies found that moderately or highly active individuals had lower risk of stroke incidence or mortality than did low-active individuals [20]. Overall, moderately active individuals had a 20 % lower risk (RR=0.80; 95 % CI, 0.74–0.86; $P < 0.001$), and highly active individuals had a 27 % lower risk of stroke incidence or mortality (RR=0.73; 95 % CI, 0.67–0.79; $P<0.001$) than low-active individuals. The 2008 Physical Activity Guidelines for Americans recommends that adults should engage in at least 150 min (2 h and 30 min) per week of moderate intensity or 75 min (1 h and 15 min) per week of vigorous-intensity aerobic physical activity, or an equivalent combination of moderate- and vigorous-intensity aerobic activity [21].

Lipids

Most but not all epidemiological studies have found an association between higher cholesterol levels and an increased risk of ischemic stroke, and they have demonstrated a benefit of lowering LDL in lowering stroke risk. One meta-analysis, for example, found that a reduction in LDL-C by 1 mmol/l (39 mg/dl) results in a decreased incidence of ischemic stroke by 16–17 % regardless of age, blood pressure, and pretrial blood lipid profile. Primary prevention guidelines for stroke recommend following the NCEP guidelines, which tailor goals and implementation of cholesterol-lowering agents based upon risk of cardiovascular event [2].

Atrial Fibrillation

Atrial fibrillation (AF) is a powerful risk factor for stroke that increases risk fivefold through all age groups. The prevalence of AF increases with age, from 1 % in the population aged under 50 years to approximately 10 % of those above 80 years. Because of the increasing prevalence with age, the percentage of strokes attributable to AF increases in older age groups, from 1.5 % at 50–59 years of age to 23.5 % at 80–89 years of age [1]. Because AF can be clinically undiagnosed, the stroke risk attributed to AF may be substantially underestimated [22]. The current American Heart Association/American Stroke Association guidelines recommend anticoagulation with either adjusted-dose warfarin (target international normalized ratio, 2.0–3.0) dabigatran, apixaban, or rivaroxaban for all high-risk patients at with nonvalvular atrial fibrillation [23]. Antiplatelet therapy is recommended for patients considered low risk for stroke.

Depression

Psychosocial stressors and depression have received less attention than other risk factors in stroke prevention efforts. There is growing evidence that these factors pose an increased risk factors for stroke. In a 2007 meta-analysis, for example, the pooled estimate for total stroke was 1.43 (95 % CI 1.17–1.75) [24]. There has been some thought that the use of antidepressant medications could be contributing to this increased risk. Results from the Women's Health Initiative prospective cohort study among postmenopausal women demonstrated that antidepressant use, specifically selective serotonin reuptake inhibitors, increased the risk of stroke by almost 45 % [25]. The findings of an association between antidepressant use and stroke have been variable, however [26].

Transient Ischemic Attacks

Approximately 15 % of all strokes are heralded by a transient ischemic attack (TIA), and they provide an important opportunity for intervention to prevent a stroke. Estimates of the prevalence of TIAs in the USA have varied widely, ranging from 1.1 to 6.3 %, depending on the specific population studied, definition of TIA, and study design [27].

There is a significant short-term risk of stroke in patients who have experienced a TIA. One of the seminal studies evaluating this involved 1,707 TIA patients seen in the emergency departments of Kaiser Permanente, Northern California. Ten percent (108 patients) had a stroke within 90 days and 5 % (91 patients) had a stroke within 2 days [28]. Other cohorts of patients with TIA have confirmed the high short-term risk of stroke after TIA, which has been shown to be as high as 10 % at 2 days and as high as 17 % at 90 days [29]. Predictors of stroke in TIA patients in the Kaiser study and another cohort study of patients from Oxford UK [30] were jointly evaluated to develop the ACBD2 scale that determines the short-term risk of stroke based on specific symptoms [31] Items on the scale include age >60, blood pressure >140/90, clinical features (unilateral weakness, 2 points, or speech impairment without weakness, 1 point), duration (>60 min, 2 points, or 10–59 min,1 point), and diabetes.

Variability in the use of brain imaging and the type of diagnostic imaging used can markedly affect estimates of the incidence and prevalence of TIAs. With increasing use of imaging in the evaluation of TIAs, especially magnetic resonance imaging (MRI), there is realization that as many as 50 % of patients with transient deficits lasting <24 h have evidence of a stroke [32].

The traditional definition of a TIA is "a sudden, focal neurological deficit of presumed vascular origin lasting <24 h" [32]. The arbitrary 24-h time window used to differentiate TIA from stroke arose in the mid-1960s when less was known about pathophysiology of cerebral ischemia. There has been a move over the last few years for a formal change in the definition of TIA that would remove the time-based portion in the traditional definition. The new proposed definition is "transient episode of neurological dysfunction caused by focal brain, spinal cord, or retinal ischemia, without acute infarction" [32]. One analysis estimated that the potential epidemiologic impact of adopting a tissue-based definition of TIA in the USA would lower annual incidence rates of TIA by 33 % and would increase the number of cases labeled as stroke by 7 % [33]. Regardless of official change in definition of TIA, the increased identification of permanent tissue injury on imaging in patients with transient deficits has already impacted current estimates of incidence and mortality.

Silent Strokes

With the increasing use of brain imaging, there is an increased recognition of "silent" strokes, which are not associated with focal clinical symptoms. Silent strokes are actually more common than clinical strokes, with prevalence estimates ranging from 6 to 28 % compared to a 3 % prevalence of clinical strokes. There is a higher prevalence of silent infarcts with increasing age [1]. These "silent infarcts" may cause memory symptoms. One cardiovascular health study evaluated 1,433 patients >65 years over a 5-year period with MRI scans. New infarctions not associated with focal neurological deficits were seen in 15.7 % subjects. The authors classified them as "covert" infarcts rather than silent because they showed decreased scores on the Modified Mini-Mental State Examination and Digit Symbol Substitution Test [34]. Similar findings were seen in the Rotterdam Scan Study, where1,015 patients underwent a neuropsychological and MRI twice an average of 3.6 years apart. Having a silent brain infarct at baseline doubled the risk of subsequent dementia (HR 2.26; 95 % CI, 1.09–4.70) and was associated with a steeper decline in global cognitive function [35].

Women

Women have lower age-adjusted stroke incidence than men; although each year, about 55,000 more women than men have a stroke. This is because of the larger numbers of elderly women compared to men. More women than men also die of stroke each year; in 2008 women accounted for 60.1 % of US stroke deaths [4] This differential mortality is due in part to the larger number of elderly women compared to men, but may also be partly due to a higher frequency of subarachnoid hemorrhage and a greater severity of ischemic stroke in women [36]. In addition, women are older at stroke onset on average than men (~75 years compared with 71 years) and may have poorer compensatory ability because of their older age at the time of stroke [37].

On top of the higher death rate from stroke, there are currently more women stroke survivors (2.1 million) than men (1.9 million). Most of these stroke survivors live with some disability, and it has been estimated that women spend approximately twice as many years disabled prior to death as their male counterparts [38]. Studies have also suggested worse functional outcomes after compared with men [36, 39] although it is likely that the older age at initial stroke in women largely accounts for this difference [39].

Finally, stroke also has a significant *indirect* impact on women. They significantly outnumber men as caregivers to stroke survivors. In the USA, 72 % of the caregivers are women. With the aging of the population, the global burden of stroke will increase and the mortality from stroke is expected to double in the next 25 years [9]. Because life expectancy is projected to increase more in women than men, the burden of stroke will continue to be heavier in women [40].

Outcomes

Stroke is a leading cause of major disability in adults. Living with severe disability from stroke has been considered by some to be worse than death [41]. Over 50 % of stroke survivors are functionally disabled. According to the Framingham Heart Study, among ischemic stroke survivors at 6 months who were >=65 years of age [42], 50 % had hemiparesis, 30 % were unable to walk without some assistance, 26 % were dependent in activities of daily living, 19 % had aphasia, 35 % had depressive symptoms, and 26 % were institutionalized in a nursing home. In addition to the physical and emotional toll, the cost of stroke is immense. Recent estimate of the mean lifetime cost of ischemic stroke in the USA is $140,048. This includes inpatient care, rehabilitation, and follow-up care necessary for lasting deficits (1999 dollars). This direct medical cost is estimated to increase by 238 % between 2010 and 2030, which is the largest relative increase of all cardiovascular diseases [10].

Conclusion

The prevalence of stroke in the USA is high and its cost will increase as the population ages. In addition, stroke incidence and mortality will increase in less developed countries due to changing lifestyles and population characteristics. The health burden from stroke will be tremendous and will further tax healthcare resources here in the USA and across the world. However, improvement in control of vascular risk factors could help offset the ominous stroke projections. One analysis, using the Archimedes model, estimated that if everyone received 11 recommended prevention activities, such as aspirin if their 10-year MI risk ≥ 10 %, lowering BP to 140/90 in nondiabetic people, lowering HgbA1C to <7.0 in diabetics, or reducing weight to body mass index <30 kg/m^2, and they achieved feasible improvements in their vascular risk factor status, strokes would be reduced 20 % in the next 30 years [37, 43]. For stroke that does occur, optimizing management will be critical to reduce disability and maximize functional outcomes.

References

1. Roger VL, Go AS, Lloyd-Jones DM, Benjamin EJ, Berry JD, Borden WB, et al. Heart disease and stroke statistics—2012 update: a report from the American Heart Association. Circulation. 2012;125:e2–220.
2. Goldstein LB, Bushnell CD, Adams RJ, Appel LJ. Braun LT. Chaturvedi S. et al. Guidelines for the primary prevention of stroke: a guideline for healthcare professionals from the American Heart Association/American Stroke Association. Stroke. 2011;42:517–84.
3. Howard VJ, Kleindorfer DO, Judd SE, McClure LA. Safford MM. Rhodes JD, et al. Disparities in stroke incidence contributing to disparities in stroke mortality. Ann Neurol. 2011;69: 619–27.

4. Rich DQ, Gaziano JM, Kurth T. Geographic patterns in overall and specific cardiovascular disease incidence in apparently healthy men in the United States. Stroke. 2007;38:2221–7.
5. WHO. The global burden of disease: 2004 update, WHO Press, Switzerland, http://www.who.int/healthinfo/global_burden_disease/GBD_report_2004update_full.pdf (accessed March 25, 2013).
6. Strong K, Mathers C, Bonita R. Preventing stroke: saving lives around the world. Lancet Neurol. 2007;6:182–7.
7. Feigin VL. Stroke in developing countries: can the epidemic be stopped and outcomes improved? Lancet Neurol. 2007;6:94–7.
8. Ovbiagele B, Nguyen-Huynh MN. Stroke epidemiology: advancing our understanding of disease mechanism and therapy. Neurotherapeutics. 2011;8:319–29.
9. Warlow C, Sudlow C, Dennis M, Wardlaw J, Sandercock P. Stroke. Lancet. 2003;362: 1211–24.
10. Heidenreich PA, Trogdon JG, Khavjou OA, Butler J, Dracup K, Ezekowitz MD, et al. Forecasting the future of cardiovascular disease in the United States: a policy statement from the American Heart Association. Circulation. 2011;123:933–44.
11. Elkins JS, Johnston SC. Thirty-year projections for deaths from ischemic stroke in the United States. Stroke. 2003;34:2109–12.
12. Longstreth Jr WT, Tirschwell DL. Editorial comment—The next 30 years of stroke for patients, providers, planners, and politicians. Stroke. 2003;34:2113.
13. O'Donnell MJ, Xavier D, Liu L, Zhang H, Chin SL, Rao-Melacini P, et al. Risk factors for ischaemic and intracerebral haemorrhagic stroke in 22 countries (the interstroke study): a case-control study. Lancet. 2010;376:112–23.
14. Law MR, Morris JK, Wald NJ. Use of blood pressure lowering drugs in the prevention of cardiovascular disease: meta-analysis of 147 randomised trials in the context of expectations from prospective epidemiological studies. BMJ. 2009;338:b1665.
15. Lewington S, Clarke R, Qizilbash N, Peto R, Collins R. Age-specific relevance of usual blood pressure to vascular mortality: a meta-analysis of individual data for one million adults in 61 prospective studies. Lancet. 2002;360:1903–13.
16. Brown A, Reynolds LR, Bruemmer D. Intensive glycemic control and cardiovascular disease: an update. Nat Rev Cardiol. 2010;7:369–75.
17. Gaede P, Lund-Andersen H, Parving HH, Pedersen O. Effect of a multifactorial intervention on mortality in type 2 diabetes. N Engl J Med. 2008;358:580–91.
18. Whitlock G, Lewington S, Sherliker P, Clarke R, Emberson J, Halsey J, et al. Body-mass index and cause-specific mortality in 900 000 adults: collaborative analyses of 57 prospective studies. Lancet. 2009;373:1083–96.
19. Kuklina EV, Tong X, George MG, Bansil P. Epidemiology and prevention of stroke: a worldwide perspective. Expert Rev Neurother. 2012;12:199–208.
20. Lee CD, Folsom AR, Blair SN. Physical activity and stroke risk: a meta-analysis. Stroke. 2003;34:2475–81.
21. Physical activity guidelines advisory committee report. US Dept of health and human services, Washington, DC. Available at http://www.Health.Gov/paguidelines/
22. Elijovich L, Josephson SA, Fung GL, Smith WS. Intermittent atrial fibrillation may account for a large proportion of otherwise cryptogenic stroke: a study of 30-day cardiac event monitors. J Stroke Cerebrovasc Dis. 2009;18:185–9.
23. Furie KL, Goldstein LB, Albers GW, et al. Science Advisory: Oral Antithrombotic Agents for the Prevention of stroke in Nonvalvular Atrial Fibrillation, A Science Advisory for Healthcare Professionals From the American Heart Association/American Stroke Association. Stroke 2012;43:3442–3453.
24. Van der Kooy K, van Hout H, Marwijk H, Marten H, Stehouwer C, Beekman A. Depression and the risk for cardiovascular diseases: systematic review and meta analysis. Int J Geriatr Psychiatry. 2007;22:613–26.
25. Smoller JW, Allison M, Cochrane BB, Curb JD, Perlis RH, Robinson JG, et al. Antidepressant use and risk of incident cardiovascular morbidity and mortality among postmenopausal women in the women's health initiative study. Arch Intern Med. 2009;169:2128–39.

26. Salaycik KJ, Kelly-Hayes M, Beiser A, Nguyen AH, Brady SM, Kase CS, et al. Depressive symptoms and risk of stroke: the Framingham study. Stroke. 2007;38:16–21.
27. Johnston SC, Fayad PB, Gorelick PB, Hanley DF, Shwayder P, van Husen D, et al. Prevalence and knowledge of transient ischemic attack among US adults. Neurology. 2003;60:1429–34.
28. Johnston SC, Gress DR, Browner WS, Sidney S. Short-term prognosis after emergency department diagnosis of TIA. JAMA. 2000;284:2901–6.
29. Giles MF, Rothwell PM. Risk of stroke early after transient ischaemic attack: a systematic review and meta-analysis. Lancet Neurol. 2007;6:1063–72.
30. Rothwell PM, Giles MF, Flossmann E, Lovelock CE, Redgrave JN, Warlow CP, et al. A simple score (ABCD) to identify individuals at high early risk of stroke after transient ischaemic attack. Lancet. 2005;366:29–36.
31. Johnston SC, Rothwell PM, Nguyen-Huynh MN, Giles MF, Elkins JS, Bernstein AL, et al. Validation and refinement of scores to predict very early stroke risk after transient ischaemic attack. Lancet. 2007;369:283–92.
32. Easton JD, Saver JL, Albers GW, Alberts MJ, Chaturvedi S, Feldmann E, et al. Definition and evaluation of transient ischemic attack: a scientific statement for healthcare professionals from the American Heart Association/American Stroke Association stroke council; council on cardiovascular surgery and anesthesia; council on cardiovascular radiology and intervention; council on cardiovascular nursing; and the interdisciplinary council on peripheral vascular disease. The American academy of neurology affirms the value of this statement as an educational tool for neurologists. Stroke. 2009;40:2276–93.
33. Ovbiagele B, Kidwell CS, Saver JL. Epidemiological impact in the United States of a tissue-based definition of transient ischemic attack. Stroke. 2003;34:919–24.
34. Longstreth Jr WT, Dulberg C, Manolio TA, Lewis MR, Beauchamp NJ Jr, O'Leary D, et al. Incidence, manifestations, and predictors of brain infarcts defined by serial cranial magnetic resonance imaging in the elderly: the cardiovascular health study. Stroke. 2002;33:2376–82.
35. Vermeer SE, Prins ND, den Heijer T, Hofman A, Koudstaal PJ, Breteler MM. Silent brain infarcts and the risk of dementia and cognitive decline. N Engl J Med. 2003;348:1215–22.
36. Roquer J, Campello AR, Gomis M. Sex differences in first-ever acute stroke. Stroke. 2003;34:1581–5.
37. Petrea RE, Beiser AS, Seshadri S, Kelly-Hayes M, Kase CS, Wolf PA. Gender differences in stroke incidence and poststroke disability in the Framingham heart study. Stroke. 2009;40:1032–7.
38. Guralnik JM, LaCroix AZ, Branch LG, Kasl SV, Wallace RB. Morbidity and disability in older persons in the years prior to death. Am J Public Health. 1991;81:443–7.
39. Kapral MK, Fang J, Hill MD, Silver F, Richards J, Jaigobin C, et al. Sex differences in stroke care and outcomes: results from the registry of the Canadian stroke network. Stroke. 2005;36:809–14.
40. Murray CJ, Lopez AD. Alternative projections of mortality and disability by cause 1990–2020: global burden of disease study. Lancet. 1997;349:1498–504.
41. Solomon NA, Glick HA, Russo CJ, Lee J, Schulman KA. Patient preferences for stroke outcomes. Stroke. 1994;25:1721–5.
42. Kelly-Hayes M, Beiser A, Kase CS, Scaramucci A, D'Agostino RB, Wolf PA. The influence of gender and age on disability following ischemic stroke: the Framingham study. J Stroke Cerebrovasc Dis. 2003;12:119–26.
43. Kahn R, Robertson RM, Smith R, Eddy D. The impact of prevention on reducing the burden of cardiovascular disease. Circulation. 2008;118:576–85.

Chapter 2
Types of Strokes

Joao Gomes and Ari Marc Wachsman

Key Points

- There are two main types of strokes: ischemic and hemorrhagic.
- Ischemic strokes are far more common than hemorrhagic strokes.
- The brain has a blood supply which is fairly consistent between individuals.
- Ischemic strokes can be due to large-vessel atherosclerosis, aortocardioembolism, small-vessel occlusion, other determined causes, and undetermined causes.
- Hemorrhagic strokes are most often due to hypertension but may be caused by specific blood vessel abnormalities and other medical problems.
- The clinical impact of a stroke depends largely on the stroke's location in the brain, whether it is ischemic or hemorrhagic, and the size/severity of the stroke itself.

Keywords Stroke • Transient ischemic attack • Ischemic • Hemorrhagic • Infarct • Cerebrovascular • Aneurysm • Arteriovenous malformation • Subarachnoid hemorrhage

Abbreviations

CAA   Cerebral Amyloid Angiopathy
ICH   Intracerebral Hemorrhages
SAH   Subarachnoid Hemorrhage

J. Gomes, M.D.
Cerebrovascular Center, Cleveland Clinic, 9500 Euclid Ave, S80, Cleveland, OH 44195, USA
e-mail: gomesj@ccf.org

A.M. Wachsman, M.D. (✉)
Neurological Institute, Cleveland Clinic, 9500 Euclid Ave, Unit H22, Cleveland, OH 44195, USA
e-mail: wachsma@ccf.org

M.L. Corrigan et al. (eds.), *Handbook of Clinical Nutrition and Stroke*,
Nutrition and Health, DOI 10.1007/978-1-62703-380-0_2,
© Springer Science+Business Media New York 2013

Introduction

The word "stroke" is taken in this brief summary and by most healthcare practitioners to describe damage to the neuraxis (i.e., the brain and spinal cord) resulting from any and all abnormalities in its blood supply. "Stroke" means many things to different people, but universally inspires a certain visceral response. Comprised of about 100 billion neurons and a trillion glia [1] packed into about 3 pounds of tissue, the brain houses our consciousness, our accumulated experiences parsed and encoded by the paired temporal lobes, and stored in a network encompassing the entire brain. The brain enables our every movement and every breath. Stroke remains the leading cause of disability in the United States [2] and is the country's fourth leading cause of death [3].

Stroke has contributed to our present understanding of the brain more than any other disease. The numerous ways in which neurologic deficits appear when one area of the brain or another is damaged were noted by physicians as early as ancient Egypt, but it was not until fairly recently that advancements in histopathology, neurophysiology, and neuroimaging informed centuries of clinical observation and forever transformed the field of neuroscience. The great revelation in the second half of the nineteenth century has been that the brain is organized into different regions with different cell types, and the pattern is relatively uniform among human beings. In other words, two right-handed people with lesions in a given region of the left hemisphere will reliably manifest the same kind of speech difficulty. Similarly, the anatomy of the arteries and veins serving the brain is much the same between individuals, so blockage of a particular artery will cause a fairly predictable constellation of physical findings. Hence, generations of neurologists have been taught "we learn the brain, stroke by stroke."

With this in mind, it may be surprising how little is known about the various types of stroke by most non-stroke physicians and allied health professionals. One can speculate on potential reasons for this—such as perceived complexity of the subject, sociocultural stigma, or simple fear of the disease under discussion—but it seems clear that anyone engaged in the care or rehabilitation of stroke patients should be familiar with the classification of stroke subtypes and their respective etiologies, especially in this age of life-saving and brain-saving stroke treatment and specialized inpatient units devoted to the unique needs of this population.

Ischemic Strokes

By far, the most common type of stroke is the so-called ischemic stroke or cerebral infarction. According to recent data released by the American Heart Association, 87 % of strokes are classified as ischemic [4] (see Fig. 2.1). Infarcts occur as a result of insufficient or interrupted flow of blood to an area of the brain, typically caused by blockage of an artery (though "venous infarcts," discussed below, may cause similar phenomena).

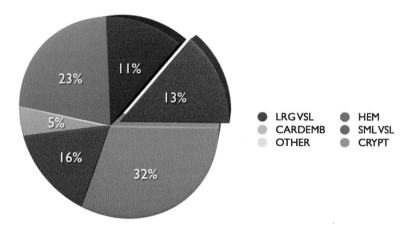

Fig. 2.1 Stroke subtype and annual incidence. Ischemic stroke in *blue* and hemorrhagic stroke in *red*. *LRG VSL* large vessel, *HEM* hemorrhagic, *CARDEMB* cardioembolic, *SML VSL* small vessel, *CRYPT* cryptogenic

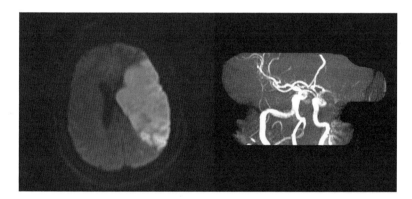

Fig. 2.2 MRI of the brain showing acute ischemic stroke in the distribution of the left middle cerebral artery territory (*left*). MR angiography shows cutoff of the left MCA in a patient with atrial fibrillation

In brief, brain tissue must be supplied with oxygen, glucose, and other vital materials by the constant influx of blood at a rate of about 50–54 ml of blood per 100 g of brain tissue per minute [5]. Brain cells deprived of adequate blood flow (cerebral blood flow [CBF] below 15–20 ml blood flow/100 g tissue/min) [6] will become ischemic; their membrane pumps will begin to fail, intracellular processes will break down, and the brain tissue becomes swollen. Importantly, the ischemic brain tissue may still be salvageable if perfusion can be restored at this point [7]. If the hypoperfusion worsens (i.e., CBF <8–10 ml/100 g/min) [7], this tissue at risk will become irreversibly damaged with cell death proceeding within 4–8 min. This event is referred to as an ischemic stroke (see Fig. 2.2).

Damage to brain tissue will occur initially in the region contiguous to the blocked artery (the so-called infarct core [6]), while a penumbra of at-risk tissue surrounding this region remains viable for some time following onset of ictus and with timely intervention may respond to efforts to restore blood flow to the region.

A Review of Relevant Anatomy

Arteries supplying blood to the brain are all branches of the large brachiocephalic arteries that stem from the aorta. The common carotid arteries on either side ascend the anterior neck and bifurcate around the level of the angle of the mandible, into the internal and external carotid arteries [8] The external carotid arteries give off branches that supply the structures of the anterior neck and most of the head and face with blood, with the notable exception of the brain. The internal carotids, by contrast, ascend the neck, enter the skull, and through their intracranial branches will then perfuse most of the anterior 2/3 of the brain, including the entire frontal and parietal lobes and most of the temporal lobes. The internal carotid arteries and their tributaries constitute the so-called anterior circulation [8].

The posterior circulation (or vertebrobasilar system) is composed of two arteries, the right and left vertebral arteries, which are branches of the subclavian arteries arising from the aorta. These ascend laterally and posteriorly within the vertebral foramen and loop over the transverse process of the C1 vertebra to enter the skull, ascending the ventral surface of the medulla oblongata as it ascends the foramen magnum [8]. The vertebral arteries then merge to form the basilar artery at the level of the pons. The basilar artery continues to ascend and bifurcates at the level of the midbrain to parent the right and left posterior cerebral arteries. Through perforating branches, the vertebrobasilar system perfuses the brainstem, cerebellum, thalamus, occipital lobe, and part of the temporal lobe [9].

At the base of the skull, shortly after the large arteries enter the cranial cavity, the major arteries join to form anastomoses in a pattern shared to some degree by all humans—the so-called Circle of Willis (CoW—see Fig. 2.3), formed by arteries which communicate between the anterior and posterior systems and between the left and right sides of the brain [9]. Distal to the CoW, the major named cerebral arteries emerge to perfuse the brain: the anterior and middle cerebral arteries from the anterior circulation and the posterior cerebral arteries from the bifurcation at the top of the basilar artery, linked by the anterior and posterior communicating arteries, respectively [9].

There are a number of ways in which ischemic strokes can occur, and the various etiologies often result in different clinical presentations and characteristic appearance of the lesion on imaging. Several subclassification schemes for ischemic strokes have been proposed over the last four decades [10], including the Harvard Stroke Registry (1978) [11], Oxfordshire Community Stroke Project (1993) [12], TOAST (or "Trial of Org 10172 in Acute Stroke Treatment") (1992) [13], SSS-TOAST (2005) [14], A-S-C-O, or "phenotypic" (2009) [15], and the Chinese

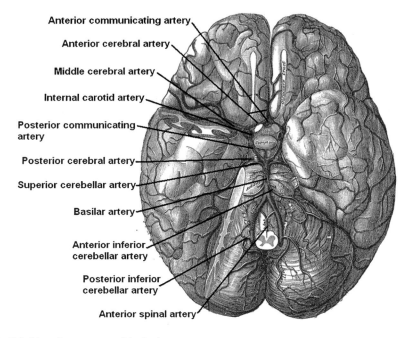

Anterior communicating artery

Anterior cerebral artery

Middle cerebral artery

Internal carotid artery

Posterior communicating artery

Posterior cerebral artery

Superior cerebellar artery

Basilar artery

Anterior inferior cerebellar artery

Posterior inferior cerebellar artery

Anterior spinal artery

Fig. 2.3 Vascular anatomy of the brain

Ischemic Stroke Subclassification (2011) [16]. The TOAST classification is the most widely used and includes (1) *large-vessel atherothrombosis* (12.9 % of ischemic strokes), (2) *cardioembolism* (36.5 %), (3) *small-vessel disease* (18.4 %), (4) *other determined causes* (6 %), and (5) *undetermined causes*, which includes cases invoking more than one primary mechanism (26.4–42.3 %) [17].

Large-Vessel Atherothrombosis

This mechanism refers to the formation of lipid-laden atherosclerotic plaques on the inner wall of a large vessel and can affect both extracranial and intracranial arteries [18]. The most common sites for formation of atherosclerotic plaques include the bifurcations of the common carotid arteries, the origins of the vertebral arteries, and the course of the middle cerebral artery prior to its trifurcation [19]. Atherosclerotic plaques involving the cerebral vasculature are associated with the same risk factors as those which form elsewhere in the body, i.e., high blood pressure, diabetes mellitus, and dyslipidemia, among others [20]. They tend to form gradually over a prolonged time course, and the brain is able to adjust for gradual reductions in CBF without leading to infarcts until some critical level of stenosis is reached [21].

Table 2.1
Common sources of cardioembolic strokes

I.	Valvular disease
	A. Mitral stenosis
	B. Mitral annular calcification
	C. Bacterial endocarditis
	D. Nonbacterial endocarditis (i.e., thrombotic)
II.	Abnormal heart rhythms
	A. Atrial fibrillation
III.	Ischemic heart disease
	A. Mural thrombi
	B. Left ventricular aneurysms
IV.	Septal wall abnormalities
	A. Atrial septal defect
	B. Patent foramen ovale
V.	Cardiomyopathies
	A. Alcohol related
	B. Myocarditis
	C. Amyloidosis
VI.	Other
	A. Myxomas
	B. Fibroelastomas

Depending on the arteries affected and the lesion's location within the course of the affected artery, the acuity of the process, and the presence or absence of anastomoses, this mechanism typically results in a single large territorial stroke [22]. In the case of so-called atheroembolism, a thrombus that has formed on the wall of a particular vessel may break apart and shed pieces of clot which are swept downstream and lodge in smaller arterial branches, resulting in multiple smaller strokes within the expected territory of the parent vessel [23].

Cardioembolism

In much the same way that blood clots forming in situ within atherosclerotic large arteries can lead to ischemic stroke, blood clots forming within the heart can break loose, enter the circulation, and lodge downstream in a cerebral artery. Clots can form within the heart due to intracardiac stasis of blood (often due to paroxysmal supraventricular arrhythmias, most commonly atrial fibrillation [24]) or adhering to a thrombogenic device or lesion (such as an implanted prosthetic valve [25]). Table 2.1 includes common cardiac sources of emboli.

On neuroimaging, cardioembolic strokes tend to occur in more than one arterial distribution, often favor the anterior circulation [26], and can be bilateral; acute strokes involving both the right and left anterior circulation can be thought of as embolic until proven otherwise [27]. Here, too, if the embolus is large, it will lodge in a large artery and result in a correspondingly large stroke; this kind of stroke, distressingly common, is also associated with a higher risk of poststroke bleeding (hemorrhagic conversion) [28]. In some cases the "shower of emboli" occurs when an intracardiac thrombus fragments and a large number of small thrombi enter the cerebral circulation, resulting in a characteristic scattershot appearance on neuroimaging of many small acute infarcts in most or all of the brain's arterial territories [29].

Some authorities include in this category strokes resulting from thromboemboli originating from aortic arch atheroma, while others characterize such strokes as resulting from large-artery atheroembolism [30]. While the distinction may be academic to healthcare providers who are not stroke epidemiologists, choosing the appropriate treatment for a particular patient—i.e., antiplatelet agents vs. anticoagulation or surgery—may depend on this distinction.

Small-Vessel Disease

This mechanism refers to occlusive disease involving the microcirculation of the brain—the unnamed small arteries and arterioles which take off from the named intracerebral parent vessels. The classical etiology of this stroke subtype is lipohyalinotic changes in the walls of these vessels [31], but increasingly microatheromatous disease has been recognized as an important contributing pathology [32]. Common locations for small-vessel disease include deep areas of the hemispheric white matter (such as the corona radiata); the region of white matter known as the internal capsule, adjacent to the proximal middle cerebral artery and supplied with blood by its penetrating branches; the pons in the mid-brainstem, supplied by penetrators arising from the basilar artery; and the thalamus, reliant primarily on branches of the posterior cerebral arteries [33].

Infarctions of these typical regions are classically small (<1.5 cm) [34] and depending on the location within the brain usually produce one of the classic *lacunar syndromes:* (1) *pure motor* symptoms, usually face + arm or arm + leg, comprising 33–50 % of all small-vessel strokes [35]; (2) *pure sensory*; (3) *mixed sensorimotor*; (4) *ataxic hemiparesis*, which features weakness of one side with disproportionate clumsiness (ataxia) of the same side; and (5) *clumsy hand-dysarthria,* clumsiness of either hand, out of proportion to any weakness of the limb, combined with slurred speech [36]. Other lacunar syndromes referable to the posterior circulation have been recognized, such as hemiballism, hemichorea, and isolated dysarthria [37], but they are less commonly seen as results of acute stroke [38].

Other Causes

These include, but are not limited to, strokes caused by extracranial arterial dissections [39], strokes caused by vasospasm associated with subarachnoid hemorrhage (see below) [40], a broad array of hereditary arteriopathies with diverse pathophysiologies (such as moyamoya disease and fibromuscular dysplasia) [41], primary or parainfectious cerebral vasculitis [42], and coagulopathies (including that associated with malignancy, genetic disorders, and medical therapy) [43].

Undetermined Cause

This includes patients in whom a complete workup screening for cardiac conduction or structural abnormalities, intracranial or extracranial large-artery stenosis, coagulopathy, and other conditions has been unrevealing. Clinical situations in which a complete workup cannot be done, or has not yet been done, have also often placed in this category [44].

Also, in the regrettably common eventuality (approaching 40 % of all ischemic strokes [45]) that two likely causes for a given stroke are identified, such as in the case of a patient with comorbid atrial fibrillation and intracranial arterial stenosis, one primary cause cannot be assigned. Especially as this is such a large tranche of stroke patients, the desire for information about their outcomes and risk factors has led to the proposal of arguably more nuanced subclassification schemes such as ASCO [14] and the computer-aided SSS-TOAST [46]. These account for the presence of multiple potential etiologies or attempt to assign a level of likelihood (evident, likely, or possible) to a given etiology from those listed above.

A word should also be said about *watershed* and *borderzone (terminoterminal) strokes*, which tend to occur at the junction between two arterial territories. If a stroke develops in a region between adjacent arterial territories which share collateral circulation, such as the ipsilateral ACA and MCA, the stroke is termed watershed [47]. Borderzone infarcts occur when the infarct occurs between two arterial territories whose parent vessels do not share collateral flow [48], whether via the CoW or other regions of anastomosis (beyond the scope of this review). These are most commonly precipitated by a global or regional hemodynamic insufficiency, although they can at times be embolic [49]. For example, transient ICA occlusion and recanalization will result in a band of infarcted tissue in the borderzone between the ACA and MCA territories, furthest from the two respective parent vessels. These strokes may often be preceded by hypotension and/or hypovolemia and in post-cardiac arrest and shock patients [50].

Hemorrhagic Strokes

In this type of stroke the primary pathology is an area of bleeding causing direct damage to brain tissue. These constitute up to 10–15 % of all strokes and have a significantly higher morbidity and mortality than do ischemic strokes [51]. There are primarily two different types of hemorrhagic strokes: subarachnoid hemorrhage and intracerebral hemorrhage. In the former, blood accumulates in the potential spaces around and within the brain where cerebrospinal fluid is normally found,

Fig. 2.4 Head CT showing
left basal ganglia
intraparenchymal hemorrhage
with surrounding edema and
extension into the ventricular
system

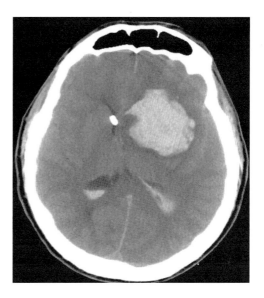

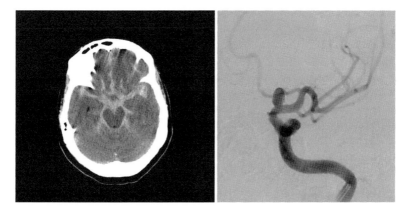

Fig. 2.5 Head CT showing diffuse subarachnoid hemorrhage in the basal cisterns (*left*). Digital
subtraction angiography demonstrating left internal carotid artery aneurysm (*right*)

whereas in the latter the extravasation of blood occurs directly into the parenchyma
(see Figs. 2.4 and 2.5) [52].

Intracranial hemorrhages are associated with the following etiologies.

Hypertension

Most intracerebral hemorrhages (ICH) are associated with rupture of an artery in
the setting of acute or chronic arterial hypertension, which increases risk of spontaneous ICH two- to sixfold [53]. This has been attributed to the presence of

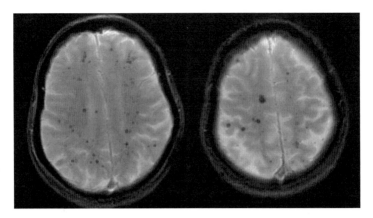

Fig. 2.6 Brain MRI showing multiple lobar microbleeds as a result of cerebral amyloid angiopathy

lipohyalinotic changes within the small arteries or the formation of microaneurysmal outpouchings (Charcot-Bouchard aneurysms) [54], which weaken the arterial wall. It should be noted that systemic hypertension is often caused by ICH as the body attempts to overcome raised intracranial pressure to perfuse the brain, and may not necessarily be the causative etiology in some ICH patients presenting to the Emergency Department [55].

The most common sites of hypertensive hemorrhages are the paired deep gray-matter structures referred to as the basal ganglia (putamen and lentiform nuclei as well as caudate nuclei); the thalamus; the pons; the cerebellum; and larger lobar hemorrhages affecting the cerebral hemispheres [56]. These will cause different presentations with varying degrees of neurologic compromise depending on size and location.

A significant proportion of hypertensive hemorrhages occur in the setting of suboptimal adherence to a medical antihypertensive regimen, such as the abrupt discontinuation of a blood pressure medication due to an inability to afford the medication, or as a result of illicit catecholaminergic drug use, such as cocaine or methamphetamine [57]. Such cases illustrate on a daily basis the myriad social and cultural issues that accompany the ICH patient in the neuro-ICU and beyond.

Cerebral Amyloid Angiopathy

This is a disease characterized by deposition of fibrillary proteins in the walls of arterioles, making them stiff and brittle and predisposing them to rupture. These characteristically occur at the junction of the gray and white matter in the cerebral hemisphere and therefore typically present as lobar bleeds [58]. This etiology of intracranial hemorrhage is commonly seen in the elderly and is often diagnosed when an MRI of the brain discloses the existence of multiple microbleeds, which were previously undetected (see Fig. 2.6). Cerebral amyloid angiopathy (CAA) typically occurs sporadically, though hereditary forms have been described. Because of the superficial location of the amyloid depositions, patients with CAA may also present with subarachnoid hemorrhage [59].

Bleeding Diathesis-Associated Hemorrhage

Patients may suffer intraparenchymal hemorrhages in the setting of bleeding disorders either due to a primary factor deficiency such as hemophilia A, an acquired factor deficiency such as that seen in hepatic failure, thrombocytopenia with its diverse causes, or disseminated intravascular coagulation [60].

Therapeutic Anticoagulation

A rather large subset of patients with ICH present with clotting dysfunction from use of anticoagulants, usually for primary or secondary prevention of cardioembolic stroke in the setting of valvular heart disease or atrial fibrillation. Patients also may be on anticoagulation therapy for deep vein thrombosis and/or pulmonary embolism, thrombophilia secondary to neoplastic disease, coagulopathy associated with rheumatologic conditions such as systemic lupus erythematosus, or due to intrinsic sporadic or hereditary coagulopathies [61]. The use of antiplatelet agents such as aspirin and/or clopidogrel, common in the outpatient treatment and secondary prevention of ischemic stroke, also confers a small but statistically significant risk of intracranial hemorrhage [62].

Hemorrhage in the Setting of a Vascular Malformation

The presence of certain abnormalities of the blood vessels within the brain or on its surface carries an increased risk of intracranial hemorrhage. These abnormalities include ruptured aneurysms (typically leading to subarachnoid hemorrhages), arteriovenous malformations (especially in the presence of venous aneurysms), dural arteriovenous fistulas, or cavernous angiomas. Rarely, intraparenchymal hemorrhages may occur due to dissection of intracranial arteries, in the form of a pseudoaneurysm [63].

Hemorrhagic Conversion of Ischemic Stroke

Hemorrhages in this category may occur after administration of thrombolytic drugs for acute stroke treatment, or in the setting of a large territorial stroke. The latter occurs more commonly in the setting of cardioembolic strokes, which tend to be larger [28]. Furthermore, when a thrombus embolizes to the brain, it will usually be broken up after some time by the body's intrinsic process of thrombolysis, and blood flow will be restored to that region [64]. This is often after the point at which the blood vessels themselves have become ischemic and friable, leading to rupture of the vessel wall and extravasation of blood when hydrostatic pressure is restored. A small amount of pete-chial hemorrhage within a territorial stroke is not unexpected and may not significantly affect outcomes [65], but large, devastating lobar hemorrhages can occur as well.

Hemorrhage Due to Cerebral Venous Thrombosis

If a patient develops a blood clot in a superficial or deep cerebral vein or venous sinus, hydrostatic pressure will increase upstream of the venous side of the capil-lary bed until ultimately water is forced through the capillary walls and into the interstitium of the adjacent brain tissue reliant on the affected vein for normal fluid balance [66]. This process can cause edema and tissue dysfunction leading to vari-able neurologic deficits, altered sensorium, and seizures. If this continues unabated, hemorrhagic necrosis and vasogenic edema can develop in the affected area. This is sometimes referred to as venous infarction, though unlike true ischemic stroke, arte-rial supply may not be compromised [67].

Other Causes

Intraparenchymal hemorrhages may also occur in the setting of neoplastic disease, both in primary brain tumors and metastatic disease [68]. Indeed, acute neurologic deficits found to be due to a hemorrhagic metastasis may often be the initial present-ing sign of the disease's existence. Additional causes within this category include hemorrhage due to sympathomimetic drugs such as cocaine (often ascribed to hypertension, as above); those due to head trauma with blunt or penetrating brain injury; and those due to systemic or primary cerebral arteriopathy (i.e., moyamoya), primary CNS or systemic vasculitis, infectious vasculitis, and infective endocarditis (i.e., due to rupture of a mycotic aneurysm) [69].

Subarachnoid Hemorrhage

Subarachnoid hemorrhage (SAH) is defined as bleeding into the subarachnoid space, between the pia mater—the delicate lining directly adherent to the surface of the brain—and the arachnoid membrane which overlies it. This space is usually occupied only by a small quantity of clear, colorless cerebrospinal fluid (CSF), which among other functions cushions the brain from injury and plays a key role in autoregulation of cerebral blood flow at the arteriolar level [70]. When blood is introduced to this space, it causes marked painful irritation of the meninges and may obstruct the normal flow of CSF. (see Fig. 2.5) [70, 71]. Craniocerebral trauma is overall the most common cause of SAH, while aneurysm rupture (saccular or berry) accounts for over 80 % of nontraumatic SAH [72]. Other less common etiologies include perimesencephalic (presumably venous) hemorrhages, arterial dissections, vascular malformations, drug abuse, coagulopathies, and sickle-cell disease [73].

The estimated annual incidence of SAH varies greatly with the population studied and with other demographic and geographical factors. In a recent meta-analysis the pooled incidence of SAH was 10.5 per 100,000 person-years, and in the United States alone 30,000 new cases are reported every year [74]. The relative risk of developing SAH is increased with alcohol intake, hypertension, smoking, and history of a first degree relative with SAH [74]. The prevalence of intracranial aneurysm in the general United States population is 0.5–1.0 % [74]. After an episode of aneurysmal SAH, only 80 % of patients reach the hospital alive, 30 % die during their hospital admission, and only about 16 % ultimately regain independence without cognitive deficits. Overall, less than 50 % of independent patients return to their prior level of work after SAH [75].

Hydrocephalus, vasospasm, cerebral salt wasting, stress cardiomyopathy, neurogenic pulmonary edema, and delayed cerebral ischemia are among the common complications encountered following aneurysmal SAH. Due to the need for frequent patient monitoring after the ictus and the high risk of poor neurologic outcomes and death if these conditions are not treated expectantly, patients presenting with aneurysmal SAH are best cared for in the setting of a Neurosciences Intensive Care Unit [76]. SAH patients are often young and had high functional status at baseline prior to their hemorrhage [77]; as such, of all the patients in the hospital, these patients may have the most to lose.

Conclusion

Stroke—whether ischemic or hemorrhagic—is a disease with many faces. A small-vessel lacunar infarct which involves the deep subcortical white matter may produce nothing but a subtle arm weakness, but an identical lesion located in the upper pons might result in a persistent vegetative state. One patient with paroxysmal atrial fibrillation might present with a dozen infarcts in numerous vascular territories, while another with the same arrhythmia presents instead with isolated transient vision loss. The variety in clinical manifestation can be dizzying; however, with the application of clinical data and some pathophysiology, this protean disease can be thought of as caused by just a few basic etiologies, briefly outlined above.

Due to the unique needs of this population, the stroke patient requires a high level of specialized care, which must be provided by an interdisciplinary team. A good working knowledge of the fundamentals of neuroanatomy and cerebrovascular anatomy is crucial to caring for this patient population and to preventing future events.

References

1. Lamberti E, Ross L, Taub E, editors. Thieme atlas of anatomy: head and neuroanatomy. 1st ed. New York: Thieme; 2007. p. 176.
2. Ifejika-Jones NL, Barrett AM. Rehabilitation—emerging technologies, innovative therapies, and future objectives. Neurotherapeutics. 2011;8(3):452–62.
3. Towfighi A, Saver JL. Stroke declines from third to fourth leading cause of death in the United States: historical perspective and challenges ahead. Stroke. 2011;42(8):2351–5.
4. Roger VL, for the American Heart Association Statistics Committee and Stroke Statistics Subcommittee, et al. Executive summary: heart disease and stroke statistics—2012 update: a report from the American Heart Association. Circulation. 2012;125(1):188–97.
5. Torbey MT, Bhardwaj A. Cerebral blood flow physiology and monitoring. In: Suarez JI, editor. Critical care neurology and neurosurgery. Totowa, NJ: Humana; 2004. p. 23.
6. Astrup J, Sisejo BK, Symon L. Thresholds in cerebral ischemia—the ischemic penumbra. Stroke. 1981;12(6):723–5.
7. Hossmann KA. Viability thresholds and the penumbra of focal ischemia. Ann Neurol. 1994;36(4):557–65.
8. Victor M. Adams and Victor's principles of neurology. Chapter 34: Cerebrovascular diseases. 7th ed. New York: McGraw Hill; 2001. p. 829–31.
9. Cereda C, Carrera E. Posterior cerebral artery territory infarctions. Front Neurol Neurosci. 2012;30:128–31.
10. Chen PH, Gao S, Wang YJ, Xu AD, Li YS, Wang D. Classifying ischemic stroke, from TOAST to CISS. CNS Neurosci Ther. 2012;18(6):452–6. doi:10.1111/j.1755-5949.2011.00292.x.
11. Mohr JP, Caplan LR, Melski JW, Goldstein RJ, Duncan GW, Kistler JP, et al. The Harvard Cooperative Stroke Registry: a prospective registry. Neurology. 1978;28(8):754–62.
12. Lindley RI, Warlow CP, Wardlaw JM, Dennis MS, Slattery J, Sandercock PA. Interobserver reliability of a clinical classification of acute cerebral infarction. Stroke. 1993;24(12): 1801–4.
13. Adams HP, for the TOAST Investigators, et al. Classification of subtype of acute ischemic stroke. Stroke. 1993;24:35–41.
14. Ay H, Furie KL, et al. An evidence-based causative classification system for acute ischemic stroke. Ann Neurol. 2005;58:688–97.
15. Marnane M, Duggan CA, et al. Stroke subtype classification to mechanism specific and undetermined categories by TOAST, ASCO, and causative classification system. Stroke. 2010;41:1579–86.
16. Gao S, Wang YJ, Xu AD, Li YS, Wang DZ. Chinese ischemic stroke subclassification. Front Neurol. 2011;2:6.
17. Adams HP, Bendixen BH, Kapelle LJ, for the TOAST Investigators, et al. Classification of subtype of acute ischemic stroke. Stroke. 1993;24:35–7.
18. Rovira A, Grivé E, Rovira A, Alvarez-Sabin J. Distribution territories and causative mechanisms of ischemic stroke. Eur Radiol. 2005;15(3):416–26.
19. Derdeyn CP. Mechanisms of ischemic stroke secondary to large artery atherosclerotic disease. Neuroimaging Clin N Am. 2007;17(3):303–11. vii–viii.
20. Luitse MJ, Biessels GJ, Rutten GE, Kappelle LJ. Diabetes, hyperglycaemia, and acute ischaemic stroke. Lancet Neurol. 2012;11(3):261–71.
21. Klijn CJ, Kappelle LJ. Haemodynamic stroke: clinical features, prognosis, and management. Lancet Neurol. 2010;9(10):1008–17.
22. Arenillas JF, Alvarez-Sabín J. Basic mechanisms in intracranial large-artery atherosclerosis: advances and challenges. Cerebrovasc Dis. 2005;20 Suppl 2:75–83.
23. Rapp JH, Pan XM, Yu B, Swanson RA, Higashida RT, Simpson P, et al. Cerebral ischemia and infarction from atheroemboli <100 micron in size. Stroke. 2003;34(8):1976–80.
24. Olsson SB, Halperin JL. Prevention of stroke in patients with atrial fibrillation. Semin Vasc Med. 2005;5(3):285–92.

25. Verheugt FW. Anticoagulation after artificial valve replacement with or without atrial fibrillation: how much is really needed? Thromb Haemost. 1999;82 Suppl 1:130–5.
26. Chung EM, Hague JP, Chanrion MA, Ramnarine KV, Katsogridakis E, Evans DH. Embolus trajectory through a physical replica of the major cerebral arteries. Stroke. 2010;41(4): 647–52.
27. Takahashi K, Kobayashi S, Matui R, Yamaguchi S, Yamashita K. The differences of clinical parameters between small multiple ischemic lesions and single lesion detected by diffusion-weighted MRI. Acta Neurol Scand. 2002;106(1):24–9.
28. Molina CA, Montaner J, Abilleira S, Ibarra B, Romero F, Arenillas JF, et al. Timing of spontaneous recanalization and risk of hemorrhagic transformation in acute cardioembolic stroke. Stroke. 2001;32(5):1079–84.
29. Cho AH, Kim JS, Jeon SB, Kwon SU, Lee DH, Kang DW. Mechanism of multiple infarcts in multiple cerebral circulations on diffusion-weighted imaging. J Neurol. 2007;254(7):924–30.
30. Doufekias E, Segal AZ, Kizer JR. Cardiogenic and aortogenic brain embolism. J Am Coll Cardiol. 2008;51(11):1049–59.
31. Schmal M, Marini C, Carolei A, Di Napoli M, Kessels F, Lodder J. Different vascular risk factor profiles among cortical infarcts, small deep infarcts, and primary intracerebral haemorrhage point to different types of underlying vasculopathy. A study from the L'Aquila Stroke Registry. Cerebrovasc Dis. 1998;8(1):14–9.
32. Ogata J, Yamanishi H, Ishibashi-Ueda H. Review: role of cerebral vessels in ischaemic injury of the brain. Neuropathol Appl Neurobiol. 2011;37(1):40–55.
33. Nah HW, Kang DW, Kwon SU, Kim JS. Diversity of single small subcortical infarctions according to infarct location and parent artery disease: analysis of indicators for small vessel disease and atherosclerosis. Stroke. 2010;41(12):2822–7.
34. Koch S, McClendon MS, Bhatia R. Imaging evolution of acute lacunar infarction: leukoaraiosis or lacune? Neurology. 2011;77(11):1091–5.
35. De Reuck J, De Groote L, Van Maele G. The classic lacunar syndromes: clinical and neuroimaging correlates. Eur J Neurol. 2008;15(7):681–4.
36. Arboix A, López-Grau M, Casasnovas C, García-Eroles L, Massons J, Balcells M. Clinical study of 39 patients with atypical lacunar syndrome. J Neurol Neurosurg Psychiatry. 2006; 77(3):381–4.
37. Victor M. Adams and Victor's principles of neurology. Chap 34: Cerebrovascular diseases. 7th ed. New York: McGraw Hill; 2001. p. 847.
38. Debette S, Leys D. Cervical-artery dissections: predisposing factors, diagnosis, and outcome. Lancet Neurol. 2009;8(7):668–78.
39. Vergouwen MD, Participants in the International Multi-Disciplinary Consensus Conference on the Critical Care Management of Subarachnoid Hemorrhage. Vasospasm versus delayed cerebral ischemia as an outcome event in clinical trials and observational studies. Neurocrit Care. 2011;15(2):308–11.
40. Starke RM, Crowley RW, Maltenfort M, Jabbour PM, Gonzalez LF, Tjoumakaris SI, et al. Moyamoya disorder in the United States. Neurosurgery. 2012;71(1):93–9.
41. Pugin D, Copin JC, Goodyear MC, Landis T, Gasche Y. Persisting vasculitis after pneumococcal meningitis. Neurocrit Care. 2006;4(3):237–40.
42. Ferro JM, Massaro AR, Mas JL. Aetiological diagnosis of ischaemic stroke in young adults. Lancet Neurol. 2010;9(11):1085–96.
43. Amarenco P. Underlying pathology of stroke of unknown cause (cryptogenic stroke). Cerebrovasc Dis. 2009;27 Suppl 1:97–103.
44. Marnane M, Duggan CA, et al. Stroke subtype classification to mechanism specific and undetermined categories by TOAST, ASCO, and causative classification system. Stroke. 2010;41:1584.
45. Wolf ME, Sauer T, Alonso A, Hennerici MG. Comparison of the new ASCO classification with the TOAST classification in a population with acute ischemic stroke. J Neurol. 2012;259(7):1284–9.

46. Paciaroni M, Agnelli G, Caso V, Bogousslavsky J, editors. Manifestations of stroke. Front Neurol Neurosci. Basel: Karger; 2012. 30:181–184.
47. D'Amore C, Paciaroni M. Border-zone and watershed infarctions. Front Neurol Neurosci. 2012;30:181–4.
48. Mangla R, Kolar B, Almast J, Ekholm SE. Border zone infarcts: pathophysiologic and imaging characteristics. Radiographics. 2011;31(5):1201–14.
49. Gutierrez LG, Rovira A, Portela LA, Leite Cda C, Lucato LT. CT and MR in non-neonatal hypoxic-ischemic encephalopathy: radiological findings with pathophysiological correlations. Neuroradiology. 2010;52(11):949–76.
50. Gebel JM, Broderick JP. Intracerebral hemorrhage. Neurol Clin. 2000;18(2):419–38.
51. Dupont SA, Wijdicks EF, Lanzino G, Rabinstein AA. Aneurysmal subarachnoid hemorrhage: an overview for the practicing neurologist. Semin Neurol. 2010;30(5):545–54.
52. Elliott J, Smith M. The acute management of intracerebral hemorrhage: a clinical review. Anesth Analg. 2010;110(5):1419–27.
53. Challa VR, Moody DM, Bell MA. The Charcôt-Bouchard aneurysm controversy: impact of a new histologic technique. J Neuropathol Exp Neurol. 1992;51(3):264–71.
54. Hocker S, Morales-Vidal S, Schneck MJ. Management of arterial blood pressure in acute ischemic and hemorrhagic stroke. Neurol Clin. 2010;28(4):863–86.
55. Kase CS. Intracerebral haemorrhage. Baillieres Clin Neurol. 1995;4(2):247–78.
56. Green RM, Kelly KM, Gabrielsen T, Levine SR, Vanderzant C. Multiple intracerebral hemorrhages after smoking "crack" cocaine. Stroke. 1990;21(6):957–62.
57. Pezzini A, Padovani A. Cerebral amyloid angiopathy-related hemorrhages. Neurol Sci. 2008;29 Suppl 2:S260–3.
58. Haan J, Maat-Schieman ML, Roos RA. Clinical aspects of cerebral amyloid angiopathy. Dementia. 1994;5(3–4):210–3.
59. del Zoppo GJ, Mori E. Hematologic causes of intracerebral hemorrhage and their treatment. Neurosurg Clin N Am. 1992;3(3):637–58.
60. Rolfe S, Papadopoulos S, Cabral KP. Controversies of anticoagulation reversal in life-threatening bleeds. J Pharm Pract. 2010;23(3):217–25.
61. Soo YO, Yang SR, et al. Risk vs. benefit of anti-thrombotic therapy in ischaemic stroke patients with cerebral microbleeds. J Neurol. 2008;255(11):1679–86.
62. Krings T, Choi IS. The many faces of intracranial arterial dissections. Interv Neuroradiol. 2010;16(2):151–60.
63. Di Tullio MR, Homma S. Mechanisms of cardioembolic stroke. Curr Cardiol Rep. 2002; 4(2):141–8.
64. Babikian VL, Kase CS, Pessin MS, Norrving B, Gorelick PB. Intracerebral hemorrhage in stroke patients anticoagulated with heparin. Stroke. 1989;20(11):1500–3.
65. Nguyen J, Nishimura N, Fetcho RN, Iadecola C, Schaffer CB. Occlusion of cortical ascending venules causes blood flow decreases, reversals in flow direction, and vessel dilation in upstream capillaries. J Cereb Blood Flow Metab. 2011;31(11):2243–54.
66. Masuhr F, Mehraein S, Einhäupl K. Cerebral venous and sinus thrombosis. J Neurol. 2004;251(1):11–23.
67. Sagduyu A, Sirin H, Mulayim S, Bademkiran F, Yunten N, Kitis O, et al. Cerebral cortical and deep venous thrombosis without sinus thrombosis: clinical MRI correlates. Acta Neurol Scand. 2006;114(4):254–60.
68. Rogers LR. Cerebrovascular complications in cancer patients. Neurol Clin. 2003;21(1): 167–92.
69. Burke GM, Burke AM, Sherma AK, Hurley MC, Batjer HH, Bendok BR. Moyamoya disease: a summary. Neurosurg Focus. 2009;26(4):E11.
70. Pollay M. Overview of the CSF dual outflow system. Acta Neurochir Suppl. 2012;113: 47–50.
71. Ostergaard JR. Headache as a warning symptom of impending aneurysmal subarachnoid haemorrhage. Cephalalgia. 1991;11(1):53–5.

72. Cuvinciuc V, Viguier A, Calviere L, Raposo N, Larrue V, Cognard C, et al. Isolated acute nontraumatic cortical subarachnoid hemorrhage. AJNR Am J Neuroradiol. 2010;31(8): 1355–62.
73. Anson JA, Koshy M, Ferguson L, Crowell RM. Subarachnoid hemorrhage in sickle-cell disease. J Neurosurg. 1991;75(4):552–8.
74. Diringer MN, Bleck TP, for the Neurocritical Care Society, et al. Critical care management of patients following aneurysmal subarachnoid hemorrhage: recommendations from the Neurocritical Care Society's Multidisciplinary Consensus Conference. Neurocrit Care. 2011;15(2):211–40.
75. Zacharia BE, Hickman ZL, Grobelny BT, DeRosa P, Kotchetkov I, Ducruet AF, et al. Epidemiology of aneurysmal subarachnoid hemorrhage. Neurosurg Clin N Am. 2010;21(2): 221–33.
76. Bederson JB, Awad IA, Wiebers DO, Piepgras D, Haley Jr EC, Brott T, et al. Recommendations for the management of patients with unruptured intracranial aneurysms: a statement for healthcare professionals from the Stroke Council of the American Heart Association. Circulation. 2000;102(18):2300–8.
77. Rinkel GJ, Algra A. Long-term outcomes of patients with aneurysmal subarachnoid haemorrhage. Lancet Neurol. 2011;10(4):349–56.
78. Wijdicks EF, Kallmes DF, Manno EM, Fulgham JR, Piepgras DG. Subarachnoid hemorrhage: neurointensive care and aneurysm repair. Mayo Clin Proc. 2005;80(4):550–9.
79. de Rooij NK, Linn FH, van der Plas JA, Algra A, Rinkel GJ. Incidence of subarachnoid haemorrhage: a systematic review with emphasis on region, age, gender and time trends. J Neurol Neurosurg Psychiatry. 2007;78(12):1365–72.

Chapter 3
Stroke Risk Factors

Gursimran S. Kochhar, Jennifer F.T. Jue, and Craig Nielsen

Key Points

- Stroke risk factors can be divided into situational risk factors (generally non-modifiable), medical risk factors, and lifestyle risk factors (both potentially modifiable).
- Hypertension and atrial fibrillation are the two most modifiable medical risk factors.
- The increased incidence of obesity in the United States may result in an increased incidence of stroke.
- Patients with multiple risk factors are best addressed with a multifactorial team-based approach that focuses on counseling regarding lifestyle risk factors and appropriate medication use regarding known medical risk factors.

Keywords Stroke • Risk factors • Modifiable • Lifestyle • Hypertension • Atrial fibrillation

Abbreviations

ADA	American Diabetes Association
AF	Atrial Fibrillation
ALLHAT	Antihypertensive and Lipid Lowering Treatment to Prevent Heart Attack Trial
CARASIL	Cerebral Autosomal Recessive Arteriopathy with Subcortical Infarcts and Leukoencephalopathy

G.S. Kochhar, M.D. • J.F.T. Jue, M.D. • C. Nielsen, M.D. (✉)
Department of Internal Medicine, Cleveland Clinic Foundation, 9500 Euclid Avenue,
Cleveland, OH 44195, USA
e-mail: kochhag@ccf.org; juej@ccf.org; nielsec@ccf.org

M.L. Corrigan et al. (eds.), *Handbook of Clinical Nutrition and Stroke*,
Nutrition and Health, DOI 10.1007/978-1-62703-380-0_3,
© Springer Science+Business Media New York 2013

CAS   Carotid Artery Stenosis
HDL   High Density of Lipoprotein
LDL   Low-Density Lipoprotein
MELAS   Mitochondrial Myopathy, Encephalopathy, Lactacidosis, and Stroke
OSA   Obstructive Sleep Apnea
SHEP   Systolic Hypertension in the Elderly Program
UKPDS   United Kingdom Prospective Diabetes Study
WHR   Waist-to-Hip Ratio

Introduction

A stroke, which may be defined as a reduction in cerebral blood flow to a region of
the brain in association with a vascular injury, is the second leading cause of death
worldwide, fourth leading cause in the United States, and a leading cause of disability [1, 2]. Strokes may be broadly classified as ischemic (approximately 85 % of
cases) or hemorrhagic (15 % of cases), depending upon the underlying pathophysiologic mechanism. Ischemic stroke is characterized by an insufficient perfusion to a part of the brain resulting from occlusion or stenosis of a cerebral
vessel. Hemorrhagic stroke, by contrast, results from the rupture of an intracranial
blood vessel. Risk factors for stroke are generally divided into non-modifiable
and modifiable factors with various levels of evidence supporting the modifiability
of each. We have chosen to look at stroke risk factors in the following way—
situational risk factors (generally non-modifiable), medical risk factors, and lifestyle risk factors (both potentially modifiable)—see Table 3.1. This chapter provides
a brief overview of some of these risk factors and their association with stroke.

Situational Risk Factors

Age

Age is one of the most important non-modifiable risk factors. For every 10 years
after the age of 55 years, the stroke rate doubles in both men and women [3]. More
than half of all strokes occur in people over age 75 and more than 80 % of strokes
occur in ages over age 65 [4, 5].

Gender

Studies have shown that men have a higher incidence of ischemic stroke up until age
85 years, and then the incidence increases for women over age 85 years due to the
fact that women live longer than men [6]. Consequently, women have a later average

Table 3.1
Stroke risk factors

Situational risk factors
• Age
• Gender
• Race/ethnicity
• Genetic factors
• Socioeconomic factors
• Family history
Medical risk factors
• Hypertension
• Atrial fibrillation
• Diabetes
• Hyperlipidemia
• Hypercoagulable conditions
• Carotid artery disease
• Aortic arch atheromas
• Transient ischemic attacks (TIA)
• Medication use (e.g., oral contraceptive pills (OCPs))
• Obstructive sleep apnea
• Mood disorders
Lifestyle risk factors
• Tobacco use
• Alcohol use
• Diet
• Exercise
• Obesity

onset of stroke at 75 years, while the average onset for men is age 71 years. The lifetime risk of stroke is also higher in women aged 55–75 years at 1 in 5 versus 1 in 6 for men as shown in the Framingham Heart Study [7].

Sex differences in stroke exist and have been studied by investigating the role of estrogen and testosterone as well as risk factors unique to women such as the use of OCP, HRT, and pregnancy. For example, one study found that women with the onset of menopause before age 42 had twice the stroke risk compared to all other women [8].

Family History

Family history of stroke has generally been felt to increase the risk of stroke. Family history studies, twin studies, and those looking at specific genes have had varying results. The Framingham Study from 2010 which is a two-generation, community-based prospective cohort study showed that documented parental stroke by age 65 was associated with a threefold increase in risk of stroke in the offspring [9]. There are likely genetic factors associated with stroke since the study adjusted for conventional stroke risk factors which would be indicative of shared environmental factors. Other studies have shown that family history of stroke is an independent risk factor for lacunar stroke especially in younger patients, again suggestive of genetic factors [10].

However, contrary to previous belief, in one of the most comprehensive family history studies to date published in Circulation Cardiovascular Genetics in 2011 which used a prospective, population-based approach to compare relative heritability of transient ischemic attack and stroke versus acute coronary syndrome, it showed that ischemic stroke usually has a relatively low heritability, while myocardial infarction had moderate heritability with more clustering within families [11]. The findings were independent of age, gender, smoking, and stroke subtype. These results may affect the impact of family history in the calculation of scores for stroke risk in the future.

Genetics

Most cases of stroke are multifactorial with no identified patterns of heritability. However, there are known common single gene disorders associated with stroke which usually present at a younger age, under age 40. For example, CADASIL— cerebral autosomal dominant arteriopathy with subcortical infarcts and leukoencephalopathy, which is caused by mutations of the human NOTCH3 gene, presents at age 30–60 years. CARASIL—cerebral autosomal recessive arteriopathy with subcortical infarcts and leukoencephalopathy—presents at an earlier age at 25–35 years. Moyamoya disease found in East Asian populations with a female predominance has a familial pattern in 12 % of cases [12]. Other disorders include the glycosphingolipid storage disorder, Fabry disease, sickle-cell anemia, homocystinuria, MELAS (mitochondrial myopathy, encephalopathy, lactacidosis, and stroke), Marfan syndrome, and Ehlers–Danlos syndrome [12].

Race and Ethnicity

There are racial disparities in the risk factors that contribute to stroke. For example, African Americans and Hispanics have increased risk factor prevalence of hypertension and diabetes, while whites are more affected by atrial fibrillation and coronary artery disease [13]. According to CDC reports, African Americans are at highest risk of stroke death compared to all other race/ethnic minorities in the United States. This is due to a higher stroke incidence among African Americans by almost double when compared to whites, but they have similar case-fatality rates [14]. African Americans less than 55 years old had a two- to fivefold higher risk than whites, but they had similar rates at older ages [15]. Recent studies have shown that the racial disparity is widening with a decreasing incidence of ischemic strokes among whites but no change among African Americans [16]. The Reasons for Geographic and Racial Differences in Stroke (REGARDS) Study is an ongoing national, population-based longitudinal study of 30,000 black and white adults over the age of 45 years whose aim is to investigate the racial and geographic disparities in the development of stroke.

Socioeconomic Factors

A study has been done to show that approximately half of the racial disparity in stroke risk for people between ages 45 and 65 years is attributable to traditional risk factors (such as systolic blood pressure) and the additional risk attributable to socio-economic factors [17]. Socioeconomic disparity was studied by stratifying subjects by poverty status, and results showed that 39 % of excess stroke incidence risk in African Americans could be explained by community socioeconomic status [15].

Lifestyle Risk Factors

Physical Activity

The American Heart Association (AHA) recommends 30 minutes a day of moderate exercise to decrease recurrence of ischemic stroke [18]. In both the Framingham Study cohort and the Northern Manhattan Study, a prospective cohort study in older, urban-dwelling, multiethnic, stroke-free individuals, it was shown that moderate-to-heavy intensity physical activity was protective against risk of ischemic stroke among men [18, 19]. The 2004 AHA guidelines on stroke prevention recommend aerobic activity 3–7 days a week with an intensity level 50–80 % of maximum heart rate for a duration of 20–60 min per session or multiple 10 min sessions [20]. There are also studies that show benefit of physical activity in women [21]. Patients who exceeded the recommended AHA/Centers for Disease Control and Prevention (CDC) and National Institutes of Health guideline activity level had significantly lower risk, and the study showed that men and women who ran ≥8 km/day were at 60 % lower risk than those who ran <2 km/day [22].

Obesity

In 2009–2010, an estimated 35.5 % of adult men and 35.8 % of adult women in the USA were obese with no significant change from 2003 to 2008 according to results from the 2009–2010 National Health and Nutrition Examination [23]. Although one of the national health objectives is to reduce the prevalence of obesity among adults, data shows that obesity is trending upwards. Abdominal obesity measured as increased waist-to-hip ratio (WHR) has been found to be associated with a greater risk of stroke in men and women in all race/ethnic groups [24]. In addition, some studies have concluded that markers of abdominal adiposity such as WHR, waist circumference, and waist-to-stature ratio were better predictors of TIA and stroke than BMI with a greater effect among young people [24]. With obesity on the rise, increasing numbers of people will be at risk for stroke (see Chap. 8).

Diet

Poor diet is one of the potentially modifiable risk factors for stroke. Oxidative stress and systemic inflammation have been shown by studies to be involved in the pathogenesis of ischemic stroke [25]. As a result, increased consumption of fruits and vegetables which contain phytochemicals with antioxidant properties such as vitamin C, vitamin E, carotenoids, and flavonoids has been shown in epidemiological studies to decrease risk of stroke [26]. In addition to fruits and vegetables, a wide range of antioxidant-rich foods including whole grains and tea were evaluated in a prospective Swedish cohort study and shown to decrease stroke risk in women with no previous history of stroke [25]. Other diet measures to reduce stroke risk include following the Dietary Approaches to Stop Hypertension (DASH), a diet high in fruits and vegetables, moderate in low-fat dairy products, and low in animal protein [27].

Alcohol Consumption

Many studies have been conducted investigating the effect of alcohol on stroke, and the results are controversial. Some studies have shown a linear positive association between alcohol use and hemorrhagic stroke, while some have shown a J-shaped curve for risk of ischemic stroke, with a protective effect for low-to-moderate consumption and increased risk at higher exposure [28]. Drinking less than 12–24 g/day, which is equivalent to one or two drinks per day, had the lowest risk, while those drinking more than 60 g/day or five drinks per day were at highest risk [28]. Chronic heavy drinking and binge drinking with alcohol intoxication increase risk of stroke by way of increasing blood pressure, triggering cardiac arrhythmias and hypercoagulability [29]. As a result, current public health recommendations state that men should consume less than two drinks a day and for women to consume less than one drink per day.

Cigarette Smoking

Recent statistics show 21.2 % of men and 17.5 % of women are cigarette smokers [30]. Cigarette smoking has been shown to have an increased risk of total hemorrhagic stroke, intracranial hemorrhage, and subarachnoid hemorrhage in both men and women. In one study looking at women aged 15–49 years, there was a dose–response relationship—adjusted odds ratio (OR) increased with increasing number of cigarettes smoked per day: OR 2.2 for 1–10 cigarettes/day, 2.5 for 11–20 cigarettes/day, 4.3 for 21–39 cigarettes/day, and 9.1 for 40 or more cigarettes/day [31]. The Framingham Study showed that stroke risk decreased significantly by 2 years and was at the level of nonsmokers by 5 years after cessation of cigarette smoking [32].

Medical Risk Factors

Hypertension

Hypertension is one of the most important modifiable risk factor for prevention of first stroke [33]. Blood pressure control can be achieved in most patients through use of one or two different blood pressure lowering medications. The seventh report of joint national committee on prevention, evaluation, and treatment of high blood pressure (JNC7) guidelines recommends lowering blood pressure to less than 140/90 mmHg (or 130/80 mmHg in individuals with diabetes) [34]. Overall, antihypertensive therapy is associated with a 35–44 % reduction in incidence of stroke [35]. Different types of medication either used alone or in combination have shown to reduce the risk of stroke. The Systolic Hypertension in the Elderly Program (SHEP) trial found 36 % reduction in the incidence of stroke with treatment with a thiazide diuretic with or without beta blocker in patients over age 60 with isolated systolic hypertension [36]. The results from the Antihypertensive and Lipid-Lowering Treatment to Prevent Heart Attack Trial (ALLHAT), a randomized, double-blind trial with 24,316 participants, showed superiority of diuretic based over alpha-blocker-based antihypertensive treatment for the prevention of stroke and cardiovascular disease [37]. A meta-analysis of 18 long-term randomized trials found that both diuretics (hazard ratio, 0.49; 95 % CI, 0.39–0.62) and beta blockers (hazard ratio, 0.71; 95 % CI, 0.59–0.86) were effective in preventing stroke [38].

The treatment of patients with hypertension is beneficial in both younger and elderly patients. It is now well established that blood pressure lowering is not only effective for the primary prevention of stroke and other cardiovascular disorders but also effective for prevention of recurrent stroke. Despite beneficial effects of lowering blood pressure, only 25 % of the hypertensive populations worldwide achieve adequate blood pressure control [39]. Lack of diagnosis and inadequate treatment are particularly evident in minority populations and in the elderly. The challenge now is to effectively implement strategies for the control of blood pressure and to individualize therapy.

Atrial Fibrillation

Atrial fibrillation (AF) is another well-documented risk factor for stroke [40]. AF is common among the elderly as the incidence of AF increases with age. Approximately 6–10 % of people age 75 and over have AF [41]. Anticoagulation therapies remain the main agent for stroke prevention in patients with AF.

Randomized clinical trials have shown warfarin to reduce overall risk of stroke by 68 % with a 1 % increase in risk of major bleeds [42]. Aspirin alone has shown to decrease risk by 20 % [43]. To help the clinician risk stratify patients who need anticoagulation therapy, a risk stratification model has been developed known as the CHADS2 score [44]. It derives its name from C for congestive heart failure, H for hypertension, A for age, D for diabetes, and S2 for prior stroke or transient ischemic attack. The score gives 1 point for each variable and 2 points for prior stroke. Any patients with score 2 or above will benefit from anticoagulation therapy provided no other major contraindications are present to anticoagulation.

Despite many obvious benefits, warfarin therapy is often underused in patients with atrial fibrillation. According to some estimates only about 50 % of patients with AFib who are candidates of warfarin therapy actually receive warfarin, especially in elderly [45]. Recently newer anticoagulants like Dabigatran were approved in October 2010 by Food and Drug Administration (FDA). Its advantages over warfarin include fewer drug interactions and reduced need to monitor PT/INR and a potential disadvantage being we do not yet have a simple antidote if someone develops life-threatening bleed [46].

Diabetes

Individuals with type 2 diabetes are considered high risk for vascular events. As per the Adult Treatment Panel III (ATP III) of the National Cholesterol Education Program, patients with type 2 diabetes have a 20 % likelihood of a major vascular event including stroke in 10 years [47]. As per American Diabetes Association, a total of 25.8 million Americans have diabetes as of January 2011[48]. Due to development of cardiovascular disease at an earlier age in individuals with diabetes, the American Diabetes Association (ADA) recommends a multifactorial approach to management of type 2 diabetes. As noted in the hypertension paragraph, the target levels of blood pressure are more stringent in patients with diabetes than general population. Many trials have compared the effect on stroke and other cardiovascular outcomes of tight control of blood glucose and blood pressure. In the United Kingdom Prospective Diabetes Study (UKPDS) Group, tight blood pressure control (mean BP achieved 144/82 mmHg) showed 44 % reduction in fatal and nonfatal stroke, compared with more liberal control (mean BP achieved 154/87 mmHg) [49]. For the same reason current recommendations are to achieve blood pressures of 130/80 or less, in individuals with diabetes.

Good glycemic control is an important factor regarding the prevention of cardio-vascular morbidity and mortality in patients with diabetes. Ideally the glucose target is near-normal glycemic control with avoidance of hypoglycemia. The UKPDS has shown that good glycemic control reduces risk of stroke in this population of newly diagnosed patients with type 2 diabetes [49]. Current guidelines from ADA recommend target Hba1c levels to be less than 7 for optimal management of diabetes and its complications. Insulin treatment should be considered as soon as treatment with oral agents fails to achieve the target Hba1c or there is end-organ damage despite oral therapy (see Chap. 6).

Dyslipidemia

Existing evidence shows no clear relationship between total cholesterol levels and overall stroke risk, but we now do know that low levels of low-density lipoprotein (LDL) have a positive relationship with risk of ischemic stroke [50]. Also high levels of high density of lipoprotein (HDL) are considered to be protective against stroke [51]. A compelling body of evidence documents that lipid-lowering agents reduce major cardiovascular events in both secondary and primary prevention. Statins are approved by Food and Drug Administration (FDA) for prevention of ischemic stroke in patients with coronary artery disease. The evidence for lipid reduction in diabetes mellitus in relation to vascular disease is mainly derived from subgroup analyses of large clinical trials, which included patients with diabetes. The Collaborative Atrovastatin Diabetes Study (CARDS) is a recent trial, which evaluated statin, which is class of medication known as HMG-CoA reductase inhibitors (hydroxymethylglutaryl-CoA reductase) therapy exclusively in diabetes in the primary prevention of vascular events. A total of 2,838 people with type 2 diabetes were randomized to a statin or placebo. The trial was stopped prematurely because the prespecified stopping rule for efficacy was met. In people with diabetes treated with statin, the primary combined end point of acute coronary events, coronary revascularization, or stroke was reduced by 37 % (hazard ratio, 0.63; 95 % CI, 0.48–0.83) [52]. In particular, stroke was significantly reduced by 48 % [52].

In a meta-analysis of nine trials including 70,070 patients, statin treatment resulted in 21 % relative risk reduction of stroke and 0.9 % of absolute risk reduction [53]. Non-statin lipid-modifying agents like niacin and ezetimibe also may offer stroke protection, although definitive evidence is lacking. In summary, lipid-modifying medications can reduce the risk of stroke in patients with coronary heart disease (see Chap. 7).

Asymptomatic Carotid Stenosis

Carotid artery stenosis (CAS) is an increasingly recognized condition in patients with stroke. CAS incidence increases with age—CAS of 50 % or greater is found in about 5–10 % of general population older than 65 years [54]. Individuals with asymptomatic CAS of 50–99 % have an annual risk of 1–3 % for a stroke [55]. However, the appropriate management of asymptomatic CAS is a controversial and is a topic of further research. Lately some studies suggest combining both surgical and medical approaches, that is, combining carotid endarterectomy with medical therapy over just medical therapy alone [56].

Obstructive Sleep Apnea

Obstructive sleep apnea (OSA) is a medical disorder characterized by repetitive interruption of ventilation during sleep caused by collapse of pharyngeal airway or central nervous system dysfunction. A Sleep study or polysomnogram (PSG) remains the gold standard for diagnoses. OSA affects an estimated 15 million adults Americans [57]. OSA is now a well-documented risk factor for stroke. A recent analysis from more than 6,000 adults participating in the Sleep Heart Health Study showed that hypopneas accompanied by oxyhemoglobin desaturation of more than 4 % were associated with prevalent cardiovascular disease and stroke [58]. Habitual snoring and daytime sleepiness are also risk factors for stroke [59]. Treatment of OSA is individualized and includes noninvasive positive airway pressure ventilation. A variety of surgical interventions and prosthetic oral devices are available.

Hypercoagulability

Hypercoagulable states can increase the risk of stroke. When large (≥4 mm) aortic arch plaques are found in the setting of hypercoagulability, stroke risk is increased possibly due to a higher embolic potential [60].

Thrombophilias such as factor V Leiden, prothrombin G20210A gene mutation, and homocysteine metabolism abnormalities increase the risk for myocardial infarction and ischemic stroke, especially among younger patients and women [61]. Routine testing for thrombophilia in most patients with acute ischemic stroke is not necessary. Although one in seven patients with a first episode of acute ischemic stroke test positive for one of the inherited thrombophilias, the relationship is likely to be coincidental rather than causal in most cases [62].

In the Antiphospholipid Antibodies in Stroke Study (APASS), anticardiolipin antibodies appear to be an independent risk factor with 9.7 % of ischemic stroke patients and 4.3 % of control subjects who were anticardiolipin positive [63]. As a result, there is a potential role for antiplatelet therapy or anticoagulation in this population.

Depression

Depression is associated with a significantly increased risk of stroke morbidity and mortality as shown in several studies [64]. It has been associated with inflammatory factors such as CRP, IL-1, and IL-6 that may increase risk of stroke. Risk is also increased possibly due to association of depression with poor health behaviors and obesity as well as other major comorbidities such as diabetes and hypertension.

Conclusion

Despite substantial advances for treatment of patients with acute stroke, primary stroke prevention remains the best means for reducing the burden stroke places on the patient, their family, and our health-care resources. We believe the medical literature shows that there are many factors that increase an individual's risk of stroke and many of these risk factors are potentially modifiable. Approaching a patient with multiple risk factors is best addressed with a multifactorial team-based approach that focuses on appropriate counseling regarding lifestyle risk factors (e.g., diet, exercise, tobacco and alcohol use) and appropriate medication use and compliance regarding known medical risk factors (e.g., hypertension, atrial fibrillation)

References

1. Murphy S, Xu J, Kochanek K. http://www.cdc.gov/nchs/fastats/lcod.htm. 2012;60(4)(4).
2. Del Zoppo GJ, Saver JL, Jauch EC, Adams Jr HP, American Heart Association Stroke Council. Expansion of the time window for treatment of acute ischemic stroke with intravenous tissue plasminogen activator: a science advisory from the American Heart Association/American Stroke Association. Stroke. 2009;40(8):2945–8.
3. Rojas JI, Zurru MC, Romano M, Patrucco L, Cristiano E. Acute ischemic stroke and transient ischemic attack in the very old-risk factor profile and stroke subtype between patients older than 80 years and patients aged less than 80 years. Eur J Neurol. 2007;14(8):895–9.
4. Chen RL, Balami JS, Esiri MM, Chen LK, Buchan AM. Ischemic stroke in the elderly: an overview of evidence. Nat Rev Neurol. 2010;6(5):256–65.
5. Feigin VL, Lawes CM, Bennett DA, Anderson CS. Stroke epidemiology: a review of population-based studies of incidence, prevalence, and case-fatality in the late 20th century. Lancet Neurol. 2003;2(1):43–53.
6. Petrea RE, Beiser AS, Seshadri S, Kelly-Hayes M, Kase CS, Wolf PA. Gender differences in stroke incidence and poststroke disability in the Framingham heart study. Stroke. 2009; 40(4):1032–7.
7. Seshadri S, Beiser A, Kelly-Hayes M, Kase CS, Au R, Kannel WB, et al. The lifetime risk of stroke: estimates from the Framingham study. Stroke. 2006;37(2):345–50.

8. Lisabeth LD, Beiser AS, Brown DL, Murabito JM, Kelly-Hayes M, Wolf PA. Age at natural menopause and risk of ischemic stroke: the Framingham heart study. Stroke. 2009;40(4): 1044–9.
9. Seshadri S, Beiser A, Pikula A, Himali JJ, Kelly-Hayes M, Debette S, et al. Parental occurrence of stroke and risk of stroke in their children: the Framingham study. Circulation. 2010;121(11):1304–12.
10. Knottnerus IL, Gielen M, Lodder J, Rouhl RP, Staals J, Vlietinck R, et al. Family history of stroke is an independent risk factor for lacunar stroke subtype with asymptomatic lacunar infarcts at younger ages. Stroke. 2011;42(5):1196–200.
11. Banerjee A, Silver LE, Heneghan C, Welch SJ, Mehta Z, Banning AP, et al. Relative familial clustering of cerebral versus coronary ischemic events. Circ Cardiovasc Genet. 2011;4(4): 390–6.
12. Francis J, Raghunathan S, Khanna P. The role of genetics in stroke. Postgrad Med J. 2007;83(983):590–5.
13. Sacco RL, Boden-Albala B, Abel G, Lin IF, Elkind M, Hauser WA, et al. Race-ethnic disparities in the impact of stroke risk factors: the northern Manhattan stroke study. Stroke. 2001;32(8):1725–31.
14. Kissela B, Schneider A, Kleindorfer D, Khoury J, Miller R, Alwell K, et al. Stroke in a biracial population: the excess burden of stroke among blacks. Stroke. 2004;35(2):426–31.
15. Kleindorfer D. Sociodemographic groups at risk: race/ethnicity. Stroke. 2009;40(3 Suppl): S75–8.
16. Kleindorfer DO, Khoury J, Moomaw CJ, Alwell K, Woo D, Flaherty ML, et al. Stroke incidence is decreasing in whites but not in blacks: a population-based estimate of temporal trends in stroke incidence from the Greater Cincinnati/Northern Kentucky Stroke Study. Stroke. 2010;41(7):1326–31.
17. Howard G, Cushman M, Kissela BM, Kleindorfer DO, McClure LA, Safford MM, et al. Traditional risk factors as the underlying cause of racial disparities in stroke: lessons from the half-full (empty?) glass. Stroke. 2011;42(12):3369–75.
18. Sacco RL, Adams R, Albers G, Alberts MJ, Benavente O, Furie K, et al. Guidelines for prevention of stroke in patients with ischemic stroke or transient ischemic attack: a statement for healthcare professionals from the American Heart Association/American Stroke Association Council on Stroke: co-sponsored by the Council on Cardiovascular Radiology and Intervention: the American Academy of Neurology affirms the value of this guideline. Stroke. 2006; 37(2):577–617.
19. Landau WM, Willey JZ, Elkind MS. Physical activity and risk of ischemic stroke in the Northern Manhattan study. Neurology. 2010;75(1):94. author reply 94.
20. Nelson ME, Rejeski WJ, Blair SN, Duncan PW, Judge JO, King AC, et al. Physical activity and public health in older adults: recommendation from the American College of Sports Medicine and the American Heart Association. Circulation. 2007;116(9):1094–105.
21. Sattelmair JR, Kurth T, Buring JE, Lee IM. Physical activity and risk of stroke in women. Stroke. 2010;41(6):1243–50.
22. Williams PT. Reduction in incident stroke risk with vigorous physical activity: evidence from 7.7-year follow-up of the national runners' health study. Stroke. 2009;40(5):1921–3.
23. Flegal KM, Carroll MD, Kit BK, Ogden CL. Prevalence of obesity and trends in the distribution of body mass index among US adults, 1999–2010. JAMA. 2012;307(5):491–7.
24. Suk SH, Sacco RL, Boden-Albala B, Cheun JF, Pittman JG, Elkind MS, et al. Abdominal obesity and risk of ischemic stroke: the Northern Manhattan stroke study. Stroke. 2003;34(7): 1586–92.
25. Rautiainen S, Larsson S, Virtamo J, Wolk A. Total antioxidant capacity of diet and risk of stroke: a population-based prospective cohort of women. Stroke. 2012;43(2):335–40.
26. He FJ, Nowson CA, MacGregor GA. Fruit and vegetable consumption and stroke: meta-analysis of cohort studies. Lancet. 2006;367(9507):320–6.
27. Fung TT, Chiuve SE, McCullough ML, Rexrode KM, Logroscino G, Hu FB. Adherence to a DASH-style diet and risk of coronary heart disease and stroke in women. Arch Intern Med. 2008;168(7):713–20.

28. Patra J, Taylor B, Irving H, Roerecke M, Baliunas D, Mohapatra S, et al. Alcohol consumption and the risk of morbidity and mortality for different stroke types—a systematic review and meta-analysis. BMC Public Health. 2010;10:258.
29. Zakhari S. Alcohol and the cardiovascular system: molecular mechanisms for beneficial and harmful action. Alcohol Health Res World. 1997;21(1):21–9.
30. Roger VL, Go AS, Lloyd-Jones DM, Benjamin EJ, Berry JD, Borden WB, et al. Heart disease and stroke statistics—2012 update: a report from the American Heart Association. Circulation. 2012;125(1):e2–220.
31. Bhat VM, Cole JW, Sorkin JD, Wozniak MA, Malarcher AM, Giles WH, et al. Dose-response relationship between cigarette smoking and risk of ischemic stroke in young women. Stroke. 2008;39(9):2439–43.
32. Wolf PA, D'Agostino RB, Kannel WB, Bonita R, Belanger AJ. Cigarette smoking as a risk factor for stroke. The Framingham study. JAMA. 1988;259(7):1025–9.
33. Vasan RS, Beiser A, Seshadri S, Larson MG, Kannel WB, D'Agostino RB, et al. Residual lifetime risk for developing hypertension in middle-aged women and men: the Framingham heart study. JAMA. 2002;287(8):1003–10.
34. Chobanian AV, Bakris GL, Black HR, Cushman WC, Green LA, Izzo Jr JL, et al. Seventh report of the Joint National Committee on prevention, detection, evaluation, and treatment of high blood pressure. Hypertension. 2003;42(6):1206–52.
35. Neal B, MacMahon S, Chapman N, Blood Pressure Lowering Treatment Trialists' Collaboration. Effects of ACE inhibitors, calcium antagonists, and other blood-pressure-lowering drugs: results of prospectively designed overviews of randomised trials. Blood Pressure Lowering Treatment Trialists' Collaboration. Lancet. 2000;356(9246):1955–64.
36. SHEP Cooperative Research Group. Prevention of stroke by antihypertensive drug treatment in older persons with isolated systolic hypertension. Final results of the Systolic Hypertension in the Elderly Program (SHEP). JAMA. 1991;265(24):3255–64.
37. Flack JM, Nasser SA. Antihypertensive and lipid-lowering treatment to prevent heart attack trial (ALLHAT). The Antihypertensive and lipid-lowering treatment to prevent heart attack trial (ALLHAT). Major outcomes in high-risk hypertensive patients randomized to angiotensin-converting enzyme inhibitor or calcium channel blocker vs. diuretic. Curr Hypertens Rep. 2003;5(3):189–91.
38. Psaty BM, Smith NL, Siscovick DS, Koepsell TD, Weiss NS, Heckbert SR, et al. Health outcomes associated with antihypertensive therapies used as first-line agents. A systematic review and meta-analysis. JAMA. 1997;277(9):739–45.
39. Cutler DM, Long G, Berndt ER, Royer J, Fournier AA, Sasser A, et al. The value of antihypertensive drugs: a perspective on medical innovation. Health Aff (Millwood). 2007;26(1):97–110.
40. Wolf PA, Abbott RD, Kannel WB. Atrial fibrillation as an independent risk factor for stroke: the Framingham study. Stroke. 1991;22(8):983–8.
41. Sudlow M, Thomson R, Thwaites B, Rodgers H, Kenny RA. Prevalence of atrial fibrillation and eligibility for anticoagulants in the community. Lancet. 1998;352(9135):1167–71.
42. Feinberg WM. Anticoagulation for prevention of stroke. Neurology. 1998;51(3 Suppl 3):S20–2.
43. van Walraven C, Hart RG, Singer DE, Laupacis A, Connolly S, Petersen P, et al. Oral anticoagulants vs. aspirin in nonvalvular atrial fibrillation: an individual patient meta-analysis. JAMA. 2002;288(19):2441–8.
44. Gage BF, Waterman AD, Shannon W, Boechler M, Rich MW, Radford MJ. Validation of clinical classification schemes for predicting stroke: results from the National Registry of Atrial Fibrillation. JAMA. 2001;285(22):2864–70.
45. Hart RG. Warfarin in atrial fibrillation: underused in the elderly, often inappropriately used in the young. Heart. 1999;82(5):539–40.
46. Abraham ME, Marcy TR. Warfarin versus dabigatran: comparing the old with the new. Consult Pharm. 2012;27(2):121–4.
47. National Cholesterol Education Program (NCEP). Expert Panel on Detection, Evaluation, and Treatment of High Blood Cholesterol in Adults (Adult Treatment Panel III). Third Report of

the National Cholesterol Education Program (NCEP) expert panel on detection, evaluation, and treatment of high blood cholesterol in adults (Adult Treatment Panel III) final report. Circulation. 2002;106(25):3143–421.

48. Centers for disease control and prevention. 2011 National Diabetes Fact Sheet. 2011; Available at: http://www.cdc.gov/diabetes/pubs/factsheet11.htm#citation.

49. UK Prospective Diabetes Study (UKPDS) Group. Effect of intensive blood-glucose control with metformin on complications in overweight patients with type 2 diabetes (UKPDS 34). Lancet. 1998;352(9131):854–65.

50. Leppala JM, Virtamo J, Fogelholm R, Albanes D, Heinonen OP. Different risk factors for different stroke subtypes: association of blood pressure, cholesterol, and antioxidants. Stroke. 1999;30(12):2535–40.

51. Soyama Y, Miura K, Morikawa Y, Nishijo M, Nakanishi Y, Naruse Y, et al. High-density lipoprotein cholesterol and risk of stroke in Japanese men and women: the Oyabe study. Stroke. 2003;34(4):863–8.

52. Colhoun HM, Betteridge DJ, Durrington PN, Hitman GA, Neil HA, Livingstone SJ, et al. Primary prevention of cardiovascular disease with atorvastatin in type 2 diabetes in the Collaborative Atorvastatin Diabetes Study (CARDS): multicentre randomised placebo-controlled trial. Lancet. 2004;364(9435):685–96.

53. Amarenco P, Tonkin AM. Statins for stroke prevention: disappointment and hope. Circulation. 2004;109(23 Suppl 1):III44–9.

54. O'Leary DH, Polak JF, Kronmal RA, Kittner SJ, Bond MG, Wolfson Jr SK, et al. Distribution and correlates of sonographically detected carotid artery disease in the Cardiovascular Health Study. The CHS Collaborative Research Group. Stroke. 1992;23(12):1752–60.

55. Autret A, Pourcelot L, Saudeau D, Marchal C, Bertrand P, de Boisvilliers S. Stroke risk in patients with carotid stenosis. Lancet. 1987;1(8538):888–90.

56. Roffi M, Sievert H, Gray WA, White CJ, Torsello G, Cao P, et al. Carotid artery stenting versus surgery: adequate comparisons? Lancet Neurol. 2010;9(4):339–41. author reply 341–2.

57. Somers VK, White DP, Amin R, Abraham WT, Costa F, Culebras A, et al. Sleep apnea and cardiovascular disease: an American Heart Association/American College of Cardiology Foundation Scientific Statement from the American Heart Association Council for High Blood Pressure Research Professional Education Committee, Council on Clinical Cardiology, Stroke Council, and Council On Cardiovascular Nursing. In collaboration with the National Heart, Lung, and Blood Institute National Center on Sleep Disorders Research (National Institutes of Health). Circulation. 2008;118(10):1080–111.

58. Punjabi NM, Newman AB, Young TB, Resnick HE, Sanders MH. Sleep-disordered breathing and cardiovascular disease: an outcome-based definition of hypopneas. Am J Respir Crit Care Med. 2008;177(10):1150–5.

59. Partinen M, Palomaki H. Snoring and cerebral infarction. Lancet. 1985;2(8468):1325–6.

60. Di Tullio MR, Homma S, Jin Z, Sacco RL. Aortic atherosclerosis, hypercoagulability, and stroke the APRIS (aortic plaque and risk of ischemic stroke) study. J Am Coll Cardiol. 2008;52(10):855–61.

61. Kim RJ, Becker RC. Association between factor V Leiden, prothrombin G20210A, and methylenetetrahydrofolate reductase C677T mutations and events of the arterial circulatory system: a meta-analysis of published studies. Am Heart J. 2003;146(6):948–57.

62. Hankey GJ, Eikelboom JW, van Bockxmeer FM, Lofthouse E, Staples N, Baker RI. Inherited thrombophilia in ischemic stroke and its pathogenic subtypes. Stroke. 2001;32(8):1793–9.

63. The Antiphospholipid Antibodies in Stroke Study (APASS) Group. Anticardiolipin antibodies are an independent risk factor for first ischemic stroke. Neurology. 1993;43(10):2069–73.

64. Pan A, Sun Q, Okereke OI, Rexrode KM, Hu FB. Depression and risk of stroke morbidity and mortality: a meta-analysis and systematic review. JAMA. 2011;306(11):1241–9.

Chapter 4
Perspectives and Approach to Stroke Prevention and Therapy

Bassel Raad and Michael De Georgia

Key Points

- Stroke is the second leading cause of death globally and in countries with high or middle income. Worldwide, 15 million strokes happen annually and they account for around 5.5 million deaths or nearly 10 % of all deaths per year.
- The prevalence of stroke is expected to increase in the future as the aging population continues to grow.
- The WHO developed a stepwise approach to stroke surveillance (STEPS-stroke) in order to collect epidemiologic data on stroke worldwide and improvise better preventive measures in disadvantaged societies.
- A stroke is a vascular accident of the central nervous system that leads to sudden death of brain cells due to inadequate blood flow. It is a heterogeneous disease that can be divided into two broad categories: ischemic and hemorrhagic strokes.
- Age, sex, race, and heredity are non-modifiable risk factors for stroke. However, the following risk factors (hypertension, atrial fibrillation, diabetes mellitus, dyslipidemia, carotid artery disease, smoking, alcoholism, physical inactivity, obesity, drug abuse) are among the modifiable ones.
- Age is the single most important risk factor for strokes, and hypertension is the most important modifiable one.
- The role of antiplatelet agents like aspirin, clopidogrel, and dipyridamole in primary stroke prevention has not been well defined yet, but in terms of secondary prevention, they seem to be moderately effective in preventing recurrent strokes.
- Recombinant tissue plasminogen activator (r-tPA) is currently the mainstay therapy for acute ischemic strokes. If administered in the first 4.5 h after stroke onset,

B. Raad, M.D. (✉) • M. De Georgia, M.D.
Department of Neurology, University Hospitals Case Medical Center,
11100 Euclid Avenue, Hanna House Room Number: 512, Cleveland, OH, USA
e-mail: bassel.raad@uhhospitals.org

M.L. Corrigan et al. (eds.), *Handbook of Clinical Nutrition and Stroke*,
Nutrition and Health, DOI 10.1007/978-1-62703-380-0_4,
© Springer Science+Business Media New York 2013

it may result in 30 % more likelihood of patients having minimal or no disability at 3 months after the stroke.
- For large artery occlusion strokes, the American Heart Association recommends using intra-arterial fibrinolytic therapy in the first 3–6 h window after stroke as an alternative to intravenous therapy.
- Recent advances in the interventional management of acute strokes led to the development of new ways to mechanically disrupt blood clots or retrieve them from the arteries.

Keywords Global stroke burden • WHO STEPS • Ischemic stroke • Intracerebral hemorrhage • Subarachnoid hemorrhage • Framingham risk score • Recombinant tissue plasminogen activator (r-tPA) • Thrombolysis

Abbreviations

ACAS	Asymptomatic Carotid Atherosclerosis Study
CRP	C-Reactive Protein
DALYs	Disability-Adjusted Life Years)
HTN	Hypertension
LDL-C	Low-Density Lipoprotein Cholesterol
r-tPA	Recombinant Tissue Plasminogen Activator
STEPS	Stepwise Approach to Stroke Surveillance
TIAs	Transient Ischemic Attacks

Introduction

Stroke is the second leading cause of death globally and in countries with high or middle income. It is, however, the sixth leading cause of mortality in low-income countries (due to prevalence of other diseases like HIV, malaria, and diarrheal illnesses in these countries) [1]. Preliminary data for 2010 from Centers for Disease Control and Prevention suggests that stroke is the fourth leading cause of death in the USA [2]. Stroke remains also the leading cause of long-term disability in the USA [3]. Worldwide, 15 million strokes happen annually and they account for around 5.5 million deaths or nearly 10 % of all deaths per year [4]. More than 700,000 stroke incidents occur annually in the USA with one third of new stroke patients dying each year and less than a half regaining their independence [5]. Overall, Blacks and Hispanic Americans have higher stroke incidence and mortality rates than age-matched Whites. The prevalence of stroke is expected to increase in the future as the aging population continues to grow and more than 800 million people will be above 65 years of age by 2025 [6]. While the incidence of stroke, between 1970 and 2008, decreased by around 40 % (163–94 per 100,000 person years) in high-income countries, it increased by more than 100 % (52–117 per

STEPS Stroke diagram   The following diagram illustrates the general concept of the WHO STEPwise approach

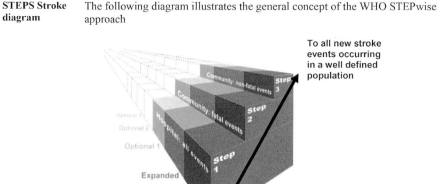

Fig. 4.1 The WHO STEPS Diagram. Reproduced with permission from [9]

100,000 person years) in low- and middle-income countries [7]. The striking change in developing countries is likely due to urbanization, change in nutrition with over-consumption of calories, and increased prevalence of metabolic syndrome [8].

Global Burden of Stroke and Surveillance Methods

The assessment of the true burden of stroke including incidence, prevalence, and mortality rates faces multiple difficulties, and most of the current data is based on epidemiologic studies done in high-income countries. Reporting of even the very basic epidemiological data like mortality is only done in less than one third of the countries worldwide [4]. The number of patients with strokes is expected to increase in the future because of the demographic changes mentioned above and the inadequate control of major stroke risk factors. This is mainly true in low- and middle-income countries where two thirds of the world strokes occur. For this reason, the World Health Organization (WHO) developed a stepwise approach to stroke surveillance (STEPS-stroke) in order to collect epidemiologic data on stroke worldwide and improvise better preventive measures in disadvantaged societies. This surveillance approach collects data from three major types of stroke patients: those admitted to the hospital, those with fatal events outside the hospital, and those with nonfatal events in the community; see Fig. 4.1 [9]. Similarly, stroke risk factors surveillance is done in a stepwise approach that includes at the most basic level demographic data self-reported by patients. The second level of surveillance includes data obtained from physical examination like weight, blood pressure, and body mass index. The third tier of surveillance is more readily available from high-income countries and includes data obtained from laboratory measurements like serum glucose and cholesterol levels. Based on the WHO approach, multiple studies assessed and still continue to assess the global burden of stroke on morbidity and mortality in different countries. The loss incurred from stroke is measured in DALYs (disability-adjusted life years) which combines the years of life lost from premature death and the years of life lived with disability [10–12]. In multiple studies, stroke was found to contribute to around 43.7 million lost DALY's per year worldwide. This only represents around nine to ten times the number of global stroke incidents annually because the majority of strokes occur in the elderly population. Low- and middle-income countries have up to ten times higher mortality rates and DALYs loss than high-income countries. The impact of stroke on lost DALYs seems to be more predicted by national per capita income than any other comorbidity associated with stroke, including cardiovascular disease, smoking, or hypertension [11].

What Is a Stroke?

A stroke is a vascular accident of the central nervous system that leads to sudden death of brain cells due to inadequate blood flow. According to the WHO definition (2005), stroke is defined as the rapid development of clinical signs and symptoms of a focal neurological disturbance lasting more than 24 h or leading to death with no apparent cause other than vascular origin. The classic symptoms of stroke include sudden loss of vision, speech impairment, unilateral numbness, weakness, or paralysis. Other symptoms may include memory loss, impaired reasoning ability, coma, or death. Stroke is a heterogeneous disease that can be divided into two broad categories:

1. Ischemic strokes: caused by arterial occlusion from thrombosis or embolism (account for 50–85 % of all strokes worldwide) [7].
2. Hemorrhagic strokes: caused by subarachnoid hemorrhage or intracerebral hemorrhage and account for 1–7 % and 7–27 %, respectively, of all strokes worldwide [7].

According to Bath and Lee [13], the mortality rates of the different types of strokes at days 30, 1 year, and 5 years in percentages are as follows in Table 4.1 [13].

Table 4.1
Stroke subtypes mortality rates in percentages at different time intervals from stroke onset

	30 days	1 year	5 years
Ischemic stroke	10	23	52
Intracerebral hemorrhage	52	62	70
Subarachnoid hemorrhage	45	48	52

Reproduced from *British Medical Journal*, Philip M. W. Bath, Kennedy R. Lees, 320: 920, 2000, with permission from BMJ Publishing Group Ltd

Ischemic strokes are preceded in about one third of the cases by transient ischemic attacks (TIAs) which result from transient reduction or blockage of blood flow to a specific area in the brain. The symptoms from TIAs which are similar to stroke symptoms generally last less than 24 h.

Risk Factors for Ischemic Strokes and Prevention Measures

Ischemic strokes represent the biggest public burden among all strokes subtypes; therefore in this chapter, we will focus mainly on the risk factors, preventive measures, and treatment of ischemic strokes. (Unless otherwise specified, the word stroke in the rest of this chapter will refer to ischemic strokes mainly.)

Despite the advances in acute stroke therapy in the last two decades, prevention remains a cornerstone in stroke treatment. Prevention is usually started when risk factors for stroke exist in a person. It is very important to start prevention before strokes happen (primary prevention) and to start/continue this prevention after strokes occur (secondary prevention).

Non-modifiable Risk Factors

Some risk factors for stroke are non-modifiable like age, sex, race, and heredity; however, they help identifying individuals at highest risk of stroke which prompts for more vigorous treatment of the modifiable risk factors. Age is the single most important risk factor for stroke [14]. For each 10 years after the age 55, stroke risk more than doubles for both men and women [15]. Men have a 1.25 times greater risk of strokes compared to women, but the risk equates or may reverse after the age 85. Overall, African Americans, Hispanics, and Chinese or Japanese races have higher risks of strokes than White Americans. Individuals with a paternal or maternal family history of stroke also are more predisposed to have strokes [16].

Modifiable Risk Factors: These Are Discussed in Depth in Chaps. 3, 6, 7, and 8

Hypertension

Hypertension (HTN) is the most important modifiable risk factor for stroke [14]. Hypertensive patients have a relative risk of 4 for cerebrovascular accidents compared to normal controls. However, the impact of hypertension decreases with age and nearly vanishes at 90 years of age. The current guidelines recommend using oral antihypertensives to keep BP <140/90 mmHg [17]. If heart failure, renal insufficiency, diabetes mellitus exist, the goal is BP <135/85 mmHg. Controlling blood pressure with antihypertensives results in 35–45 % reduction in the relative stroke risk [17].

Atrial Fibrillation

Atrial fibrillation is the second most important modifiable risk factor for stroke after hypertension, and it affects up to 2.2 million Americans [14]. Overall, half of all embolic strokes are due to atrial fibrillation which imposes a yearly 4.5 % risk of stroke without treatment [18]. The current guidelines recommend treating atrial fibrillation with oral anticoagulants (warfarin) to target an INR=2–3 [17]. This results in stroke relative risk reduction of 68 % [19]. Other oral anticoagulants, like dabigatran, may also be used and have been shown to have a similar efficacy profile to that of warfarin.

Diabetes Mellitus

Patients with diabetes mellitus have increased prevalence of atherosclerosis, coronary artery disease (CAD), obesity, dyslipidemia, and hypertension [20]. According to the Framingham study, diabetes mellitus confers an independent relative risk of 2 for ischemic strokes [14]. In other epidemiological studies, the relative risk ranged between 1.8 and 6 for ischemic strokes [20]. According to the National Stroke Association and American Heart Association, the recommended target for fasting blood sugar is below 126 mg/dL in diabetics with HBA1C below 7 %. Also if there is associated dyslipidemia with diabetes, the recommended low density lipoprotein (LDL) level is below 100 mg/dL [20].

Dyslipidemia

Hyperlipidemia has been clearly associated with an increased risk of CAD and extracranial carotid atherosclerosis [21]. However, whether dyslipidemia is a risk factor for stroke remains unknown. Recent trials have shown a reduction in the stroke risk with HMG-CoA reductase inhibitors (statins) [22]. The American Heart Association recommends managing dyslipidemia with a combination of lifestyle modification with or without the use of oral lipid-lowering drugs (statins, bile resins, fibrates, niacin). The goals for low-density lipoprotein cholesterol (LDL-C) are as follows:

- LDL-C <160 mg/dL if ≤1 risk factor is present
- LDL-C <130 mg/dL if ≥2 risk factors are present and the 10-year CHD risk is <20 % (using Framingham score)

- LDL-C <100 mg/dL if ≥2 risk factors are present and the 10-year CHD risk is ≥20 % or if patient has diabetes

  The goals for HDL are above 40 mg/dL in men and above 50 mg/dL in women.

  Although elevated serum triglycerides (TG) have not been yet correlated to increased stroke risk, it is recommended to keep the fasting TG level below 150 mg/dL [22].

Smoking

Cigarette smoking is recognized as a major risk factor for stroke and confers a relative risk of stroke that is nearly double the risk without smoking [23]. The risk does not change significantly between heavy and moderate smokers and even it is present in passive smokers. Smoking cessation is associated with progressive decrease in the risk of stroke and, per the Framingham study, it levels down to that of nonsmokers 5 years after complete smoking cessation. Current recommendations suggest complete cessation of smoking and avoidance of exposure to second-hand smoke.

Alcohol Consumption

It seems there is a dose-dependent relationship between alcohol consumption and stroke [24]. In fact, epidemiologic studies revealed a J-shaped curve for the association between alcohol consumption doses and the risk of ischemic strokes [24]. Heavy drinking (>60 g ethanol/day) increases the incidence of all types of strokes [25], but moderate alcohol consumption (up to two drinks per day) seems to have a protective effect [26].

Physical Activity

Regular physical activity has been well established to have protective role in ischemic strokes [27]. In the Framingham study, moderate physical activity reduced the relative risk of strokes in males to 0.41 [27]. The Nurses' Health Study showed an inverse relationship between stroke and physical activity in middle-age women [28]. The optimal amount of exercise that has a protective effect on stroke is at least 30 min of activity at 40–60 % of maximum capacity most of the week days. Vigorous exercise does not seem to confer further protection when compared to moderate exercise.

Obesity

Obesity has been defined as body mass index (BMI) >30 kg/m^2 and is a well-established risk factor for cardiovascular disease, hypertension, diabetes, and dyslipidemia [19]. Beyond its effect on these factors, it is not known whether obesity is an independent risk factor for stroke. Up to 30 % of people in the USA meet the criteria for obesity [29]. In the Nurses' Health Study which followed 116,759 women for 16 years, there was a higher risk of stroke at BMI >27 compared to lower BMIs, and the risk got higher as the BMI increased [30]. Other studies did not show a relationship between higher BMI and stroke [31]. Body adiposity may be more closely related to stroke risk than BMI and is measured by the waist/hip circumference. The current recommendations target a BMI of 18.5–24.9 kg/m^2, and when BMI >25 kg/m^2, it is desirable to keep the waist circumference at the iliac crest below 40 in. in men and below 35 in. in women [32].

Homocysteine

Homocysteine levels in the blood are affected by genetic factors and by the intake of vitamin B12 and folate. These vitamins are cofactors in the reaction that changes homocysteine to methionine. Some studies have shown an inverse relationship between homocysteine levels and the intake of these vitamins [33]. Other studies have shown it as an independent risk factor for coronary and carotid atherosclerotic disease [34]. The higher the level of homocysteine in serum, the higher the stroke risk is [35]. It is now known that homocysteine is atherogenic and prothrombotic which plausibly explains its role in strokes. Although the supplemental intake of vitamins B6, B12, and folate may decrease the levels of homocysteine in blood, large randomized controlled trials did not show a benefit from these supplemental vitamins in preventing recurrent strokes [36].

Biomarkers

The inflammatory biomarker C-reactive protein (CRP) has been associated with a twofold increase in the risk of strokes at high serum levels [37]. The Framingham study showed an increase in stroke incidence in patients with high fibrinogen levels. Also fibrinogen was associated with progression of carotid atherosclerosis and stroke recurrence [38]. Some studies have associated high levels of the lipoprotein-associated phospholipase A2 (Lp-PLA2) with increased stroke risk independent of the existence of dyslipidemia [39]. The risk of stroke increases further in patients with high levels of both CRP and (Lp-PLA2) [39].

Carotid Artery Disease

Although there are multiple large trials that addressed the risks of stroke from carotid artery disease, the optimal management of this vascular condition remains a controversial topic especially when it is still asymptomatic. The Asymptomatic Carotid Atherosclerosis Study (ACAS) has been the largest trial done on asymptomatic carotid disease, and it randomized patients with more than 60 % stenosis to medical treatment versus surgical management with prophylactic carotid endarterectomy [40]. It showed that the risk of stroke from carotid disease is around 11.8 % at 5 years when medical treatment is employed alone. The risk of stroke drops to 6.4 % at 5 years when surgery is added to medical management [40]. The difference between the two management arms was statistically significant especially for men but not for women. Because the surgical risks are in most centers higher than those reported by the ACAS study group, the decision on surgical versus medical management of asymptomatic stenosis is still controversial.

For symptomatic carotid stenosis, the benefit of surgery is clearer especially when the stenosis is severe. This is illustrated mainly in the North American Carotid Endarterectomy Trial (NASCET) which showed a 5-year risk reduction from 32.3 to 15.8 % with surgery compared to medical therapy in patients with severe carotid stenosis (70–99 %) [41]. There was also a 5-year risk reduction from 22 to 15.7 % with surgery compared to medical therapy in patients with moderate carotid stenosis (50–69 %) [41]. The current recommendation for severe and symptomatic carotid stenosis is to implement both surgical and medical management. If the patient is high surgical risk, then stenting of the carotid artery can be done and is as effective as surgery in preventing recurrent strokes. For symptomatic and moderate stenosis, the current guidelines recommend medical therapy with or without surgery (which also remains controversial) [32].

Illicit Drugs

Multiple drugs have been linked to the development of strokes, and cocaine has the biggest social burden among all drugs. Others include heroin, LSD, marijuana, PCP, sympathomimetic decongestants, and cold remedies. These drugs possibly are linked more to hemorrhagic than ischemic strokes [42].

Miscellaneous Cardiac Risk Factors

All of the following cardiac conditions may be risk factors for embolic strokes including left ventricular failure, acute myocardial infarction, left ventricular or atrial septal aneurysm, patent foramen ovale (PFO), and bacterial endocarditis [20]. Aside from recommendation on using oral antiplatelet agents, the role of anticoagulation with vitamin K inhibitors is still controversial in these conditions. Another important risk factor for ischemic embolic strokes is aortic arch atheroma which may have a risk of embolism up to 12 % per year if it is >4 mm thick, is ulcerated, or has a mobile component. In these cases, the recommended approach is to treat with oral vitamin K inhibitors like warfarin [20].

Antiplatelet Agents in Primary and Secondary Stroke Prevention

Aspirin 50–325 mg/day

Aspirin has a well-established role in the primary prevention of myocardial infarction. In fact, the American Heart Association recommends starting aspirin treatment in all patients with evidence of CAD, diabetes mellitus, and peripheral vascular disease (including carotid artery disease) or those with a Framingham 10-year risk score of at least 10 % for prediction of cardiovascular disease [43]. However, the role of aspirin in primary stroke prevention has not been well defined yet, and most studies have shown absence of stroke risk reduction with this treatment and absence of effect on the severity of first ever stroke. In terms of secondary prevention, aspirin seems to be moderately effective in preventing recurrent strokes. A meta-analysis of 21 trials done on aspirin therapy versus placebo in patients with a prior history of stroke revealed that aspirin reduces stroke occurrence by about one fifth per year (stroke risk per year: with aspirin [2.08 %], without aspirin [2.54 %]) [44]. It is recommended to treat all stroke survivors with aspirin 50–325 mg daily.

Dipyridamole

Most studies that compared dipyridamole to aspirin in secondary stroke prevention showed similar efficacy rates between the two medications [45]. The use of combination aspirin and dipyridamole was shown in the European Stroke Prevention Study to reduce stroke risk slightly better than aspirin alone [46]. Current guidelines recommend using the combination of aspirin and dipyridamole as an option instead of aspirin alone, but the regimen has the disadvantage of twice daily dosing and more side effects like headache, gastric upset, diarrhea, and gastrointestinal bleeding [47].

Thienopyridines

When compared to aspirin, both ticlopidine and clopidogrel have similar or slightly better efficacy in prevention of recurrent strokes. The use of ticlopidine, however, is limited by its side effect profile (diarrhea, neutropenia, TTP). A clopidogrel dose of 75 mg daily was shown to have an absolute risk reduction in stroke recurrence of 0.9 % when compared to aspirin 325 mg daily [48]. The current recommendations consider clopidogrel an option for treatment instead of aspirin, mainly in cases of aspirin intolerance.

Acute Stroke Management

The acute management of ischemic strokes underwent major and significant changes in the last 15 years after thrombolysis was approved as part of the treatment regimen. Thrombolysis was used for acute myocardial infarction since the 1960s. However, because of the inability to differentiate between ischemic and hemorrhagic strokes, thrombolysis was not a possible option for strokes at that time. Classically, acute stroke care consisted of symptom management, antiplatelet agents, institution of preventive care, and acute rehabilitation. Later, the advent of computed tomography in the 1980s made the differentiation between ischemic and hemorrhagic strokes possible, and this prompted the start of thrombolysis trials in the early 1990s. To date, major, multicenter trials on intravenous and intra-arterial thrombolysis have been conducted and published. These trials changed dramatically our approach to acute stroke care in the last decade. Recombinant tissue plasminogen activator (r-tPA) is currently the mainstay therapy for acute ischemic strokes. It was approved for use based on results of the National Institute of Neurological Disorders and Stroke (NINDS) trial [49]. These results showed that intravenous administration of r-tPA in the first 3 h of a stroke results in 30 % more likelihood of patients having minimal or no disability at 3 months after the stroke. Other trials done to extend the window of intravenous r-tPA beyond 3 h showed that benefit from r-tPA could still be gained up to 4.5 h from stroke onset [50]. Currently, intravenous r-tPA at 0.9 mg/kg is used worldwide for acute stroke therapy, and the American Heart Association recommends using it up to a maximum window of 4.5 h from stroke onset. Overall, intravenous thrombolysis is more likely to be of benefit with smaller strokes than larger ones which involve major artery or major vessel branch occlusion. This prompted the need for intra-arterial delivery of thrombolytics in order to target the clot directly with a high concentration of the medication. The PROACT II trial [51] and the Japanese MELT trial [52] studied the effect of intra-arterially delivered pro-urokinase (r-proUK) on major strokes. They found better arterial recanalization rates and better patient outcome at 3 months after stroke. Currently, the American Heart Association recommends using intra-arterial fibrinolytic therapy in the 3–6 h window after large artery occlusion strokes as an alternative to intravenous therapy. Unfortunately, the availability of intra-arterial thrombolysis remains a challenge in most developing world countries because it is associated with high costs and is a relatively new therapy. In addition, recent advances in the interventional management of acute strokes led to development of new ways to mechanically disrupt blood clots or retrieve them from the arteries.

These methods are used in many tertiary care stroke centers in North America and Europe with promising results that will likely be validated in ongoing and future clinical trials.

Summary

Stroke is the fourth leading cause of death in the USA and the second worldwide. It is also a leading cause of long-term disability which makes it a major global health burden. Due to the difficulty in obtaining epidemiologic and surveillance studies on strokes in low- or middle-income societies, the WHO developed a stepwise approach to stroke surveillance (STEPS-stroke). STEPS-stroke aims at global implementation of stroke preventive measures to reduce the incidence and prevalence of stroke worldwide. Different stroke risk factors exist and while age is the single most important non-modifiable risk factor, hypertension and atrial fibrillation remain the most important modifiable ones. In addition to risk factors control, primary and secondary stroke preventions employ the use of antiplatelet agents or oral anticoagulants in the case of atrial fibrillation. The management of acute strokes underwent major advances in the last 15 years with the introduction of thrombolysis and arterial recanalization procedures. Despite the promising results of these acute stroke management methods, they are still not widely available in most low- or moderate-income world countries.

References

1. World Health Organization. The 10 leading causes of death by broad income group 2008 [Internet]. 2011 [updated 2011 June]. Available from: http://www.who.int/mediacentre/fact-sheets/fs310/en/#.T_dfxOjZSW0
2. Murphy SL, Xu JQ, Kochanek KD. Deaths: preliminary data for 2010. National vital statistics reports; vol. 60 no. 4. Hyattsville, MD: National Center for Health Statistics; 2012. Available from: http://www.cdc.gov/nchs/data/nvsr/nvsr60/nvsr60_04.pdf
3. Lloyd-Jones D, Adams R, Carnethon M, De Simone G, Ferguson TB, Flegal K, et al. American Heart Association: Heart disease and stroke. Statistics 2009. Update. Circulation. 2009;119: e1–161.
4. World Health Organization. World health report 2004: changing history [Internet]. 2004. Available from: http://www.who.int/whr/2004/en/
5. World Health Organization. The world health report 2002: reducing risks, promoting healthy life [Internet]. 2002. Available from: http://www.who.int/whr/2002/en/
6. United Nations. World population prospects: the 2006 revision, Volume III: Analytical Report [Internet]. 2006. Available from: http://www.un.org/esa/population/publications/WPP2006Rev Vol_III/WPP2006RevVol_III_final.pdf
7. Feigin VL, Lawes CM, Bennett DA, Braker-Collo SL, Parag V. Worldwide stroke incidence and early case fatality reported in 56 population-based studies: a systematic review. Lancet Neurol. 2009;8:355–69.
8. Lock K, Smith RD, Dangour AD, Keogh-Brown M, Pigatto G, Hawkes C, et al. Health, agricultural, and economic effects of adoption of healthy diet recommendations. Lancet. 2010;376: 1699–709.

9. World Health Organization. WHO STEPS stroke manual: the WHO STEPwise approach to stroke surveillance 2006 [Internet]. Available from: http://www.who.int/chp/steps/stroke/manual/en/index.html. Accessed 22 Sept 2007.

10. Murray CJL, Lopez AD. The global burden of disease: a comprehensive assessment of mortality and disability from diseases, injuries, and risk factors in 1990 and projected to 2020. Cambridge, MA: Harvard University Press; 1996. p. 1996.

11. Johnston SC, Mendis S, Mathers CD. Global variation in stroke burden and mortality: estimates from monitoring, surveillance, and modeling. Lancet Neurol. 2009;8:345–54.

12. Strong K, Mathers C, Bonita R. Preventing stroke: saving lives around the world. Lancet Neurol. 2007;6:182–7.

13. Bath P, Lees K. ABC of arterial and venous disease. Acute stroke. BMJ. 2000;320:920–3.

14. Sacco RL, Benjamin EJ, Broderick JP, Dyken M, Easton JD, Feinberg WM, et al. American Heart Association Prevention Conference IV. Prevention and rehabilitation of stroke. Risk factors. Stroke. 1997;28:1507–17.

15. Wolf PA, D'Agostino RB, O'Neal MA, Sytkowski P, Kase CS, Belanger AJ, et al. Secular trends in stroke incidence and mortality: the Framingham Study. Stroke. 1992;23:1551–5.

16. Kiely DK, Wolf PA, Cupples LA, Beiser AS, Myers RH, et al. Familial aggregation of stroke: the Framingham Study. Stroke. 1993;24:1366–71.

17. Goldstein LB, Adams R, Alberts MJ, Appel LJ, Brass LM, Bushnell CD, et al. Primary prevention of ischemic stroke: a guideline from the American Heart Association/American Stroke Association Stroke Council. Stroke. 2006;37:1583–633.

18. Risk factors for stroke and efficacy of antithrombotic therapy in atrial fibrillation. Analysis of pooled data from five randomized controlled trials. Arch Intern Med. 1994;154(13):1449–57.

19. Goldstein LB, Adams R, Becker K, Furberg CD, Gorelick PB, Hademenos G, et al. Primary prevention of ischemic stroke. Stroke. 2001;32(1):280–99.

20. Akopov S, Cohen SN. Preventing stroke: a review of current guidelines. J Am Med Dir Assoc. 2003;4(5 Suppl):S127–32.

21. Heiss G, Sharrett AR, Barnes R, Chambless LE, Szklo M, Alzola C. Carotid atherosclerosis measured by B-mode ultrasound in populations: associations with cardiovascular risk factors in the ARIC study. Am J Epidemiol. 1991;134(3):250–6.

22. Gorelick PB, Mazzone T. Plasma lipids and stroke. J Cardiovasc Risk. 1999;6:217–21.

23. Shinton R, Beevers G. Meta-analysis of relation between cigarette smoking and stroke. BMJ. 1989;298:789–94.

24. Camargo Jr CA. Moderate alcohol consumption and stroke: the epidemiologic evidence. Stroke. 1989;20:1611–26.

25. Lindegard B, Hillbom M. Associations between brain infarction, diabetes and alcoholism: observations from the Gothenburg population cohort study. Acta Neurol Scand. 1987;75: 195–200.

26. Sacco RL, Elkind M, Boden-Albala B, Lin IF, Kargman DE, Hauser WA. The protective effect of moderate alcohol consumption on ischemic stroke. JAMA. 1999;281(1):53–60.

27. Kiely DK, Wolf PA, Cupples LA, Beiser AS, Kannel WB. Physical activity and stroke risk: the Framingham Study. Am J Epidemiol. 1994;140(7):608–20.

28. Manson JE, Willett WC, Stampfer MJ, Colditz GA, Hunter DJ, Hankinson SE, et al. Body weight and mortality among women. N Engl J Med. 1995;333(11):677–85.

29. Hedley AA, Ogden CL, Johnson CL, Carroll MD, Curtin LR, Flegal KM. Prevalence of overweight and obesity among US children, adolescents, and adults, 1999–2002. JAMA. 2004; 291(23):2847–50.

30. Rexrode KM, Hennekens CH, Willett WC, Colditz GA, Stampfer MJ, Rich-Edwards JW, et al. A prospective study of body mass index, weight change, and risk of stroke in women. JAMA. 1997;277(19):1539–45.

31. Walker SP, Rimm EB, Ascherio A, Kawachi I, Stampfer MJ, Willett WC. Body size and fat distribution as predictors of stroke among US men. Am J Epidemiol. 1996;144:1143–50.

32. Sacco RL, Adams R, Albers G, et al. Guidelines for prevention of stroke in patients with ischemic stroke or transient ischemic attack. Stroke. 2006;37(2):577–617.

33. Collaboration HLT. Lowering blood homocysteine with folic acid based supplements: meta-analysis of randomised trials. BMJ. 1998;316(7135):894–8.
34. Stampfer MJ, Malinow MR, Willett WC, et al. A prospective study of plasma homocyst(e)ine and risk of myocardial infarction in US physicians. JAMA. 1992;268(7):877–81.
35. Perry IJ, Morris RW, Ebrahim SB, Shaper AG, Refsum H, Ueland PM. Prospective study of serum total homocysteine concentration and risk of stroke in middle-aged British men. Lancet. 1995;346(8987):1395–8.
36. Toole JF, Malinow MR, Chambless LE, et al. Lowering homocysteine in patients with ischemic stroke to prevent recurrent stroke, myocardial infarction, and death: the Vitamin Intervention for Stroke Prevention (VISP) randomized controlled trial. JAMA. 2004; 291(5):565–75.
37. Kaplan RC, McGinn AP, Baird AE, et al. Inflammation and hemostasis biomarkers for predicting stroke in postmenopausal women: the Women's Health Initiative Observational Study. J Stroke Cerebrovasc Dis. 2008;17(6):344–55.
38. Ernst E, Resch KL. Fibrinogen as a cardiovascular risk factor: a meta-analysis and review of the literature. Ann Intern Med. 1993;118(12):956–63.
39. Ballantyne CM, Hoogeveen RC, Bang H, et al. Lipoprotein-associated phospholipase A2, high-sensitivity C-reactive protein, and risk for incident ischemic stroke in middle-aged men and women in the Atherosclerosis Risk in Communities (ARIC) study. Arch Intern Med. 2005;165(21):2479–84.
40. Endarterectomy for asymptomatic carotid artery stenosis. Executive Committee for the Asymptomatic Carotid Atherosclerosis Study. JAMA. 1995;273(18):1421–8.
41. Barnett HJM, Taylor DW, Eliasziw M, et al. Benefit of carotid endarterectomy in patients with symptomatic moderate or severe stenosis. N Engl J Med. 1998;339(20):1415–25.
42. Sloan MA, Kittner SJ, Rigamonti D, Price TR. Occurrence of stroke associated with use/abuse of drugs. Neurology. 1991;41(9):1358–64.
43. Members WC, Redberg RF, Benjamin EJ, et al. AHA/ACCF 2009 performance measures for primary prevention of cardiovascular disease in adults. Circulation. 2009;120(13):1296–336.
44. Antithrombotic Trialists C. Aspirin in the primary and secondary prevention of vascular disease: collaborative meta-analysis of individual participant data from randomised trials. Lancet. 2009;373(9678):1849–60.
45. Straus SE, Majumdar SR, McAlister FA. New evidence for stroke prevention. JAMA. 2002;288:1388–95.
46. Diener HC, Cunha L, Forbes C, Sivenius J, Smets P, Lowenthal A. European Stroke Prevention Study 2. Dipyridamole and acetylsalicylic acid in the secondary prevention of stroke. J Neurol Sci. 1996;143(1–2):1–13.
47. Hart RG, Bailey RD. An assessment of guidelines for prevention of ischemic stroke. Neurology. 2002;59(7):977–82.
48. A randomised, blinded, trial of clopidogrel versus aspirin in patients at risk of ischaemic events (CAPRIE). The Lancet. 1996;348(9038):1329–39.
49. Tissue plasminogen activator for acute ischemic stroke. The National Institute of Neurological Disorders and Stroke rt-PA Stroke Study Group. N Engl J Med. 1995;333(24):1581–7.
50. Hacke W, Kaste M, Bluhmki E, et al. Thrombolysis with alteplase 3 to 4.5 hours after acute ischemic stroke. N Engl J Med. 2008;359(13):1317–29.
51. Furlan A, Higashida R, Wechsler L, Gent M, Rowley H, Kase C, et al. Intra-arterial prourokinase for acute ischemic stroke. The PROACT II study: a randomized controlled trial. Prolyse in acute cerebral thromboembolism. JAMA. 1999;282(21):2003–11.
52. Ogawa A, Mori E, Minematsu K, et al. Randomized trial of intraarterial infusion of urokinase within 6 hours of middle cerebral artery stroke. Stroke. 2007;38(10):2633–9.

Part II
Health-Related Risk Factors
for Stroke

Chapter 5
Diabetes Mellitus Prevention and Treatment

Andrea Vegh Dunn and Kavita Nyalakonda

Key Points

- Diabetes is a complex syndrome characterized by hyperglycemia that is associated with an increased risk of microvascular and macrovascular complications.
- Preventing these complications including stroke entails a multifaceted approach that should involve combined treatment of hypertension, hyperlipidemia, and hyperglycemia.
- Treatment should involve a multidisciplinary approach including both medical nutrition therapy (MNT) and pharmacologic therapy.
- MNT should focus on both carbohydrates and a general healthy eating pattern to reduce the risk of cardiovascular disease.
- Algorithms are available to provide guidance to clinicians for use of oral or injectable medications in the treatment of glycemia.

Keywords Type 2 diabetes • Diabetes prevention • Stroke prevention • Medical nutrition therapy • Carbohydrates • Pharmacotherapy for diabetes

Abbreviations

AACE	American Association of Clinical Endocrinologists
ACE	American College of Endocrinology
ACCORD	Action in Diabetes Vascular Disease-Preterex and Diamicron
ACCORD	Action to Control Cardiovascular Risk in Diabetes

A.V. Dunn, R.D., L.D., C.D.E. (✉) • K. Nyalakonda, M.D.
Cleveland Clinic, Richard E. Jacobs Health Center,
33100 Cleveland Clinic Blvd., Avon, OH 44011, USA
e-mail: dm2rdcde@gmail.com; nyalakk@ccf.org

M.L. Corrigan et al. (eds.), *Handbook of Clinical Nutrition and Stroke*,
Nutrition and Health, DOI 10.1007/978-1-62703-380-0_5,
© Springer Science+Business Media New York 2013

ADA   American Diabetes Association
AHA   American Heart Association
ASA   American Stroke Association
DCCT   Diabetes Control and Complications Trial
GIP   Glucose-dependent Insulinotropic Polypeptide
MNT   Medical Nutrition Therapy
TZDs   Thiazolidinediones
UKPDS   UK Prospective Diabetes Study
VADT   Veterans Affairs Diabetes Trial

Introduction

Approximately 8.3% of the US population (25.8 million) is affected by diabetes [1]. About 7 million of this number is undiagnosed and unaware they have the disease. The risk of diabetes increases as we age, and among those 65 years of age or older, 26.9% have diabetes (10.9 million) [1]. Diabetes is a major cause of heart disease and stroke. Adults with diabetes have two to four times higher rates of death from heart disease than adults without diabetes. The risk for stroke is also two to four times higher among people with diabetes [1]. In 2004, among people aged 65 years or older, heart disease was noted on 68% of diabetes-related death certificates, and stroke was noted on 16% of diabetes-related death certificates. Overall, diabetes is the seventh leading cause of death in the United States [1].

In addition to those with diabetes (type 1 or type 2), it is estimated that 79 million Americans aged 20 years or older have prediabetes [1]. Those with prediabetes have blood glucose levels that are higher than normal but not high enough to be classified as diabetes. Not only is prediabetes a risk factor for developing type 2 diabetes, but blood glucose numbers in the prediabetes range also put individuals at risk for cardiovascular disease (CVD) and stroke. Diagnostic criteria for diabetes and prediabetes are listed in Table 5.1 [2].

Goals of Therapy in Diabetes and Prevention of Stroke

Diabetes is a complex syndrome characterized by hyperglycemia. It is associated with an increased risk of microvascular (retinopathy, nephropathy, neuropathy) and macrovascular complications. Other atherogenic risk factors are highly prevalent in patients with diabetes including hypertension, hyperlipidemia, and obesity. Numerous studies have shown that diabetes independently increases the risk of stroke [3–6]. The indications for treatment of diabetes are to relieve acute symptoms of hyperglycemia and to prevent chronic complications associated with long-standing elevation of blood glucose. It has clearly been shown that in both patients with type 1 and type 2 diabetes, microvascular complications can be reduced with

Table 5.1
Blood glucose at diagnosis of prediabetes and diabetes [2]

Diagnosis of prediabetes
Fasting plasma glucose 100–125 mg/dl
Or
2-h plasma glucose 140–199 mg/dl during an oral glucose tolerance test
Or
A1c 5.7–6.4%
Diagnosis of diabetes
Fasting plasma glucose ≥126 mg/dl[a]
Or
2-h plasma glucose ≥200 g/dl during an oral glucose tolerance test[a]
Or
A1c ≥6.5%[a]
Or
A random plasma glucose of ≥200 mg/dl in a patient with classic symptoms of hyperglycemia

[a]Should be confirmed by repeat testing in the absence of unequivocal hyperglycemia

intensive glycemic control, which aims to achieve blood glucose values as close to the normal range as possible [7, 8]. In the diabetes control and complications trial (DCCT), the goals of intensive therapy included preprandial blood glucose values between 70 and 120 mg/dl and postprandial blood glucose values of less than 180 mg/dl [7]. In the UK Prospective Diabetes Study (UKPDS), the goals of intensive therapy included fasting plasma glucose of less than 6 mmol/L and preprandial glucose concentrations of 4–7 mmol/L [8].

The risk of macrovascular complications including stroke can also be decreased in persons with diabetes. The Steno-2 study randomized 160 patients with type 2 diabetes and persistent microalbuminuria to receive conventional multifactorial treatment or intensive therapy consistent with the American Diabetes Association (ADA) guidelines at that time [9]. Intensified targets included hemoglobin A1c (A1c) less than 6.5%, total cholesterol less than 175 mg/dl, triglyceride level less than 150 mg/dl, and blood pressure less than 130/80 mmHg. All patients received a renin-angiotensin system blocker and low-dose aspirin. The mean treatment period was 7.8 years. After the initial trial ended, patients were observed for an additional mean 5.5 years in a follow-up study. After an average of 13.3 years, there was a 59% reduction in relative risk for the cardiovascular event composite and a 13% reduction in absolute risk of death from cardiovascular causes in patients that had received intensive therapy. There were 30 strokes in the conventional therapy group compared to 6 in the intensive therapy group.

Studies have also shown that modifying a single cardiovascular risk factor in patients with diabetes can be beneficial. Intensified treatment of hypertension in patients with diabetes reduces the risk of stroke [10–12]. The UKPDS assigned hypertensive patients with type 2 diabetes to either tight blood pressure control (aiming for a blood pressure < 150/85) or less tight control (aiming for a blood pressure < 180/105 mmHg). The tight blood pressure control group achieved an average blood pressure of 144/82 mmHg, while the less tight control group had a mean blood pressure of 154/87. There was a 44% reduction in risk of stroke in the tight control group [10]. In the Action to Control Cardiovascular Risk in Diabetes (ACCORD) study, 4,733 patients were assigned to intensive blood pressure therapy (aiming for a systolic pressure < 120 mmHg) or conventional therapy (aiming for a systolic pressure < 140 mmHg) and achieved a systolic blood pressure of 119.3 and 133.5 mmHg, respectively [12]. There was no significant difference seen in the rate of the primary composite outcome of nonfatal myocardial infarction, nonfatal stroke, or death from cardiovascular causes, but intensive blood pressure therapy did reduce the risk of total stroke (hazard ratio, 0.59; 95% CI, 0.39–0.89; $P = 0.01$).

Statins have also been shown to be beneficial in the reduction of stroke risk in patients with type 2 diabetes [13–15]. Subanalysis of the Treating to New Targets (TNT) study looked at the effect of atorvastatin 80 mg/day versus atorvastatin 10 mg/day in patients with coronary heart disease and type 2 diabetes [15]. Patients were followed for a median of 4.9 years. Mean LDL cholesterol levels were 98.6 mg/dl with atorvastatin 10 mg and 77.0 mg/dl with atorvastatin 80 mg. There was a significant decrease in time to cerebrovascular event in the atorvastatin 80 mg group (0.69 [0.48–0.98], $P = 0.037$).

Although treating diabetes with a multifactorial intervention is effective in decreasing stroke risk, it is less clear whether improving glycemic control alone has such beneficial effects. The DCCT investigated the effects of intensified glycemic control in patients with type 1 diabetes. The DCCT randomized 1,441 patients with type 1 diabetes to either conventional insulin therapy or intensive insulin therapy for a mean of 6.5 years. Conventional therapy consisted of 1–2 daily injections of insulin with the goal of preventing symptoms of hyperglycemia or hypoglycemia. Intensive insulin therapy consisted of three or more daily insulin injections or use of an external insulin pump with the goal of achieving blood glucose values between 70 and120 mg/dl before meals and less than 180 mg/dl after meals. The study compared the effects of standard control of blood glucose versus intensive control on the vascular and neurologic complications of diabetes. The Epidemiology of Diabetes Interventions and Complications (EDIC) study was an observational follow-up study to assess the long-term outcomes in participants of the DCCT. Intensive therapy reduced the risk of any CVD event by 42% and the risk of nonfatal MI, stroke, or death by 57% [16]. The number of strokes that were observed overall was small with five nonfatal cerebrovascular events in the conventional therapy group and one in the intensive therapy group.

UKPDS was a prospective study of subjects with newly diagnosed type 2 diabetes randomized to intensive glycemic treatment or conventional therapy. A 10-year observational follow-up study demonstrated a reduction in cardiovascular events, but there was no significant change in stroke [17]. Three large randomized clinical trials were conducted to investigate the effect of intensive glycemic control on cardiovascular events in subjects with type 2 diabetes: ACCORD, Action in Diabetes

Table 5.2

Recommendations for the primary prevention of stroke in adults with diabetes

Class 1: level A recommendations
- Control of hypertension as recommended by the Seventh Report of the Joint National Committee on Prevention, Detection, Evaluation and Treatment of High Blood Pressure (JNC 7) guidelines
- Use of an ace inhibitor or angiotensin II receptor blocker for hypertension is beneficial
- Treatment with a statin is recommended for primary prevention of stroke

Class IIb: level B recommendations
- Aspirin may be reasonable in those with high CVD risk
- Fibrate monotherapy may be considered

Class III: level B recommendations
- The addition of a fibrate to a statin is not useful for decreasing stroke risk

and Vascular Disease-Preterex and Diamicron Modified Release Controlled Evaluation (ADVANCE), and the Veterans Affairs Diabetes Trial (VADT). These trials studied individuals who had more advanced diabetes and significant risk for cardiovascular disease. None of these studies showed a difference in macrovascular events including stroke with more intensive therapy [18–20].

The American Heart Association (AHA)/American Stroke Association (ASA) Guidelines for the primary prevention of stroke concluded that there is insufficient evidence to demonstrate that improved glycemic control reduces the risk of stroke [21]. The AHA/ASA guidelines recommend a multifaceted approach focusing on treatment of hypertension and dyslipidemia. A summary of these recommendations for the primary prevention of stroke in adults with diabetes is listed in Table 5.2 [21]. Although there is limited data demonstrating reduction in stroke risk with intensive glycemic control, the general goal of an A1c <7% is reasonable [22, 23].

Goals of Nutrition Therapy in Diabetes and Prevention of Stroke

Lifestyle modification including dietary changes, exercise, and weight loss is a key intervention in the management of diabetes and prediabetes. In fact, studies, such as the Diabetes Prevention Program, [24] have shown that people with prediabetes who lose at least 7% of their weight and include at least 150 min of physical activity/week can prevent or delay type 2 diabetes and in some cases return their blood glucose levels to normal. This prevention or delay of diabetes with lifestyle intervention can persist for at least 10 years [25].

Medical nutrition therapy (MNT) provided by a registered dietitian (RD) is recommended for all individuals with type 1 and type 2 diabetes. Research reports sustained improvements in hemoglobin A1C at 12 months and longer with long-term follow-up encounters (1–5 individual sessions or a series of 6–12 group sessions initially with one annual follow-up yearly) with an RD [26]. MNT goals for both type 1 and type 2 diabetes are similar: to achieve and maintain glucose levels in the target range set by the managing health-care provider. Food intake (focusing on carbohydrate), medication, metabolic control (glycemia, lipids, and blood pressure), anthropometric measurements, and physical activity should be assessed by the RD to help individualize the nutrition prescription, goals, and intervention. Research does not support any one specific diabetic diet, ADA diet, or an ideal percentage of energy from macronutrients for persons with diabetes [2, 27]. Adequacy of intake based on the dietary reference intakes (DRI) for healthy adults should be encouraged [28].

Since persons with diabetes have the equivalent cardiovascular disease risk as persons with preexisting CVD and no diabetes, any MNT interventions for diabetes need to address this risk [29]. Nutritional interventions in the treatment of cardiovascular disease in people with diabetes have been studied. Improved measures of endothelial health, improved serum lipid profile, and reductions in blood pressure were noted in studies based on currently accepted guidelines, low-fat diets and the consumption of specific fatty acids, combination drug and diet therapies, Mediterranean diets, and reduced sodium diets. Further research is needed on the effect of high-protein diets, low-glycemic index diets, phytosterol consumption, and vitamin supplements [30].

The AHA has committed itself to the following impact goal: by 2020, to improve the cardiovascular health of all Americans by 20% while reducing deaths from cardiovascular diseases and stroke by 20% [31].

To achieve the AHA goals, the concept of "ideal cardiovascular health" has been defined by the presence of ideal health behaviors:

- Nonsmoking
- Body mass index <25 kg/m^2
- Physical activity at goal levels
- Pursuit of a diet consistent with current guideline recommendations (choosing four out of the five recommendations from Table 5.3) and ideal health factors
- Untreated total cholesterol <200 mg/dl
- Untreated blood pressure <120/<80 mmHg
- Fasting blood glucose <100 mg/dl [32]

Some of the above health behaviors such as smoking, weight, exercise, alcohol use, and diet have been further defined in studies that looked at prevention of cardiovascular disease and stroke in both men and women [33–35] and have also been associated with decreased risk for developing type 2 diabetes [36]. These studies determine the minimal physical activity for adults as participation in 30 min or more of moderate to vigorous physical activity daily (on average).

Current AHA diet recommendations [32] are consistent with a dietary approaches to stop hypertension (DASH)-type eating plan (*see* Table 5.4) [37]. The AHA diet recommendations are an easy style of healthy eating to promote to patients with or without diabetes. Many patients with diabetes may be already achieving one out of the five recommendations by avoiding sugar-sweetened beverages [37].

Table 5.3

AHA diet and lifestyle recommendations revision 2006 [32]

1. Fruits and vegetables: ≥4.5 cups per day
2. Fish: ≥two 3.5-oz servings per week (preferably oily fish)
3. Fiber-rich whole grains (≥1.1 g of fiber per 10 g of carbohydrate): ≥three 1-oz-equivalent servings per day
4. Sodium: ≤1,500 mg per day
5. Sugar-sweetened beverages: ≤450 kcal (36 oz) per week

(Above based on intake goals outlined for a 2,000-kcal diet)

Table 5.4

Daily nutrient goals used in the DASH studies [37]
(for a 2,100 cal eating plan)

Total fat 27% of calories	Sodium 2,300 mg[a]
Saturated fat 6% of calories	Potassium 4,700 mg
Protein 18% of calories	Calcium 1,250 mg
Carbohydrate 55% of calories	Magnesium 500 mg
Cholesterol 150 mg	Fiber 30 g

g grams, *mg* milligrams

[a]1,500 mg sodium was a lower goal tested and found to be even better for lowering blood pressure. It was particularly effective for middle-aged and older individuals, African Americans, and those who already had high blood pressure

Both the 2006 AHA Nutrition Guidelines and the DASH-type eating plan promote variety and moderation of food choices and focus on food patterns over individual foods, supplements, and fortified foods. This coincides with the position of the Academy of Nutrition and Dietetics (formerly the American Dietetic Association) that the total diet or overall pattern of food eaten is the most important focus of a healthful eating style [38].

Carbohydrates

The Academy of Nutrition and Dietetics and the ADA have published recommendations for nutrition therapy in diabetes management [26, 39]. Both agree that the best mix of carbohydrate, protein, and fat in the diet will depend upon the individual's metabolic status and food preferences, and these must be balanced in amount for weight management to occur [26, 39]. Thus, a vegan or vegetarian diet, Mediterranean diet, DASH diet, low-fat diet, or lower carbohydrate diet may all be appropriate for the patient with diabetes. A diet or lifestyle may not be dictated by the medical world but embraced and followed by the individual with health-care team guidance. Nutrition education and counseling should be sensitive to the personal needs, willingness to change, and ability to make changes of the individual with diabetes [26, 39].

Most individuals with diabetes eat a moderate intake of carbohydrate (44–46%) [27]. The recommended daily minimum value for carbohydrate is 130 g/day based on adequate glucose for brain function. Diets too low in carbohydrate may be inadequate in vitamins, minerals, and fiber. A consistent carbohydrate diet (where the amount of carbohydrate is distributed in meals and snacks throughout the day and is consistent in amount meal to meal, day to day) may be helpful in glucose management for those that are not using adjustable mealtime insulin or pump therapy [26, 27]. A more flexible intake of carbohydrate is possible for those adjusting insulin prior to the meal or snack by using insulin-to-carbohydrate ratios. Consistent carbohydrate meal plans are beneficial in the hospital setting to optimize glycemic goals. Unfortunately, patients may only consume 43–46% of the amount that they are served as caloric intake in the hospital setting, which is suboptimal [40].

Patients who cannot accurately assess or count the carbohydrate content of their meals or snacks may have a highly varied carbohydrate intake. This may lead to wide glucose swings which can be potentially dangerous in those patients who are managing their blood glucose with insulin or other glucose-lowering agents. Assessing a patient's carbohydrate-counting knowledge and providing basic carbohydrate-counting education—whether in the hospital or outpatient setting—is a necessity. A multipaged carbohydrate-counting tool has been developed and validated [41]. This tool can assist RDs and other diabetes educators in assessing the patient's knowledge of dietary carbohydrates and serve to help prevent future hypoglycemia. This quiz covers six areas of carbohydrate knowledge—carbohydrate food recognition, carbohydrate food content, nutrition label reading, glycemic targets, hypoglycemia prevention and treatments, and carbohydrate content of meals—and may be completed in less than 15 min [41]. While some might titrate insulin doses using preprandial blood glucose values and argue against carbohydrate counting, it may assist with less hypoglycemia episodes and decrease weight gain [42].

MNT is best provided in an outpatient setting where the individual with diabetes is generally better able to focus on learning needs [28]. If diabetes education is being provided during a hospitalization, it should be started as soon as possible prior to hospital discharge.

Outpatient follow-up visits should be scheduled within a few weeks of discharge with the registered dietitian and also with diabetes education community classes as assessed by the diabetes hospital team.

Glycemic Targets in Diabetes

It is important to individualize therapy and glycemic goals for each patient. One of the primary goals of diabetes management is controlling hyperglycemia while minimizing hypoglycemia and side effects. Emphasis should be placed on treatment soon after the diagnosis of diabetes. Data suggests that achieving a target A1c early in the disease process can lead to reduction in both microvascular and macrovascular complications [7, 8]. The ADA has recommended an A1c of <7% as a reasonable goal in adults, whereas other societies have advocated lower targets [43, 44]. Younger, relatively healthy patients who have a shorter duration of diabetes will benefit from tighter control in order to prevent long-term complications [7, 8, 16, 17]. Occasional mild hypoglycemia may be an acceptable risk in this population in order to achieve optimal glycemic control. In this population, an A1c goal such as <6.5% is preferential [2, 44].

In older patients with long-standing diabetes and multiple comorbidities including CVD, the risks of trying to achieve the standard glycemic target may cause more harm than good [18]. If near normal glycemic targets cannot be achieved easily or safely in patients with advanced disease, high risk for severe hypoglycemia, risk for falls, cognitive deficits, or limited life expectancy, a less stringent A1c goal (such as <8) is appropriate in order to minimize side effects and hypoglycemia [2]. The managing health-care provider should monitor response to therapy frequently (at least every 3 months) and should not delay in advancing therapy if glycemic targets have not been achieved.

Therapeutic Agents/Medical Management of Glycemia

There has been a significant increase in the number of therapeutic agents available for the treatment of hyperglycemia in type 2 diabetes. A brief description of the more commonly used classes is given below, and Table 5.5 outlines some of the agents and their respective dosing.

Biguanides

Metformin is the primary biguanide available for treatment of type 2 diabetes. It decreases hepatic glucose production and increases insulin sensitivity peripherally [45]. It typically lowers A1c by 1–2% points [43]. Metformin is usually weight neutral or results in mild weight loss. The most common side effect of metformin is gastrointestinal symptoms including bloating and diarrhea, which often improves with continued use. Metformin should not be used in conditions that cause increased risk of lactic acidosis such as class III or IV heart failure and decreased renal function with a creatinine of ≥1.5 mg/dl in men and ≥1.4 mg/dl in women [45]. Metformin therapy is associated with a higher prevalence of vitamin B12 deficiency in as many as 4.1% taking metformin <1 year and as many as 8.1% among those taking metformin >10 years ($P = 0.3219$ for <1 year vs. >10 years) [46]. Reinstatler et al. suggest that further research be done on B12 needs in metformin therapy as the amount of B12 available in general multivitamins (6 µg) may not be enough to correct this deficiency among those with diabetes [46].

Table 5.5
Medications for the treatment of type 2 diabetes

Class	Agents	Dose range	Route	Dosing
Biguanide	Metformin	500–2,550 mg	Oral	2–3 times a day usually taken with meals
Sulfonylureas	Glyburide Glipizide Glimepiride	1.25–20 mg 2.5–40 mg 1–8 mg	Oral	1–2 times a day usually taken with meals
Meglitinides	Nateglinide Repaglinide	120–360 mg 0.5–16 mg	Oral	Nateglinide: 3 times a day with meals Repaglinide: 2–4 times a day with meals
Thiazolidinediones	Pioglitazone	15–45 mg	Oral	Once a day
Glucagon-like peptide receptor agonists	Exenatide Liraglutide	10–20 µg 0.6–1.8 mg	Subcutaneous injection	Exenatide: twice a day within 60 min before the morning and evening meal Liraglutide: once a day
Dipeptidyl peptidase-4 inhibitors	Sitagliptin Saxagliptin Linagliptin	25–100 mg 2.5–5 mg 5 mg	Oral	Once a day

Sulfonylureas

Available second generation sulfonylureas include glyburide, glipizide, and glimepiride. They are insulin secretagogues and increase insulin production independent of glucose levels. As a result, sulfonylureas can cause hypoglycemia. This is more commonly seen with glyburide [47]. The average reduction in A1c is 1–2% [42]. Sulfonylureas can also be associated with weight gain.

Meglitinides

The meglitinides include repaglinide and nateglinide. They are also insulin secretagogues but provide a more rapid, short-lived insulin output. They are most effective for controlling postprandial hyperglycemia [48]. They are often used to target postprandial hyperglycemia and are therefore dosed before each meal. On average, they lower A1c by 0.5–1.5% points when used as monotherapy [43]. As with sulfonylureas, these agents can be associated with hypoglycemia and weight gain. They are safe to use in patients with renal dysfunction.

Thiazolidinediones

Thiazolidinediones (TZDs) improve glycemic control primarily by promoting glucose uptake by muscle and adipose tissue. Several weeks of treatment are required to achieve maximal benefit. There is an average reduction in A1c of 0.5–1.4% with TZD use [43]. They are not associated with hypoglycemia. Available agents on the market are pioglitazone and rosiglitazone. The use of rosiglitazone has been restricted by the FDA as noted below. The most common adverse effects are edema and weight gain. There is also an approximately twofold increased risk of fluid retention and congestive heart failure with TZD use [49–51]. Recent evidence also indicates that TZDs may increase the risk of bone fractures [52]. Recently pioglitazone use has been associated with an increased risk of bladder cancer with long-term use and cumulative exposure [53]. There have been analyses suggesting increased risk of myocardial infarction with rosiglitazone, and the FDA has restricted the use of this agent to patients who are unable to achieve glycemic control with other therapies [54].

Glucagon-Like Peptide 1 Receptor Agonists

GLP-1 and glucose-dependent insulinotropic polypeptide (GIP) belong to a class of short-lived gut hormones known as incretins, which are released in response to ingestion of food. Secretion of these hormones is impaired in patients with type 2 diabetes [55]. Exenatide and liraglutide are GLP-1 receptor agonists that mimic the effects of GLP-1. They increase insulin production in a glucose-dependent manner, slow gastric emptying, and suppress glucagon. They lower A1c by 0.5–1.0% points [43]. They can also cause appetite suppression thereby decreasing food intake and causing some weight loss. The incidence of hypoglycemia is relatively low with these agents given stimulation of insulin is glucose dependent; however, the risk of hypoglycemia increases if used with sulfonylureas [56]. Gastrointestinal side effects are common including nausea, vomiting, and diarrhea, which may abate with continued use. Based on reports of pancreatitis in patients taking Byetta, the FDA issued a warning that Byetta should be discontinued if pancreatitis is suspected and other antidiabetic therapies should be considered in patients with a history of pancreatitis [57]. Clinical trials have also shown more cases of pancreatitis with liraglutide than with other diabetes drugs [58]. Currently these agents have to be given as subcutaneous injections. An extended release formulation of exenatide, which is administered once a week, just received FDA approval.

Dipeptidyl Peptidase-4 Inhibitors

The protease DPP-4 rapidly degrades GLP-1 and GIP, and inhibitors of DPP-4 result in an increase of GLP-1 and GIP levels [59]. Drugs in this class include sitagliptin, saxagliptin, and linagliptin. The average A1c reduction is 0.5–0.8% [43]. Sitagliptin and saxagliptin must be adjusted for renal impairment but linagliptin does not. These agents are weight neutral. These drugs also include a warning about the risk of pancreatitis.

Treatment Approach

Metformin is generally accepted as first-line therapy due to proven efficacy, low-risk profile, and low cost [60, 61]. There is less agreement regarding which agents should be added if glycemic targets are not met with metformin and lifestyle changes alone. Both the ADA/European Association for the Study of Diabetes (EASD) and the American Association of Clinical Endocrinologists (AACE)/American College of Endocrinology (ACE) came out with consensus statements in 2009 outlining treatment algorithms for hyperglycemia. These algorithms differ in their approach to achieving glycemic goals.

In the AACE/ACE algorithm, the choice of therapy and the number of agents recommended are stratified by the A1c level [44]. If the initial A1c is between 7.6 and 9.0%, then dual therapy is recommended right away. If the A1c is above 9% and the patient is asymptomatic and drug-naive, then initiation of triple therapy is considered reasonable. The AACE/ACE guidelines favor incretin-based therapy over sulfonylureas and meglitinides due to their efficacy, decreased risk of hypoglycemia, and beneficial or neutral effects on weight. They also noted that TZDs are effective agents but give them lower priority due to the known potential adverse effects. If dual therapy fails, the guidelines advise that a third non-insulin agent may be reasonable if the A1c is not too far from goal.

The ADA/EASD algorithm recommends a tiered approach with escalation of therapy every 3 months if the goal A1c is not met [43]. The ADA guidelines also emphasize older agents that have been more extensively used and studied such as sulfonylureas and insulin for a second medication. If dual therapy is insufficient at achieving target glycemia, they recommend initiation or intensification of insulin [43]. Both algorithms are meant to provide guidance to clinicians, but therapies should always be individualized to a patient. When choosing a treatment regimen, one must take into account the duration of diabetes, degree of hyperglycemia, previous therapy, and costs to the patient.

Insulin Treatment

Type 2 diabetes is a progressive disease, and many patients will require insulin at some point during their disease course. Table 5.6 summarizes the various types of insulin.

The newer insulin analogues including long-acting agents levemir and glargine and the rapid-acting agents aspart, lispro, and glulisine have more beneficial action profiles compared to some of the older insulins such as NPH and regular. Levemir and glargine are relatively peakless, and therefore, the risk of hypoglycemia is less compared to NPH. Another advantage is that adequate basal levels of insulin can often be maintained with just one injection. The rapid-acting analogues have a quicker onset and shorter duration of action than regular insulin allowing them to more closely match the normal physiologic profile following meal ingestion.

Table 5.6
Various types of insulin

Type of insulin	Trade name	Onset	Peak	Duration
Rapid-acting insulin analogues		15 min	30–90 min	3–5 h
Aspart	Novolog			
Lispro	Humalog			
Glulisine	Apidra			
Short-acting insulin		30–60 min	2–3 h	5–8 h
Regular human insulin	Humulin R or Novolin R			
Long-acting insulin analogues (basal)				
Glargine	Lantus	1 h	No peak	20–26 h
Detemir	Levemir			
Intermediate-acting insulin (basal)				
NPH	Humulin N or Novolin N	1–3 h	4–10 h	12–16 h
Premixed				
70% aspart-protamine/30% aspart	Novolog mix	5–15 min	–	10–16 h
75% lispro-protamine/25% lispro	Humalog mix	5–15 min	–	10–16 h
70% NPH/30% regular	Humulin 70/30 or Novolin 70/30	30–60 min	–	10–16 h

A common approach to initiating insulin is to add a long-acting or basal insulin such as NPH, levemir, or glargine to oral medications [43]. A typical starting dose is 10 units or 0.1–0.2 units per kg at bedtime [43]. The dose can be increased by approximately 2 units every 3 days until the fasting glucose level reaches the desired target. If the fasting glucose is greater than 180, then the basal insulin dose can be increased in larger increments such as 4 units every 3 days [43].

Many agents such as TZDs, metformin, and GLP-1 agonists (exenatide is FDA approved as adjunct to insulin glargine) may complement insulin due to their mechanism of action and should be considered as a possible adjunct to insulin therapy. Both metformin and exenatide have been shown to limit or counteract insulin-induced weight gain [62, 63]. The risk/benefit profile of the combination of TZDs and insulin should be considered in each case since this combination can be associated with a higher risk of weight gain and fluid retention [44]. Insulin secretagogues (sulfonylureas and meglitinides) should be tapered and discontinued with intensification of insulin therapy (often signified by the addition of prandial insulin) as these are not considered synergistic with insulin and may increase the risk of hypoglycemia [43, 44].

If patients achieve target fasting blood sugars with the addition of basal insulin but the A1c remains above goal, then premeal blood glucose levels should be monitored. Two hour postprandial glucose levels can serve a similar purpose. If premeal or postprandial glucoses are above goal, then rapid-acting or prandial insulin should be initiated at the appropriate meals. A typical starting dose may be 3–5 units, which can be further adjusted based on the blood glucose levels.

Conclusion

Treatment for diabetes should involve a multidisciplinary approach including both MNT and pharmacotherapy and should occur soon after diagnosis. Data suggests that achieving target A1c early in the disease process can lead to reduction in both microvascular and macrovascular complications. It is important to individualize therapy and glycemic goals for each patient while minimizing hypoglycemia and side effects. When choosing a treatment regimen, one must take into account the duration of diabetes, degree of hyperglycemia, previous therapy, and costs to the patient. Nutrition education and counseling should be sensitive to the personal needs, willingness to change, and ability to make changes of the individual with diabetes. Education should take place as soon as possible in the hospital setting with scheduled follow-up as an outpatient shortly after discharge.

References

1. Centers for Disease Control and Prevention. National diabetes fact sheet: National estimates and general information on diabetes and prediabetes in the United States, 2011. Atlanta, GA: U.S. Department of Health and Human Services, Centers for Disease Control and Prevention, 2011. [cited 2012 Feb 5] Available from http://www.cdc.gov/diabetes/pubs/pdf/ndfs_2011.pdf
2. American Diabetes Association. Clinical Practice Recommendations 2012. Diabetes Care. 2012;35 Suppl 1:S12–S13
3. Abbott RD, Donahue RP, MacMahon SW, Reed DM, Yano K. Diabetes and the risk of stroke: The Honolulu Heart Program. JAMA. 1987;257:949–52.
4. Barrett-Connor E, Khaw KT. Diabetes mellitus: an independent risk factor for stroke? Am J Epidemiol. 1988;128(1):116–23.
5. Kannel WB, McGee D. Diabetes and cardiovascular disease: the framingham study. JAMA. 1979;241:2035–8.
6. Tuomilehto J, Rastenyte D, Jousilahti P, Sarti C, Vartiainen E. Diabetes mellitus as a risk factor for death from stroke: prospective study of the middle-aged finnish population. Stroke. 1996;27:210–5.
7. Diabetes Control and Complications Trial Research Group. The effect of intensive treatment of diabetes on the development and progression of long-term complications in insulin-dependent diabetes mellitus. New Engl J Med. 1993;329:977–86.
8. UK Prospective Diabetes Study (UKPDS) Group. Intensive blood-glucose control with sulphonyures or insulin compared with conventional treatment and risk of complications in patients with type 2 diabetes (UKPDS 33). The Lancet. 1998;352:837–53.
9. Gaede P, Lund-Andersen H, Parving HH, Pedersen O. Effect of a multifactorial intervention on mortality in type 2 diabetes. N Engl J Med. 2008;358:580–91.
10. UK Prospective Diabetes Study Group. Tight blood pressure control and risk of macrovascular and microvascular complications in type 2 diabetes (UKPDS 38). BMJ. 1998;317:703–13.
11. Heart Outcomes Prevention Evaluation Study Investigators. Effects of an angiotensin-converting-enzyme inhibitor, ramipril, on cardiovascular events in high-risk patients. N Engl J Med. 2000;342:145–53.
12. ACCORD Study Group. Effects of intensive blood-pressure control in type 2 diabetes mellitus. N Engl J Med. 2010;362:1575–85.
13. Heart Protection Study Collaborative Group. MRC/BHF Heart Protection Study of cholesterol lowering with simvastatin in 20, 536 high-risk individuals: a randomised placebo-controlled trial. Lancet. 2002;360:7–22.

14. Colhoun HM, Betteridge DJ, Durrington PN, Hitman GA, Neil HA, Livingstone SJ, et al. Primary prevention of cardiovascular disease with atorvastatin in type 2 diabetes in the Collaborative Atorvastatin Diabetes Study (CARDS): multicentre randomised placebo-controlled trial. Lancet. 2004;364:685–96.
15. Shepherd J, Barter P, Carmena R, Deedwania P, Fruchart JC, Haffner S, et al. Effect of lowering LDL cholesterol substantially below currently recommended levels in patients with coronary heart disease and diabetes: the Treating to New Targets (TNT) study. Diabetes Care. 2006;29:1220–6.
16. Nathan DM, Cleary PA, Backlund JY, Genuth SM, Lachin JM, Orchard TJ, et al. Intensive diabetes treatment and cardiovascular disease in patients with type 1 diabetes. N Engl J Med. 2005;353:2643–53.
17. Holman RR, Paul SK, Bethel A, Matthews DR, Neil HAW. 10-year follow-up of intensive glucose control in type 2 diabetes. N Engl J Med. 2008;359:1577–89.
18. Action to Control Cardiovascular Risk in Diabetes (ACCORD) Study Group. Effects of intensive glucose lowering in type 2 diabetes. N Engl J Med. 2008;358:2545–59.
19. ADVANCE Collaborative Group. Intensive blood glucose control and vascular outcomes in patients with type 2 diabetes. N Engl J Med. 2008;358:2560–72.
20. Duckworth W, Abraira C, Moritz T, Reda D, Emanuele N, Reaven PD, et al. Glucose control and vascular complications in veterans with type 2 diabetes. N Engl J Med. 2009;360:129–39.
21. Goldstein LB, Bushnell CD, Adams RJ, Appel LJ, Bruan LT, Chaturvedi S, et al. Guidelines for the primary prevention of stroke: a guideline for healthcare professionals from the American Heart Association/American Stroke Association. Stroke. 2011;42:517–84.
22. Skyler JS, Bergenstal R, Bonow RO, Buse J, Deedwania P, Gale EA, et al. Intensive glycemic control and the prevention of cardiovascular events: implications of the ACCORD, ADVANCE, and VA diabetes trials: a position statement of the American Diabetes Association and a scientific statement of the American College of Cardiology Foundation and the American Heart Association. Diabetes Care. 2009;32(1):187–92.
23. Furie KL, Kasner SE, Adams RJ, Albers GW, Bush RL, Fagan SC, et al. Guidelines for the prevention of stroke in patients with stroke or transient ischemic attack: a guideline for Healthcare Professionals From the American Heart Association/American Stroke Association. Stroke. 2011;42:227–76.
24. Diabetes Prevention Program Research Group. Reduction in the incidence of type 2 diabetes with lifestyle intervention or metformin. N Engl J Med. 2002;346:393–403.
25. Diabetes Prevention Program Research Group. 10-year follow-up of diabetes incidence and weight loss in the diabetes prevention program outcomes study. The Lancet. 2009;374(9702):1686–7.
26. Academy of Nutrition and Dietetics. Diabetes 1 and 2 evidence analysis project. [cited 2012 Feb 8] Available from: http://www.adaevidencelibrary.com/topic. cfm?cat=1615)
27. Franz MJ, Powers MA, Leontos C, Holzmeister KA, Kulkarni K, Monk A, et al. The evidence for medical nutrition therapy for type 1 and type 2 diabetes in adults. J Am Diet Assoc. 2010;110:1852–89.
28. Academy of Nutrition and Dietetics Nutrition Care Manual. Rationale for Nutrition Consult Order. [cited 2012 Feb 10] Available from: www.nutritioncaremanual.org/content. cfm?ncm_content_id=81039
29. Buse JB, Ginsberg HN, Barkis GL, Clark NG, Costa F, Eckel R, et al. Primary prevention of cardiovascular disease in people with diabetes mellitus: a scientific statement from the American Heart Association and the American Diabetes Association. Diabetes Care. 2007;30:162–72.
30. Academy of Nutrition and Dietetics. Diabetes 1 and 2 evidence analysis project. Diabetes and the prevention and treatment of CVD. [cited 2012 Feb 8] Available from: http://www.adaevidencelibrary.com/conclusion.cfm?conclusion_ statement_id=250604
31. American Heart Association Strategic Planning Task Force and Statistics Committee. Defining and Setting National Goals for Cardiovascular Health Promotion and Disease Reduction. The

American Heart Association's Strategic Impact Goal Through 2020 and Beyond. Lloyd-Jones DM, Hong Y, Labarthe D, Mozaffarian D, Appel LJ, Van Horn L, Greenlund K, Daniels S, Nichol G, Tomaselli GF, Arnett DK, Fonarow GC, Ho PM, Lauer MS, Masoudi FA, Robertson RM, Roger V, Schwamm LH, Sorlie P, Yancy CW, Rosamond WD. Circulation. 2010;121:586–613

32. American Heart Association Scientific Statement. Diet and Lifestyle Recommendations Revision 2006. A Scientific Statement From the American Heart Association Nutrition Committee. Lichtenstein AH, Appel LJ, Brands M, Carnethon M, Daniels S, Franch HA, Franklin B, Kris-Etherton P, Harris WS, Barbara Howard, Karanja N, Lefevre M, Rudel L, Sacks F, Van Horn L, Winston M, Wylie-Rosett J. Circulation. 2006; 114:82–96

33. Chiuve SE, McCullough ML, Sacks FM, Rimm EB. Healthy lifestyle factors in the primary prevention of coronary heart disease among men:benefits among users and nonusers of lipid-lowering and antihypertensive medications. Circulation. 2006;114:160–7.

34. Stampfer MJ, Hu FB, Manson JE, Rimm EB, Willett WC. Primary prevention of coronary heart disease in women through diet and lifestyle. N Engl J Med. 2000;343:16–22.

35. Chiuve SE, Rexrode KM, Spiegelman D, Logroscino G, Manson JE, Rimm EB. Primary prevention of stroke by healthy lifestyle. Circulation. 2008;118:947–54.

36. Hu FB, Manson JE, Stampfer MJ, Colditz G, Liu S, Solomon CG, et al. Diet, lifestyle, and the risk of type 2 diabetes mellitus in women. N Engl J Med. 2001;345:790–7.

37. Your Guide to Lowering Your Blood Pressure With DASH. [cited 2012 Feb 6] available from http://www.nhlbi.nih.gov/health/public/heart/hbp/dash/new_dash.pdf

38. Position of the American Dietetic Association. Total diet approach to communicating food and nutrition information. J Am Diet Assoc. 2007;107:1224–32.

39. Bantle JP, Wylie-Rosett J, Albright AL, American Diabetes Association, et al. Nutrition recommendations and interventions for diabetes; a position statement of the American Diabetes Association. Diabetes Care. 2008;31 Suppl 1:61–78.

40. Modic MB, Kozak A, Siedlecki SL, Nowak D, Parella D, Morris MP, et al. Do we know what our patients with diabetes are eating in the hospital? Diabetes Spectrum. 2011;24:100–6.

41. Watts SA, Anselmo JM, Kern E. Validating the adultcarbquiz: a test of carbohydrate-counting knowledge for adults with diabetes. Diabetes Spectrum. 2011;24:154–60.

42. Davis NJ, Wylie-Rosett J. Death to carbohydrate counting? Diabetes Care. 2008;31:1467–8.

43. Nathan DM, Buse JB, Davidson MB, Ferrannini E, Homan RR, Sherwin R, et al. Medical management of hyperglycemia in type 2 diabetes: a consensus algorithm for the initiation and adjustment of therapy: a consensus statement of the American Diabetes Association and the European Association for the Study of Diabetes. Diabetes Care. 2009;32(1):193–203.

44. Rodbard HW, Jellinger PS, Davidson JA, Einhorn D, Garber AJ, Grunberger G, et al. Statement by an American Association of Clinical Endocrinologists/American College of Endocrinology consensus panel on type 2 diabetes mellitus: an algorithm for glycemic control. Endocr Pract. 2009;15(6):540–59.

45. Bailey CJ, Turner RC. Drug therapy: metformin. N Engl J Med. 1996;334:574–9.

46. The National Health and Nutrition Examination Survey, 1999–2006. Association of Biochemical B12 Deficiency With Metformin Therapy and Vitamin B12 Supplements. Reinstatler L, Qi YP, Williamson RS, Garn JV, Oakley Jr GP. Diabetes Care. 2012;35:327–33

47. Gangji AS, Cukierman T, Gerstein HC, Goldsmith CH, Clase CM. A systematic review and meta-analysis of hypoglycemia and cardiovascular events: a comparison of glyburide with other secretagogues and with insulin. Diabetes Care. 2007;30:389–94.

48. Dornhorst A. Insulinotropic meglitinide analogues. The Lancet. 2001;358:1709–16.

49. Nathan DM, Buse JB, Davidson MB, Ferrannini E, Holman RR, Sherwin R, et al. Management of hyperglycemia in type 2 diabetes: a consensus algorithm for the initiation and adjustment of therapy: update regarding the thiazolidinediones. Diabetologia. 2008;51:8–11.

50. Singh S, Loke YK, Furberg CD. Thiazolidinediones and heart failure: a teloanalysis. Diabetes Care. 2007;30:2248–54.

51. Home PD, Pocock SJ, Beck-Nielsen H, Gomis R, Hanefeld M, Jones NP, et al. Rosiglitazone evaluated for cardiovascular outcomes: an interim analysis. N Engl J Med. 2007;357:28–38.

52. Schwartz AV, Sellmeyer DE, Vittinghoff E, Palermo L, Lecka-Czernik B, Feingold KR, et al. Thiazolidinedione use and bone loss in older diabetic adults. J Clin Endocrinol Metab. 2006;91:3349–54.
53. Lewis JD, Ferrara A, Peng T, Hedderson M, Bilker WB, Quesenberry Jr CP. Risk of bladder cancer among diabetic patients treated with pioglitazone: interim report of a longitudinal cohort study. Diabetes Care. 2011;34(4):916–22.
54. Bennett WL, Maruthur NM, Singh S, Segal JB, Wilson LM, Chatterjee R. Comparative effectiveness and safety of medications for type 2 diabetes: an update including new drugs and 2-drug combinations. Ann Intern Med. 2011;154:602–13.
55. Baggio LL, Drucker DJ. Biology of incretins: GLP-1 and GIP. Gastroenterology. 2007; 132:2131–57.
56. Garber AJ. Long-acting glucagon-like peptide 1 receptor agonists: a review of their efficacy and tolerability. Diabetes Care. 2011;34:S279–84.
57. US Food and Drug Administration. Safety Newsletter. Postmarketing reviews. Exenatide (marketed as Byetta): acute pancreatitis. Winter 2008;1(2). Available at: http://www.fda.gov/Drugs/DrugSafety/DrugSafetyNewsletter/ucm119034.htm#exenatide. Accessed 29 June 2012
58. US Food and Drug Administration. Briefing document. Liraglutide (injection) for the treatment of patients with type 2 diabetes. April 2009. http://www.fda.gov/ohrms/dockets/ac/09/briefing/2009-4422b2-02-NovoNordisk.pdf. Accessed 2 Jul 2012
59. Nauck MA, El-Ouaghlidi A. The therapeutic actions of DPP-IV inhibition are not mediated by glucagon-like peptide-1. Diabetologia. 2005;48:608–11.
60. Bolen S, Feldman L, Vassy J, Wilson L, Yeh H, Marinopoulos S, et al. Comparative effectiveness and safety of oral medications for type 2 diabetes mellitus. Ann Intern Med. 2007; 147:386–99.
61. Qaseem A, Humphrey LL, Sweet DE, Starkey M, Shekelle P. Oral pharmacologic treatment of type 2 diabetes mellitus: a clinical practice guideline from the American College of Physicians. Ann In tern Med. 2012;156:218–31.
62. Yki-Jarvinen H, Ryysy L, Nikkila K, Tulokas T, Vanamo R, Heikkila M, et al. Comparison of bedtime insulin regimens in patients with type 2 diabetes mellitus. Ann Intern Med. 1999;130:389–96.
63. Buse JB, Bergenstal RM, Glass LC, Heilmann CR, Lewis MS, Kwan AY, et al. Use of twice-daily exenatide in Basal insulin-treated patients with type 2 diabetes: a randomized, controlled trial. Ann Intern Med. 2011;154(2):103–12.

Suggested Readings

Diabetes Mellitus Toolkit. © 2011 Academy of Nutrition and Dietetics.
Franz MJ, Powers MA, Leontos C, Holzmeister KA, Kulkarni K, Monk A, et al. The evidence for medical nutrition therapy for type 1 and type 2 diabetes in adults. J Am Diet Assoc. 2010; 110:1852–89.
American Diabetes Association. Clinical Practice Recommendations 2012. Diabetes Care. 2012;35 Suppl 1.

Chapter 6
Hypertension/Hyperlipidemia/ Hyperhomocysteinemia and Nutrition Approaches

Katherine Patton

Key Points

- Hypertension, hyperlipidemia, and hyperhomocysteinemia are modifiable risk factors for stroke that can be controlled through dietary intervention.
- Hypertension, hyperlipidemia, and hyperhomocysteinemia contribute to athero-sclerosis, causing hardening and narrowing of artery walls, including carotid arteries which carry oxygen-rich blood to the brain.
- Hardening and narrowing of carotid arteries could result in two types of stroke: a rupture, known as intracranial hemorrhage, or a blood clot, which would cause a cerebral infarction.
- A diet low in sodium can prevent and control hypertension.
- A diet low in saturated fat, trans fat, and cholesterol can prevent and control hyperlipidemia.
- A diet that meets 100 % of recommended intake of vitamins can prevent hyperhomocysteinemia.
- The DASH Diet Eating Plan is an effective way to follow a low sodium, low-fat, and vitamin-rich diet.
- Regular physical activity reduces risk of stroke and hypertension and lowers both blood pressure and blood lipids.

Keywords Hypertension • Hyperlipidemia • Hyperhomocysteinemia • Nutrition • DASH • Diet • Physical activity

K. Patton, M.Ed., R.D., C.S.S.D., L.D. (✉)
Center for Human Nutrition—Nutrition Therapy, Cleveland Clinic, 9500 Euclid Avenue, Cleveland, OH 44195, USA
e-mail: pattonk4@ccf.org

M.L. Corrigan et al. (eds.), *Handbook of Clinical Nutrition and Stroke*,
Nutrition and Health, DOI 10.1007/978-1-62703-380-0_6,
© Springer Science+Business Media New York 2013

Abbreviations

DASH   Dietary Approaches to Stop Hypertension
DGA   Dietary Guidelines for Americans
HDL   High-Density Lipoprotein
HOPE   Heart Outcomes Prevention Evaluation
HTN   Hypertension
LDL   Low-Density Lipoprotein
NCEP   National Cholesterol Education Program
PAGA   Physical Activity Guidelines for Americans
RDA   Recommended Daily Allowance
TG   Triglycerides

Introduction

Hypertension, hyperlipidemia, and hyperhomocysteinemia are modifiable risk factors for stroke that can be controlled through dietary intervention. The commonality between hypertension, hyperlipidemia, and hyperhomocysteinemia and risk of stroke is related to atherosclerosis as each of these conditions contribute to atherosclerosis. Atherosclerosis is the build-up of plaque along artery walls resulting in hardening and narrowing of arteries. Carotid arteries carry oxygen-rich blood to the brain. Hardening or narrowing of carotid arteries can result in a rupture, known as intracranial hemorrhage, or a blood clot causing a cerebral infarction preventing oxygen-rich blood flow to the brain. The Dietary approaches to stop hypertension (DASH) eating plan is a diet that is proven to lower blood pressure, restricts dietary fats that contributes to hyperlipidemia, and incorporates micronutrients that are necessary to possibly prevent hyperhomocysteinemia; therefore the DASH eating plan is an excellent dietary intervention to prevent stroke. Regular physical activity has been shown to prevent stroke, as well as a variety of other comorbid diseases. Modifying lifestyle behaviors to include physical activity most days of the week is recommended to prevent stroke.

Facts and Statistics About Hypertension and Stroke

Hypertension (HTN) is a modifiable risk factor for cerebral infarction and intracranial hemorrhage (ICH). Hypertension is high arterial blood pressure represented by two measures of systolic blood pressure of 140 mmHg or greater and or a diastolic blood pressure of 90 mmHg or greater. HTN increases the risk for stroke is secondary to HTN causing atherosclerosis. Atherosclerosis results in hardening and narrowing of arteries which leads to blockage and weakening of the walls of blood vessels in the brain which causes them to dilate and rupture [1].

The prevalence of HTN is high and increases with age [1]. For men and women 20–34 years of age, the prevalence percentage for HTN is 13.4 % and 6.2 %, 35–44 years of age is 23.2 % and 16.5 %, 45–54 years of age is 36.2 % and 35.9 %, 55–64 years of age is 53.7 % and 55.8 %, 65–74 years old is 64.7 % and 69.6 %, and for greater than 75 years old is 64.1 % and 76.4 % [1]. According to the Centers for Disease Control and Prevention statistics from 2007 to 2008, 33 % of adults over the age of 20 have HTN which represents greater than 76 million adults [2]. Another 25 % of American adults have prehypertension [1].

Prehypertension is a systolic blood pressure of 120–139 mmHg and diastolic blood pressure between 80 and 89 mmHg [1]. Prehypertensive patients do not require antihypertensive medications; rather, lifestyle modification is encouraged. Lifestyle modification is critical in the prehypertensive stage because certain aspects of dietary intake can lead to HTN. Dietary factors that can lead to HTN are excess sodium intake, low potassium, overweight or obesity, high alcohol consumption, and suboptimal dietary intake [3]. The rise in the incidence of HTN is associated with a rise in overweight and obesity, therefore weight management is crucial in preventing HTN [4, 5].

Research shows the higher the blood pressure, the greater the risk of stroke [6]. According to one study, only 72 % of subjects knew they were diagnosed with HTN, 61 % were treated for HTN, and 35 % had a blood pressure less than 140/90 mmHg [7, 8]. Those unaware of their diagnosis, who are not treated, or have uncontrolled BP are putting themselves at risk for stroke when HTN can be controlled with lifestyle modification and medications.

Facts and Statistics About Hyperlipidemia and Stroke

The simple definition of hyperlipidemia is extra fat or lipid in the blood. The lipids that circulate in the blood are high-density lipoprotein (HDL), low-density lipoprotein (LDL), and triglycerides (TG). The total cholesterol level is composed of HDL, LDL, and TG [9]. Excess LDL in the blood is harmful because it can cling to artery walls, which contributes to atherosclerosis and increases the risk of stroke [1]. Extra HDL in the blood is positive because it helps prevent the LDL from clinging to artery walls. Elevated TG in the blood can also contribute to atherosclerosis [9].

According to the American Stroke Association's (ASA) "Guidelines for the Primary Prevention of Stroke," epidemiological research infers that high total cholesterol may be related to a higher risk of ischemic stroke, while lower total cholesterol is associated with a higher risk of hemorrhagic stroke. There is also inconclusive relationship between TG and stroke. Despite this conflicting evidence, elevated total cholesterol, LDL, and TG increase the risk for atherosclerosis and are modifiable risk factors to prevent stroke [1].

A total cholesterol greater than 200 mg/dL is elevated and a risk factor for stroke. According to the National Center for Health Statistics and National Health and Nutrition Examination Survey 2005–2008 data (NCHS/NHANES 2005–2008), greater than 33 million adults have a total cholesterol greater than 240 mg/dL [10]. A LDL cholesterol between 60 and 129 mg/dL is within normal limits. The average LDL cholesterol among American adults in 2008 was 115.2 mg/dL according to the NCHH/NHANES data [10]. Adults with a TG level greater than 150 mg/dL are at risk for stroke. A positive for American adults is that the average TG level is 137.6 mg/dL [10]. The average TG level among American men is higher at 149.4 mg/dL and lower for women, 125.5 mg/dL [10]. Many epidemiological studies show inverse relationship between HDL and ischemic stroke [11, 12]. Adults with a HDL less than 40 mg/dL are at risk for stroke. Among American adults, the average HDL is 53.3 mg/dL [10].

Facts and Statistics About Hyperhomocysteinemia and Stroke

Homocysteine is a nonessential amino acid, as the human body naturally produces it. Homocysteine is created from two different metabolic pathways which require certain B vitamins. The amount of homocysteine in the body is determined by a person's genetics and lifestyle. Human genetics control how homocysteine is processed in the body. For example, genetic defects may inhibit enzymes that play a role in homocysteine metabolism, therefore causing elevated homocysteine levels. Lifestyle factors such as dietary intake affect homocysteine levels. One dietary mechanism relates to how pyridoxine (vitamin B6), folate (vitamin B9), and cyanocobalamin (vitamin B12) work as cofactors and precursors in the metabolism of homocysteine. A deficiency of pyridoxine, folate, or cyanocobalamin can result in hyperhomocysteinemia [13].

Homocysteine has atherogenic and prothrombotic properties making elevated levels of homocysteine dangerous. One property of homocysteine is its ability to increase smooth cell proliferation and enhance collagen production [13]. A metabolite of homocysteine can attach to LDL cholesterol, therefore contributing to risk for atherosclerosis. Other problems associated with hyperhomocysteinemia are increased oxidative stress and endothelial dysfunction [13].

Hyperhomocysteinemia is associated with a two- to threefold increased risk for atherosclerotic disease, such as stroke [14–16]. More specifically, research shows both carotid artery intima-media thickness (IMT) and carotid artery stenosis are increased in those with elevated homocysteine [17–19]. A meta-analysis from the *Journal of the American Medical Association* found a 19 % reduction in stroke risk per 25 % lower homocysteine when adjusted for smoking, systolic blood pressure, and cholesterol [20]. British researcher's 2002 meta-analysis published in the *British Medical Journal* found an association between every 5 μmol/L increase in homocysteine, increased risk of stroke by 59 % and for every 3 μmol/L decrease in homocysteine, decreased risk of stroke by 24 % [21].

Certain studies have found a correlation between folate, cyanocobalamin, and pyridoxine intake and lower homocysteine levels, but a correlation between these vitamins and decreased risk of ischemic stroke is not consistent among research [22–25]. The Heart Outcomes Prevention Evaluation (HOPE 2) study has provided variable outcomes. One outcome of HOPE 2 was that subjects with a history of vascular disease or diabetes treated with a combination of folate, cyanocobalamin, and pyridoxine had a decrease in homocysteine levels, but it did not affect the end point of cardiovascular disease, myocardial infarction or stroke, but it reduced the risk of stroke by 25 % [26]. There is stronger support of B vitamins effect on the primary prevention of stroke. A 2007 meta-analysis by Wang concludes that folate supplementation ranging from 0.5 to 15 mg/day can decrease the risk of stroke in primary prevention [27]. A more recent meta-analysis found folate supplementation did result in statistically significant effect on stroke risk; however, when combined with cyanocobalamin and pyridoxine, there was a minor chance of preventing stroke in primary prevention for male subjects [28].

Goals of Therapy in HTN to Prevent Stroke

Treatment of HTN is among the most effective strategies for preventing cerebral infarction and ICH [1]. The ASA's "Guidelines for the Primary Prevention of Stroke" recommends regular BP screening, lifestyle modification, and pharmacological therapy. The ASA also recommends systolic BP <140 mmHg and diastolic <90 mmHg or systolic BP <130 mmHg and diastolic <80 mmHg for those with diabetes and chronic kidney disease. The 7th Report of the Joint National Committee on Prevention, Detection, Evaluation, and Treatment of High Blood Pressure (JNC 7) recommends BP measurement at least once every 2 years for adults with systolic BP below 120 mmHg and diastolic BP below 80 mmHg. The JNC 7 recommends an annual BP measurement for adults with systolic BP 120–139 mmHg and diastolic BP 80–99 mmHg. Lifestyle modification includes nutrition approaches, exercise, and weight management which will be discussed later in the chapter [29].

Goals of Therapy in HPL to Prevent Stroke

The primary goal of therapy for HPL in order to prevent stroke is to reduce blood lipids to within a normal range. The two most effective ways to reduce blood lipids, which is endorsed by the ASA's guidelines, is to treat with a statin and promote lifestyle changes to reduce LDL cholesterol based on the National Cholesterol Education Program (NCEP) guidelines for primary prevention of ischemic stroke for patients with coronary heart disease or diabetes. There is strong evidence to support that statins can reduce risk of stroke. For example, one meta-analysis of 26 trials including >90,000 patients showed that statins reduced risk of all strokes by

Table 6.1
Nutrient composition of the therapeutic lifestyle changes (TLC) diet [9]

Nutrient	Recommended intake
Saturated fat[a]	<7 % of total calories
Polyunsaturated fat	Up to 10 % of total calories
Monounsaturated fat	Up to 20 % of total calories
Total fat	25–35 % of total calories
Carbohydrate[b]	50–60 % of total calories
Fiber	20–30 g/day
Protein	Approximately 15 % of total calories
Cholesterol	<200 mg/day
Total calories[c]	Balance energy intake and expenditure to maintain desirable body weight/prevent weight gain

[a]*Trans* fatty acids are another LDL-raising fat should be kept at a low intake
[b]Carbohydrates should be derived predominately from foods rich in complex carbohydrates including grains, especially whole grains, fruits, and vegetables
[c]Daily energy expenditure should include at least moderate physical activity (contributing approximately 200 kcal/day)

21 %. Risk of all strokes was estimated to decrease by 15.6 % for every 10 % reduction in LDL [30]. Further discussion of pharmacological strategies to reduce stroke will be presented in a later chapter (*see* Chap. 17).

The NCEP guidelines recommend therapeutic lifestyle changes to reduce LDL cholesterol. Therapeutic lifestyle changes include diet, weight reduction, and increased physical activity. See Table 6.1 for complete breakdown of recommended macronutrient and micronutrient needs of the Therapeutic Lifestyle Changes Diet [9].

One additional treatment option in the management of HPL to prevent stroke involves another B vitamin, niacin (also known as nicotinic acid). Not only does niacin increases HDL cholesterol, but it can decrease LDL cholesterol and triglycerides [9]. The ASA opinion on niacin therapy is that it is an option for patients with low HDL cholesterol; however, there is not enough evidence to support its effect on preventing ischemic stroke. Niacin is available in prescription form and as a dietary supplement. The ASA does not recommend the dietary supplement form of niacin to treat HPL because of its risk of serious side effects and because dietary supplements are not regulated by the United States Food and Drug Administration [31].

Goals of Therapy in Hyperhomocysteinemia to Prevent Stroke

The goal of therapy in hyperhomocysteinemia is to reduce homocysteine to within normal limits of 5–15 µmol/L. Research shows that a 20–25 % relative reduction in homocysteine levels or 2.5–3.0 µmol/L reduction is correlated with a significant decrease in cardiovascular events [13]. The most studied treatment to lower

Table 6.2
RDA and tolerable upper limits for folate, cyanocobalamin, and pyridoxine [32]

Vitamin	Recommended daily allowance (µg)	Tolerable upper limit (µg)
Folate	400	1,000
Cyanocobalamin	2.4	No data to support
Pyridoxine	1,300 (ages 19–50)	1,000
	1,500 (females > 51 years old)	100,000
	1,700 (males >51 years old)	

homocysteine is through the use of B vitamins. The ASA's position on B vitamin therapy is that B vitamins may be considered, but additional studies are needed. Regardless of whether or not B vitamins will benefit or not, it is practical to first test for folate, cyanocobalamin, and pyridoxine deficiencies. If someone is deficient, then supplementation with at least recommended daily allowance (RDA) of each vitamin is warranted. See Table 6.2 for the RDA of certain B vitamins. There is no tolerable upper limit for cyanocobalamin because there is lack of data on adverse effects [32].

Nutrition and Stroke

There are challenges and opportunities when it comes to following a healthy, balanced diet to prevent stroke. It can be a challenge as there are a number of components to monitor: sodium, potassium, fat, cholesterol, alcohol, and weight. When nutrient rich, balanced meals are chosen, it will be easy to consume adequate intakes of sodium, potassium, fat, cholesterol, and alcohol in order to maintain a healthy weight.

Sodium and potassium are both minerals and also known as electrolytes, a substance that conducts electricity in the body. Other electrolytes include chloride, calcium, and magnesium. Sodium is responsible for maintaining fluid balance both in the blood and around cells, transmitting nerve impulses, and allowing muscles to work properly. Potassium is necessary to regulate heartbeat and allow muscle function. The kidneys are responsible for maintaining electrolyte balance by conserving or excreting electrolytes accordingly. Since sodium attracts fluid to maintain fluid balance, excess dietary sodium intake will increase blood volume [13]. Research has shown that low blood potassium causes sodium chloride retention. Increased blood volume puts stress on the heart to circulate more blood through blood vessels, which increases pressure in the arteries, therefore increasing blood pressure. A combination of excess sodium and inadequate potassium in the diet is a contributing factor of hypertension [13].

Another dietary component to monitor to prevent stroke is fat and cholesterol. As was mentioned earlier, hyperlipidemia can lead to atherosclerosis which is associated with increased risk of stroke; therefore, limiting total fat and cholesterol intake in the diet is crucial. Excess alcohol consumption is a risk factor for all types of stroke [33–35]. The ASA summarizes that light to moderate consumption of alcohol, mostly from wine, may reduce the risk of stroke.

The prevalence of overweight and obesity is associated with increased risk of stroke. One meta-analysis found that for subjects with body mass index (BMI) from 25 to 50 kg/m², each 5 kg/m² increase in BMI was associated with a 40 % increased risk of stroke mortality [36]. There is no research documenting the effect of weight loss on stroke outcome; however, weight loss is associated with lowering BP.

Nutrition to Prevent Stroke

The ASA's recommendation to prevent stroke through diet and nutrition is to follow the *Dietary Guidelines for Americans* (DGA) and a DASH style diet. The 2010 DGA recommends consuming less than 2,300 mg of sodium for adults ages 18–50. The recommendation decreases to less than or equal to 1,500 mg for adults 51 and older and adults of any age who are African American or have HTN, DM, or CKD. Unfortunately, on average Americans consume 3,400 mg per day according to the 2010 DGA. Americans consume sodium in their diet through table salt and processed foods. Salt is used as preservative in processed foods in order to retain moisture, improve flavor, and maintain the shelf life of the food. According to NHANES 2005–2006, the highest sources of sodium in the American diet, respectively, were yeast breads (7.3 %), chicken and chicken mixed dishes (6.8 %), pizza (6.3 %), pasta and pasta dishes (5.1 %), cold cuts (4.5 %), condiments (4.4 %), tortillas, burritos, tacos (4.1 %), sausage, hotdogs, bacon, ribs (4.1 %), and regular cheese (3.5 %) [37].

The 2010 DGA emphasizes the importance of consuming an adequate intake of potassium daily in order to prevent retention of sodium and potential for elevated blood pressure. Potassium is one of the nutrients that is under consumed in the USA, likely because it is most abundant in fruits, vegetables, and milk, which most Americans do not eat enough of. The adequate intake (AI) for potassium is 4.7 g per day for adults. Consuming at least four servings of fruits, four servings of vegetables, and 2 or 3 servings of milk or yogurt per day would meet the recommended 4.7 g per day [37].

Fat and cholesterol recommendations are also listed in the 2010 DGA. The DGA follows the Institute of Medicine's (IOM) recommendation of 20–35 % of total calories from fat which is fairly consistent with ASA's recommendation for LDL cholesterol lowering based on NCEP recommendation of 25–35 % of total calories from fat. Both the ASA and 2010 DGA recommend moderate alcohol consumption defined as up to 1 drink per day for women and up to 2 drinks for men [1, 37].

The DASH trial was a study done by the National Institutes of Health to assess the impact of certain nutrients and foods on hypertension. In the first study, subjects were adults with systolic blood pressure less than 160 mmHg and diastolic pressures of 80–95 mmHg. Of these subjects, 27 % had HTN. The study compared three eating plans: (1) similar to the typical American diet with about 3,000 mg sodium, (2) similar to the typical American diet plus extra fruits and vegetables with about 3,000 mg sodium, and (3) the DASH eating plan. The DASH eating plan consisted of 55 % of calories from carbohydrate, 18 % from protein, 27 % from total fat, 6 % of saturated fat, 150 mg cholesterol, 2,300 mg sodium, 4,700 mg potassium, 1,250 mg calcium, 500 mg magnesium, and 30 g of fiber [38]. Subjects in both the second group and the DASH group had lower blood pressure. The DASH group had the greatest effect on lowering blood pressure, especially subjects with high blood pressure.

The second DASH study compared diets effect on blood pressure with a greater sodium restriction [39]. The subjects either followed the typical American diet or the DASH eating plan. Subjects on either diet were randomized to consume either 3,300 mg, 2,300 mg, or 1,500 mg of sodium per day. A decrease in sodium intake was associated with lower blood pressure for both diets; however, blood pressure was lower for subjects on the DASH diet at each sodium level. The 1,500 mg sodium DASH group had the greatest decrease in blood pressure. From this research, the DASH diet was created [39].

The DASH diet is endorsed by the National Heart, Lung, and Blood Institute; AHA; and the 2010 DGA. Regardless of the risk factors for stroke, the DASH diet is a balanced meal plan that helps lower blood pressure and cholesterol and is associated with lower risk of certain types of cancer, heart disease, stroke, heart failure, kidney stones, and type 2 diabetes [40]. The DASH diet is broken down in to serving sizes of each of the food groups. The number of serving sizes varies according to your recommended calories per day. See Table 6.3 for recommendations based on 2,000 calories per day [41].

Physical Activity and Stroke

Physical inactivity is a modifiable risk factor associated with stroke. The benefits of physical activity are numerous and outweigh the negative outcomes. Regular physical activity reduces the risk of premature death, heart disease, stroke, high blood pressure, and type 2 diabetes; lowers blood pressure and blood lipids; and helps people maintain a healthy weight [42]. The 2008 Physical Activity Guidelines for Americans (PAGA) reports that physically active men and women have a 25–30 % lower risk of stroke or death compared to physically inactive people [42]. Physical activity's positive effect on lowering blood pressure and blood lipids as well as helping people manage their weight contributes to managing other risk factors in order to prevent stroke [43–45].

The 2008 PAGA defines physical activity as bodily movement that enhances health [42]. Types of physical activity include aerobic, muscle strengthening, and bone strengthening. Aerobic activity is defined as moving the body's large muscles in consistent manner for continued duration of time [42]. Examples of aerobic

Table 6.3
2,000 cal DASH eating plan [41]

Food group	Daily servings	Serving sizes	Examples and notes	Significance of each food group to DASH eating pattern
Grains[a]	6–8	1 slice bread 1 oz dry cereal[b] ½ cup cooked rice, pasta, or cereal	Whole wheat bread, rolls, pasta, bagel, cereal, oatmeal, brown rice	Major sources of energy and fiber
Vegetables	4–5	1 cup raw leafy vegetable ½ cup cut-up raw or cooked vegetable ½ cup vegetable juice	Broccoli, carrots, collards, green beans, green peas, kale, potatoes, tomatoes	Rich sources of potassium, magnesium, and fiber
Fruit	4–5	1 medium fruit ¼ cup dried fruit ½ cup fresh, frozen, or canned fruit ½ cup fruit juice	Apples, raisins, apricots, bananas, dates, grapes, melons, peaches, pears	Important sources of potassium, magnesium, and fiber
Fat-free or low-fat milk and milk products	2–3	1 cup milk or yogurt 1 ½oz cheese	Fat-free (skim) or low-fat (1 %) milk, cheese, yogurt, or frozen yogurt	Major sources of calcium and protein
Lean meats, poultry, and fish	6 or less	1 oz cooked meats, poultry, or fish 1 egg[c]	Select only lean; trim away visible fats; broil, roast, or poach; remove skin from poultry	Rich sources of protein and magnesium
Nuts, seeds, and legumes	4–5 per week	1/3 or 1½oz nuts 2 Tbsp peanut butter 2 Tbsp or ½oz seeds ½ cup cooked legumes (dry beans and peas)	Almonds, hazelnuts, peanuts, walnuts, sunflower seeds, kidney beans, lentils, split peas	Rich sources of energy, magnesium, protein, and fiber
Fats and oils[d]	2–3	1 tsp soft margarine 1 tsp vegetable oil 1 Tbsp mayonnaise 2 Tbsp salad dressing	Soft margarine, vegetable oil, low-fat mayonnaise, light salad dressing	The DASH study had 27 % of calories as fat, including fat in or added to foods
Sweets and added sugars	5 or less per week	1 Tbsp sugar 1 Tbsp jelly or jam ½ cup sorbet, gelatin 1 cup lemonade	Fruit-flavored gelatin, fruit punch, hard candy, jelly, maple syrup	Sweets should be low in fat

[a]Whole grains are recommended for most grain servings as a good source of fiber and nutrients

[b]Serving sizes vary between ½ cup and 1¼ cups, depending on cereal type. Check the product's Nutrition Facts label

[c]Since eggs are high in cholesterol, limit egg yolk intake to no more than four per week; two egg whites have the same amount of protein content as 1 oz of meat

[d]Fat content changes serving amount for fats and oils. For example, 1 tbsp of regular salad dressing equals 1 serving; 1 tbsp of a low-fat dressing equals one-half serving; 1 tbsp of a fat-free dressing equals zero servings

activity are brisk walking, running, bicycling, jumping rope, and swimming. Muscle strengthening activity includes resistance training and lifting weights. Muscle strengthening using weights, resistance bands, or body weight should incorporate a variety of muscle groups. Bone strengthening activity is also referred to as weight-bearing exercise because it causes a force on bones that supports bone growth and strength. Examples of bone strengthening are jumping jacks, running, brisk walking, and weight lifting [42].

The benefits of physical activity start with as little as 60 min of activity per week; however, research proves that 150 min of moderate intensity aerobic activity per week reduces the risk of chronic diseases. The 2008 PAGA recommends 150 min per week of moderate intensity physical activity or 75 min of vigorous intensity activity per week to support some overall health benefit [42]. When physical activity increases to 150–300 min of moderate intensity physical exercise per week or 75–150 min of vigorous intensity exercise per week, there is a more substantial overall health benefit [42].

The ASA's position on physical inactivity is to increase physical activity because of its correlation with decrease of stroke risk. The ASA also endorses the 2008 PAGA recommendations of at least 150 min of moderate intensity exercise per week or 75 min of vigorous intensity exercise per week [1].

Conclusion

Following a healthy balanced diet and engaging in physical activity over a lifetime are effective ways to prevent risk factors associated with stroke and stroke itself. A healthy diet and physical activity promote a strong cardiovascular system which allows blood to pump efficiently throughout the body in order to transfer nutrients to vital organs. The DASH diet plan is an excellent reference to guide a healthy, balanced diet. The 2008 PAGA offers recommendations on why and how to start exercising for persons of any age. Incorporating healthy eating and exercise habits at any age is a critical component to preventing stroke.

References

1. Guidelines for the Primary Prevention of Stroke: A Guideline for Healthcare Professionals From the American Heart Association/American Stroke Association. Stroke. 2011; 42:517–84.
2. Chiuve SE, Rexrode KM, Spiegelman D, Logroscino G, Manson JE, Rimm EB. Primary prevention of stroke by healthy lifestyle. Circulation. 2008;118:947–54.
3. Appel LJ, Brands MW, Daniels SR, Karanja N, Elmer PJ, Sacks FM. Dietary approaches to prevent and treat hypertension: a scientific statement from the American Heart Association. Hypertension. 2006;47:296–308.
4. Cutler JA, Sorlie PD, Wolz M, Thom T, Fields LE, Roccella EJ. Trends in hypertension prevalence, awareness, treatment, and control rates in United States adults between 1988–1994 and 1999–2004. Hypertension. 2008;52:818–27.

5. Baskin ML, Ard J, Franklin F, Allison DB. Prevalence of obesity in the United States. Obes Rev. 2005;6:5–7.
6. Lewington S, Clarke R, Qizilbash N, Peto R, Collins R. Age-specific relevance of usual blood pressure to vascular mortality: a meta-analysis of individual data for one million adults in 61 prospective studies. Lancet. 2002;360:1903–13.
7. Black HR, Elliott WJ, Neaton JD, Grandits G, Grambsch P, Grimm Jr RH, et al. Baseline characteristics and early blood pressure control in the CONVINCE Trial. Hypertension. 2001;37:12–8.
8. Cushman WC, Ford CE, Cutler JA, Margolis KL, Davis BR, Grimm RH, et al. Success and predictors of blood pressure control in diverse North American settings: the antihypertensive and lipid-lowering treatment to prevent heart attack trial (ALLHAT). J Clin Hypertens (Greenwich). 2002;4:393–404.
9. Grundy SM, Becker D, Clark LT, Cooper RS, Denke MA, Howard J, et al. Executive summary of the third report of the National Cholesterol Education Program (NCEP) expert panel on detection, evaluation, and treatment of high blood cholesterol in adults (adult treatment panel III). JAMA. 2001;285:2486–97.
10. Roger VL, Go AS, Lloyd-Jones DM, Adams RJ, Berry JD, Brown TM, et al. Executive summary: heart disease and stroke statistics-2011 update: a report from the American Heart Association. Circulation. 2001;123:459–63.
11. Sanossian N, Saver JL, Navab M, Ovbiagele B. High-density lipoprotein cholesterol: an emerging target for stroke treatment. Stroke. 2007;38:1104–9.
12. Lindenstrom E, Boysen G, Nyboe J. Influence of total cholesterol, high density lipoprotein cholesterol, and triglycerides on risk of cerebrovascular disease: the Copenhagen City Heart Study. BMJ. 1994;309:11–5.
13. Up to Date [Internet]. Waltham (MA):Rosenson RS, Kang DS. [cited 2011 Nov 29]. Available from: http://www.uptodate.com
14. Francescone S, Halperin JL. "Triple therapy" or triple threat? Balancing the risks of antithrombotic therapy for patients with atrial fibrillation and coronary stents. J Am Coll Cardiol. 2008;51:826–7.
15. Rubboli A, Halperin JL, Juhani Airaksinen KE, Buerke M, Eeckhout E, Freedman SB, et al. Antithrombotic therapy in patients treated with oral anticoagulation undergoing coronary artery stenting: an expert consensus document with focus on atrial fibrillation. Ann Med. 2008;40:428–36.
16. King 3rd SB, Smith Jr SC, Hirshfeld Jr JW, Jacobs AK, Morrison DA, Williams DO, et al. 2007 focused update of the ACC/AHA/SCAI 2005 guideline update for percutaneous coronary intervention: a report of the American College of Cardiology/American Heart Association Task Force on Practice Guidelines. J Am Coll Cardiol. 2008;51:172–209.
17. Doufekias E, Segal AZ, Kizer JR. Cardiogenic and aortogenic brain embolism. J Am Coll Cardiol. 2008;51:1049–59.
18. Pinto A, Tuttolomondo A, Di Raimondo D, Fernandez P, Licata G. Risk factors profile and clinical outcome of ischemic stroke patients admitted in a Department of Internal Medicine and classified by TOAST classification. Int Angiol. 2006;25:261–7.
19. Arboix A, Oliveres M, Massons J, Pujades R, Garcia-Eroles L. Early differentiation of cardioembolic from atherothrombotic cerebral infarction: a multivariate analysis. Eur J Neurol. 1999;6:677–83.
20. Clarke R, Collins R, Lewington S, Donald A, Alfthan G, Tomilehto J, et al. Homocysteine and risk of ischemic heart disease and stroke: a metaanalysis. JAMA. 2002;288:2015–2022.
21. Wald DS, Law M, Morris JK. Homocysteine and cardiovascular disease: evidence on causality from a meta-analysis. BMJ. 2002;325:1202.
22. Al-Delaimy WK, Rexrode KM, Hu FB, Albert CM, Stampfer MJ, Willett WC, et al. Folate intake and risk of stroke among women. Stroke. 2004;35:1259–63.
23. He K, Merchant A, Rimm EB, Rosner BA, Stampfer MJ, Willett WC, et al. Folate, vitamin B6, and B12 intakes in relation to risk of stroke among men. Stroke. 2004;35:169–74.

24. Van Guelpen B, Hultdin J, Johansson I, Stegmayr B, Hallmans G, Nilsson TK, et al. Folate, vitamin B12, and risk of ischemic and hemorrhagic stroke: a prospective, nested case-referent study of plasma concentrations and dietary intake. Stroke. 2005;36:1426–31.
25. Weng LC, Yeh WT, Bai CH, Chen HJ, Chuang SY, Chang HY, et al. Is ischemic stroke risk related to folate status or other nutrients correlated with folate intake? Stroke. 2008;39: 3152–8.
26. Lonn E, Yusuf S, Arnold MJ, Sheridan P, Pogue J, Micks M, et al. Homocysteine lowering with folic acid and B vitamins in vascular disease. N Engl J Med. 2006;354:1567–77.
27. Wang X, Qin X, Demirtas H, Li J, Mao G, Huo Y, et al. Efficacy of folic acid supplementation in stroke prevention: a meta-analysis. Lancet. 2007;369:1876–82.
28. Lee M, Hong KS, Chang SC, Saver LJ. Efficiency of homocysteine-lowering therapy with folic acid in stroke prevention: a meta-analysis. Stroke. 2010;41:1205–12.
29. Chobanian AV, Bakris GL, Black HR, Cushman WC, Green LA, Izzo Jr JL, et al. The Seventh Report of the Joint National Committee on Prevention, Detection, Evaluation, and Treatment of High Blood Pressure: the JNC 7 report. JAMA. 2003;289:2560–72.
30. Amarenco P, Labreuche J, Lavallee P, Touboul PJ. Statins in stroke prevention and carotid atherosclerosis: systematic review and up-to-date meta-analysis. Stroke. 2004;35:2902–9.
31. American Heart Association/American Stroke Association [Internet]. Dallas; c2012 [updated 2012 Jun 14; cited 2012 Jul 5]. Available from http://www.heart.org/HEARTORG/Conditions/Cholesterol/PreventionTreatmentofHighCholesterol/Drug-Therapy-for-Cholesterol_UCM_305632_Article.jsp
32. Food and Nutrition Information Center. National Agricultural Library. United States Department of Agriculture. Dietary Reference Intakes (DRIs): Recommended dietary allowances and adequate intakes, vitamins. Food and Nutrition Board, Institute of Medicine, National Academies. 2010. Available from: http://fnic.nal.usda.gov
33. Gill JS, Zezulka AV, Shipley MJ, Gill SK, Beevers DG. Stroke and alcohol consumption. N Engl J Med. 1986;315:1041–6.
34. Hillbom M, Numminen H, Juvela S. Recent heavy drinking of alcohol and embolic stroke. Stroke. 1999;30:2307–12.
35. Klatsky AL, Armstrong MA, Friedman GD, Sidney S. Alcohol drinking and risk of hospitalization for ischemic stroke. Am J Cardiol. 2001;88:703–6.
36. Whitlock G, Lewington S, Sherliker P, Clarke R, Emberson J, Halsey J, et al. Body-mass index and cause-specific mortality in 900,000 adults: collaborative analyses of 57 prospective studies. Lancet. 2009;373:1083–96.
37. U.S. Department of Agriculture and U.S. Department of Health and Human Services. Dietary Guidelines for Americans. 7th ed. Washington, DC: U.S. Government Printing Office; 2010.
38. Appel LJ, Moore TJ, Obarzanek E, Vollmer WM, Svetkey LP, Sacks FM, et al. A clinical trial of the effects of dietary patterns on blood pressure. DASH Collaborative Research Group. N Engl J Med. 1997;336:1117–24.
39. Svetkey LP, Sacks FM, Obarzanek E, Vollmer WM, Appel LJ, Lin PH, et al. The DASH Diet, Sodium Intake and Blood Pressure Trial (DASH-sodium): Rationale and design. J AM Diet Assoc. 1999;99(suppl):S96–S104.
40. Heller M. The DASH diet action plan. Northbrook: Grand Central; 2004.
41. U.S. Department of Health and Human Services. National Institutes of Health. National Heart, Lung, and Blood Institute. Your guide to lowering your blood pressure with DASH. 2006
42. Physical Activity Guidelines Advisory Committee Report, 2008. Washington, DC: US Department of Health and Human Services; 2008. Available at: http://www.health.gov/paguidelines/. Accessed 14 Aug 2010.
43. Manson JE, Colditz GA, Stampfer MJ, Willett WC, Krolewski AS, Rosner B, et al. A prospective study of maturity-onset diabetes mellitus and risk of coronary heart disease and stroke in women. Arch Intern Med. 1991;151:1141–7.

44. Blair SN, Kampert JB, Kohl 3rd HW, Barlow CE, Macera CA, Paffenbarger Jr RS, et al. Influences of cardiorespiratory fitness and other precursors on cardiovascular disease and all-cause mortality in men and women. JAMA. 1996;276:205–10.
45. Kokkinos PF, Holland JC, Pittaras AE, Narayan P, Dotson CO, Papademetriou V. Cardiorespiratory fitness and coronary heart disease risk factor association in women. J Am Coll Cardiol. 1995;26:358–64.

Chapter 7
Obesity and Stroke

Omer J. Deen, Sulieman Abdal Raheem, and Donald F. Kirby

Key Points

- Understand the detrimental effect of obesity prevalence in the USA.
- Identify obesity as a risk factor for stroke due to its exacerbation of hypertension, dyslipidemia, insulin resistance, and the metabolic syndrome.
- Understand how lowering the risk for obesity correlates with a lower risk for stroke.

Keywords Stroke • Obesity • Adipose • Body mass index • Nutrition • Metabolic syndrome • Hypertension • Hypercholesterolemia

Abbreviations

BMI	Body Mass Index
CDC	Centers for Disease Control and Prevention
CRP	C-Reactive Protein
HDL	High Density Lipoprotein
LDL	Low Density Lipoprotein
RACE	Receptor for Advanced Glycation End Product
TNF	Tumor Necrosis Factor

O.J. Deen, M.D. • S.A. Raheem, M.D.
Center for Human Nutrition, Digestive Disease Institute, Cleveland Clinic,
9500 Euclid Avenue/A51, Cleveland, OH 44195, USA

D.F. Kirby, M.D., F.A.C.P., F.A.C.N., F.A.C.G., A.G.A.F., C.N.S.C., C.P.N.S.
Center for Human Nutrition, Department of Gastroenterology, Cleveland Clinic,
9500 Euclid Avenue/A51, Cleveland, OH 44195, USA

M.L. Corrigan et al. (eds.), *Handbook of Clinical Nutrition and Stroke*,
Nutrition and Health, DOI 10.1007/978-1-62703-380-0_7,
© Springer Science+Business Media New York 2013

Introduction

The condition of obesity encompasses several known risk factors for stroke and can therefore increase stroke risk. Treatment of obesity can help to alleviate these individual risk factors. This chapter will discuss these risk factors and their individual contribution to an overall increased risk for stroke as well as their combined detriment in obese individuals.

Background

According to the Centers for Disease Control and Prevention (CDC), the terms "obese" and "overweight" not only signify weight beyond what is considered normal but also weight which significantly increases the likelihood of a specific set of diseases and conditions which, in turn, radically raise the incidence of stroke. In essence, excess weight or "obesity" puts patients at considerable risk for stroke, making its management crucial for decreasing morbidity and increasing quality of life (Fig. 7.1).

Defining Obesity

Is internationally the most common and reliable quantifier of a person's weight and, in effect, obesity. This index, also known as the Quetelet index, was developed by Belgium statistician Adolphe Quetelet (1796–1874) [1]. BMI is simply calculated from a person's height and weight. For example, a person whose height measures as

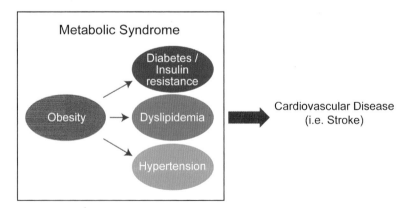

Fig. 7.1 Obesity leads to an increase in the individual risk factors which contribute to cardiovascular disease

BMI (kg/m²)	Weight Class
<18.5	Underweight
18.5-24.9	Normal
25.0-29.9	Overweight
30.0-39.9	Obese
40.0 and higher	Morbidly Obese

Fig. 7.2 Weight-based classification of corresponding BMI values

1.83 m tall and whose weight measures as 81.65 kg will calculate to have a BMI of 24.4 kg/m²:

$$BMI\ (kg/m^2) = Weight\ (kg)/Height^2\ (m^2)$$

Therefore, $24.4 = 81.65/(1.83)^2$.

With the advent of mobile applications on handheld devices, a BMI is readily accessible to patients and healthcare providers as they can simply input height and weight into a BMI calculator. Additionally, most electronic medical record software is able to calculate BMI automatically once height and weight are entered into the vital signs section.

There are other methods for quantifying weight and obesity, such as evaluating skinfold thickness, calculation of waist-to-hip circumference ratios, and other techniques such as ultrasound, computed tomography, and magnetic resonance imaging (MRI). However, BMI remains the most accessible and reliable measure for diagnosing obesity. It is generally accepted that (Fig. 7.2):

- An adult with a BMI of 25–29.9 kg/m² is overweight.
- An adult with a BMI of 30 kg/m² or higher is obese.
- An adult with a BMI of 40 kg/m² or higher is "morbidly obese."

Distribution of Adipose (Fat) Tissue

An evaluation of the adipose (fat) tissue's distribution further refines the BMI's ability to quantify weight and fat. Specifically, central adiposity (abdominal obesity) is associated with an increased risk of the obesity-related diseases and conditions (i.e., diabetes, hypertension, dyslipidemia). For these reasons, an assessment of abdominal obesity by means of waist circumference should be taken into account in addition to BMI. Unfortunately, this is not done as often as it should be in clinical practice.

Waist circumference is measured by placing a tape measure around the waist at the level of the iliac crest (Fig. 7.3). In adults with a BMI of 25–34.9 kg/m², a waist circumference greater than 102 cm (40 in.) for men and 88 cm (35 in.) for women

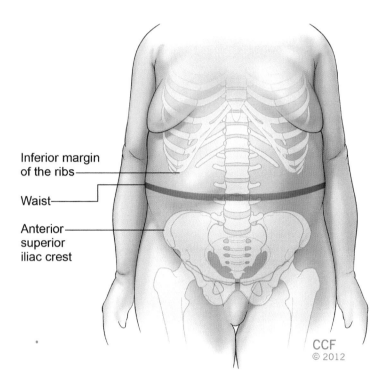

Fig. 7.3 Diagram illustrating appropriate location for waist circumference measurement. (Reprinted with permission, Cleveland Clinic Center for Medical Art & Photography ©2012. All Rights Reserved)

leads to increased risk of hypertension, type 2 diabetes, dyslipidemia, metabolic syndrome, and coronary heart disease [2]. However, in patients with a BMI greater than 35 kg/m², waist circumference measurement is less helpful as it adds little to the predictive power of the disease risk classification of BMI; almost all individuals within this BMI class also have an abnormal waist circumference.

Metabolic Syndrome

Metabolic syndrome is a term used to cluster several characteristics together which in combination and/or individually act as metabolic risk factors for type 2 diabetes, heart disease, and stroke. Three of these characteristics are necessary for a diagnosis of metabolic syndrome. These characteristics include the following

– Obesity: specifically *abdominal obesity* (defined as a waist size >94–102 cm (38–41 in.) in men or >80 cm (32 in.) in women).

- Hyperglycemia or *impaired fasting glucose* (fasting blood sugar of 100–125 mg/dL or 5.6–7 mmol/L).
- Hypertension (130/85 or higher or if you take medicine for high blood pressure).
- Hypercholesterolemia: increased fasting levels of triglycerides (>150–180 mg/dL or 1.7 mmol/L) or decreased fasting HDL cholesterol (<40 mg/dL or 1 mmol/L for men or 50 mg/dL or 1.3 mmol/L for women) or if you take medicine for high triglycerides or low HDL cholesterol.

Prevalence of Obesity

The CDC reports one-third of US adults (35.7 %) as obese and consequently, in 2008, the medical costs associated with this obesity were estimated at $147 billion [3] (Fig. 7.4). Of these adults, 5.7 % are considered "morbidly obese."

The obese population is at a higher risk for many diseases and consequently stroke. Prevalence of obesity does in fact vary with ethnicity and socioeconomic status, with non-Hispanic blacks of low socioeconomic status measuring as the most obese (Fig. 7.5). Among women specifically, increased education decreases obesity prevalence.

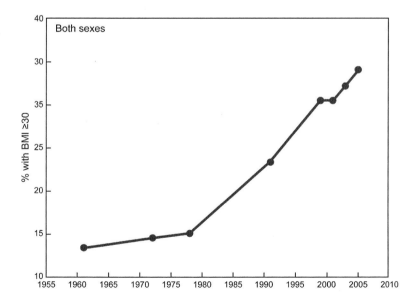

Fig. 7.4 Percentage of the population with a BMI of 30 or greater as followed over time

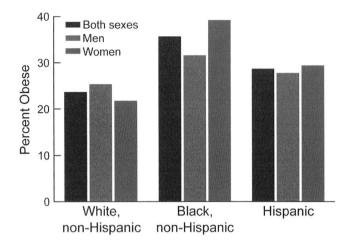

Fig. 7.5 Percent obese based on gender and ethnicity

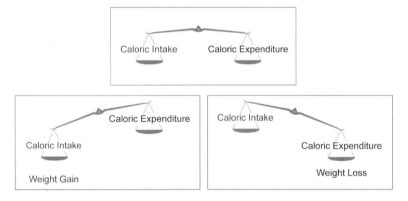

Fig. 7.6 Effect of imbalance between caloric intake and expenditure

Causes of Obesity

A myriad of factors contribute to obesity: behavior, environment, genetic factors, and certain illnesses. Behaviorally, the most relevant consideration when studying obesity is the energy imbalance occurring from caloric intake exceeding caloric expenditure resulting in weight gain. To maintain a given weight, calories expended in body functions and physical activity must match, or equal, the calories consumed in food and drink (Fig. 7.6). Any deviation results in weight loss or gain. Environment also plays a significant role in this balance of calories and thus obesity. Sedentary occupations, lack of opportunities at home for physical activity, and food choices available are all environmental factors modulating the behaviors which lead to obesity and obesity-related disease.

Genes can directly cause obesity in some disorders (i.e., Bardet-Biedl syndrome, Prader-Willi syndrome) or they may increase one's susceptibility for obesity. In the latter case, other factors from among those previously mentioned such as a caloric imbalance or poor food choice availability would be required to cause weight gain and obesity. Additionally, certain diseases and/or their medications may lead to obesity as well. For example, people suffering from hypothyroidism or others on oral steroids may gain considerable weight. Clearly, the etiology of obesity is complex and requires thorough evaluation for maintaining a healthy weight.

Obesity-Related Diseases and Conditions

Obesity and Type 2 Diabetes

The Cardiovascular Health Study (CHS), funded by the National Heart Lung and Blood Institute, demonstrated clearly that among middle- to late-aged adults, weight gain is associated with increased risk of type 2 diabetes [4]. In this prospective cohort study (1989–2007) of 4,193 men and women 65 years of age and older, measures of obesity or body adipose (fat) content were extrapolated from anthropometry and bioelectrical impedance data at baseline; anthropometry was repeated 3 years later. An outcome of incident diabetes was diagnosed by either the use of antidiabetic medication or fasting glucose levels of 126 mg/dL or greater. Participants with a greater than 10 cm increase in waist size from baseline to the third year follow-up visit were almost twice as likely to develop type 2 diabetes compared with those who gained or lost 2 cm or less.

Furthermore, a prospective (1980–2000) cohort evaluation from the Nurses' Health Study demonstrated that weight gain (and therefore, obesity) is particularly detrimental for Asians [5]. This study concluded that "the inverse association of a healthy diet with diabetes is stronger for minorities than for whites." Detailed dietary and lifestyle information for each one of the 78,419 apparently healthy female participants (75,584 whites, 801 Asians, 613 Hispanics, and 1,421 blacks) was collected every 4 years. Over 20 years, 3,844 incident cases of diabetes were documented from among this population. For each 5-unit increase in BMI, the multivariate relative risk of diabetes was 2.36 (1.83–3.04) for Asians, 2.21 (1.75–2.79) for Hispanics, 1.96 (1.93–2.00) for whites, and 1.55 (1.36–1.77) for blacks (P for interaction <0.001). Therefore, weight gain had the most detrimental effect on the Asians when considering diabetes incidence.

Obesity increases type 2 diabetes susceptibility by increasing insulin resistance. In insulin resistance, the body produces insulin, a pancreatic hormone enabling glucose utilization for energy, but does not use it properly. Thus excess glucose builds up in the bloodstream, setting the stage for diabetes. Many studies have now elucidated the mechanism for obesity's effect on insulin resistance. Adipose (fat) tissue releases increased amounts of interleukin-6 (IL-6), tumor necrosis factor-alpha

(TNF-α) [6], and C-reactive protein (CRP) [7] leading to a low level, chronic inflammatory state which further causes insulin resistance [8]. These cytokines are potentially responsible for the metabolic, hemodynamic, and hemostatic abnormalities that cluster with insulin resistance. Specifically, TNF-α and IL-6 [9, 10] inhibit the action of lipoprotein lipase [11] and stimulate lipolysis [12]. Additionally, TNF-α impairs the function of the insulin signaling pathway by effects on phosphorylation of both the insulin receptor and its substrate, IRS-1 [13, 14]. Therefore, maintaining a healthy weight and minimizing abdominal obesity becomes crucial in diabetes prevention [5].

Obesity and Dyslipidemia

Obesity may also lead to dyslipidemia, characterized by increased triglycerides, decreased high-density lipoproteins (HDL) levels, abnormal low-density lipoprotein (LDL) composition, and subsequently a low HDL–LDL ratio. An HDL–LDL of 0.3 is considered healthy, and a ratio of 0.4 ideal. A higher ratio, due to increased HDL, is desirable as this is "good cholesterol" which lowers blood cholesterol by returning it to the liver. Evaluation of the second National Health and Nutrition Educational Survey (NHANES II) data shows the increasing triglyceride levels and increasing prevalence of dyslipidemia with increasing weight and obesity class: 8.9 % for normal weight versus 19.0 % for morbidly obese (BMI over 40 kg/m^2) [15].

Secondly, while total triglyceride levels rise in obesity, HDL or "good cholesterol" levels are depressed. This depression in HDL–LDL furthers dyslipidemia. NHANES II data demonstrated a difference of 10 mg/dL in HDL between normal weight and obese men and an even greater decrease in HDL for obese women (Fig. 7.7) [16].

Obesity and Hypertension

Among the numerous other studies, the Framingham Heart study has clearly demonstrated that the age-adjusted relative risk (RR) for new hypertension was highly associated with overweight status (men: RR, 1.46; women: RR, 1.75); overweight status was defined by a BMI> or =25 with a referent group of normal-weight persons (BMI, 18.5–24.9) [17]. In other words, an elevated BMI greatly increases the risk for hypertension; for example, overweight men are at 1.46 times the risk than their normal-weight counterparts. A study of 82,473 US female nurses further corroborates these findings [18]. These female nurses aged 30–55 years old were evaluated every 2 years; specifically BMI, weight changes and incident cases of hypertension were monitored. After adjusting for variables, long-term weight gain dramatically increased the risk for hypertension. Specifically, a weight gain of

Lipoprotein Production And Interdependence

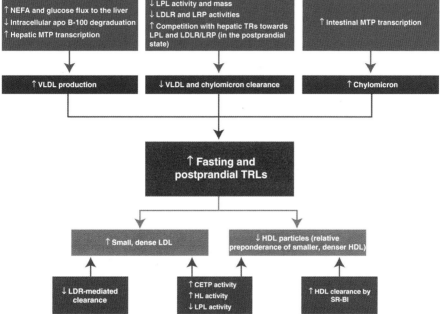

Fig. 7.7 *NEFA* nonesterified fatty acids, *LDLR* low-density lipoprotein receptors, *TRLs* triglyceride-rich lipoproteins, *LPL* lipoprotein lipase, *MTP* microsomal triglyceride transfer proteins, *VLDL* very low-density lipoproteins, *CETP* cholesteryl ester transfer protein, and *HL* hepatic lipase

5.0–9.9 kg puts the nurses at 1.74 times the risk and a weight gain of greater than 25 kg puts the nurses at 5.21 times the risk for developing hypertension. Additionally, weight loss decreased risk for hypertension; nurses with 5.0–9.9 kg weight loss decreased their risk by 15 %, and nurses with greater than 10 kg weight loss decreased their risk by 26 % for hypertension development.

Obesity leads to hypertension by increasing tubular reabsorption as glomerular filtration rate and renal plasma flow are increased in the kidney [19]. The increase in renal tubular reabsorption may be caused by a combination of hyperinsulinemia (a result of obesity-related insulin resistance), hyperactivation of the renin–angiotensin system, and perhaps physical changes in the kidney. A 2005 study published in *Hypertension* elucidated a "strong association between increasing body mass index and angiotensin-dependent control of the renal circulation" suggesting that this may be a mechanism for obesity-induced hypertension [20]. The renin–angiotensin system is the body's most important long-term blood pressure regulation system; furthermore, adipose tissue secretes all the components necessary to upregulate the renin–angiotensin system. Renin and angiotensin work together to stimulate release

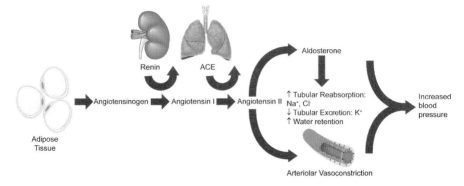

Fig. 7.8 Mechanism by which adipose tissue promotes increased blood pressure

of aldosterone, which is a very powerful vasoconstrictor, leading to large increases in blood pressure. Aldosterone also increases tubular reabsorption (the kidneys retain more salt and water), which, in effect, also raises blood pressure. In obese people, the upregulation of the renin–angiotensin control of renal circulation increases their risk of hypertension (Fig. 7.8).

Obesity and Metabolic Syndrome

Obesity significantly increases the risk for type 2 diabetes, dyslipidemia, and hypertension, presumably due its ability to induce insulin resistance and set the stage for metabolic syndrome. In addition, metabolic disease is a clustering of cardiovascular disease risk factors which markedly increases the risk of cerebrovascular accident (stroke). An analysis of the third National Health and Nutrition Examination Survey (1988–1994) determined the unadjusted and age-adjusted prevalence of metabolic syndrome in the US population to be 21.8 % and 23.7 %, respectively [21]. Thus, diagnosing obesity and metabolic disease may be instrumental in national stroke prevention (Fig. 7.1).

Metabolic Syndrome and Cardiovascular Disease

A prospective cohort study of British women aged 60–79 years old demonstrated that metabolic syndrome is positively and linearly associated with cardiovascular disease, with some confounding due to socioeconomic status and behavior (i.e., smoking, inactivity) [22]. Further evaluation of the Framingham subjects elucidated insulin resistance as a key factor in metabolic syndrome's ability to increase risk for cardiovascular disease [23]. Additionally, each one of the key characteristics (diabetic status, dyslipidemia, hypertension, abdominal obesity) of metabolic syndrome has been shown to be independently related causally to cardiovascular disease and thus stroke.

Type 2 Diabetes and Stroke

Cardiovascular disease is the primary cause of death in people with type 2 diabetes; it accounts for the greatest component of health care expenditures in diabetics [24–26]. Furthermore, people with type 2 diabetes have a 150–400 % increased risk of stroke, leading to more stroke-related dementia, stroke recurrence and stroke-related mortality [27]. Type 2 diabetes leads to microvascular disease (diabetic nephropathy, neuropathy, and retinopathy) and macrovascular disease. Macrovascular disease results in nonfatal myocardial infarction, nonfatal stroke, or death from cardiovascular causes. Adequate glycemic control is necessary to reduce the occurrence of these negative outcomes of diabetes. In fact, intensive glucose control (defined as the use of glipizide plus other drugs as required to achieve a glycated hemoglobin value of 6.5 % or less) has shown to have better efficacy in reducing both microvascular and macrovascular events (i.e., stroke) than in standard glucose control [28].

Type 2 diabetes leads to lipid-rich atherosclerotic lesions, which eventually rupture in acute vascular infarctions as found in stroke or heart attack. Presumably, the hyperglycemia, dyslipidemia, and insulin resistance of diabetes together lead to oxidative stress, protein kinase C activation, and RAGE (Receptor for Advanced Glycation End product) activation. This further leads to changes in the endothelium, which result in vasoconstriction, inflammation, and thrombosis: all elements of atherogenesis (atherosclerotic lesion formation) (Fig. 7.9) [29]. In addition to atherogenesis in type 2 diabetes, decreased fibrinolysis (dissolution of platelet aggregates) and hypercoagulability increase vascular occlusion and create the unfortunate recipe for stroke. The type 2 diabetes which increases stroke risk several fold usually occurs in the setting of metabolic syndrome found in obesity.

Dyslipidemia and Stroke

Dyslipidemia, specifically atherogenic dyslipidemia (elevated blood triglycerides, apolipoprotein B, increased small LDL particles, and a reduced level of HDL concentration), is a major risk factor for cardiovascular disease. However, the specific relationship between blood cholesterol concentration, the measure for dyslipidemia, and stroke incidence is more complex. Most of the studies evaluating this relationship do not distinguish between the various etiologic subtypes of stroke (ischemic versus hemorrhagic), weakening the ability to quantify the relationship. Specifically, atherogenic dyslipidemia is linked to increased ischemic stroke occurrence versus a

Diabetes Mellitus And Atherogenesis

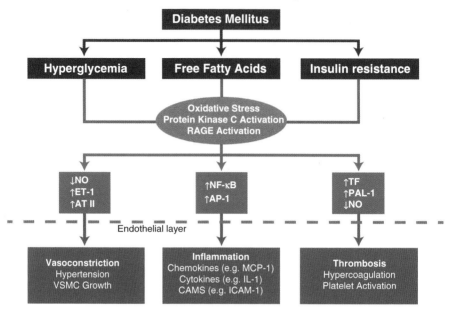

Fig. 7.9 *RAGE* receptor for advanced glycation end products, *CAMs* cell adhesion molecules, *VSMC* vascular smooth muscle cells, *NO* nitric oxide, *ET1* endothelin-1, *ATII* angiotensin II, *TF* tissue factor, *PAI*-1 plasminogen activator inhibitor (type 1), *AP*-1 activator protein-1, and *NF-kappaB* a transcription factor that regulates inflammation

conflicting link with hemorrhagic stroke [30]. The carotid atherosclerosis, which increases in dyslipidemia, consequently increases the risk of stroke.

A meta-analysis of all randomized trials testing statin drugs published before August 2003 demonstrated that administration of these agents to decrease high-LDL concentration successfully reduces stroke incidence [29]. Furthermore, each 10 % reduction in LDL concentration was estimated to reduce carotid IMT (intimal medial thickness, or thickness of artery walls) by 0.73 % per year (95 % CI, 0.27–1.19). Presumably, there is more than one mechanism by which elevated LDL concentration promotes atherogenesis. For example, these elevated concentrations lead to increased retention of small LDL particles in the vessel wall [31], increased accumulation in the foam cells of atherosclerotic plaques [32], and upregulation of the angiotensin II type I receptor [33]. In effect, the dyslipidemia resulting from obesity leads to atherogenesis and, consequently, increased stroke incidence.

Hypertension and Stroke

It is well understood that hypertension, which promotes the formation of atherosclerotic lesions and weakening of blood vessels in the brain, is the single most important treatable risk factor for stroke [34]. Studies demonstrate that reducing the blood pressure in hypertensive patients successfully lowers the risk of stroke. An analysis of 14 unconfounded randomized trials of hypertensive drugs (i.e., diuretics, beta-blockers) with 37,000 individuals over a period of 5 years demonstrated that a long-term decrease of 5-6 mm Hg in diastolic blood pressure is associated with about 35–40 % decrease in stroke incidence, thus, indicating the serious need for hypertension management in individuals at high risk for stroke [35].

In some hypertensive individuals, abnormalities in ion transport create changes in sodium, calcium, and/or proton fluxes or concentrations. These electrolyte metabolism changes enhance contractile response and further lead to hypertrophy and proliferation of vascular smooth muscle cells, a notable characteristic of atherosclerosis in large arteries [36]. Additionally, the increased stress due to elevated blood pressure weakens the delicate blood vessels of the brain, making them more susceptible to stroke.

Obesity, Metabolic Syndrome, and Stroke

Obesity or, more specifically, its resulting metabolic syndrome poses a significant risk for stroke by creating insulin resistance and often causing type 2 diabetes, dyslipidemia, and hypertension. As stated in the American Heart Association/National Heart, Lung, and Blood Institute Scientific statement, "the magnitude of the increased risk (for cardiovascular disease, and consequently stroke) can vary according to which components of the syndrome are present" [37]. Therefore, treatment of metabolic syndrome will reduce severity of stroke risk. Treatment or management varies depending on which specific phenotype of metabolic syndrome is present. For example, an individual with a large waist circumference, high triglycerides, and high fasting glucose needs to be managed differently than an individual with high blood pressure, low HDL, and high triglycerides.

Obesity and Stroke Risk Management

As previously discussed, reducing weight, and more specifically central adiposity (abdominal obesity), decreases stroke incidence and general cardiovascular disease. Cross-sectional and observational cohort evaluation of the Coronary Artery Risk Development in Young Adults Study demonstrated that abdominal obesity as measured by waist girth or waist-to-hip ratio is associated with early carotid atherosclerosis. This carotid atherosclerosis, of course, significantly increases the risk for stroke. Waist girth and waist-to-hip ratio at year 10 and subsequently in year 15 predicted carotid artery calcification (atherosclerosis) as measure by computed tomography. As mentioned earlier, stroke risk reduction must also address other individual risk factors present, such as type 2 diabetes, dyslipidemia, and hypertension [38].

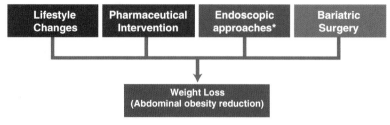

*Not currently FDA approved in the US

Fig. 7.10 Multipronged approach to abdominal obesity reduction

Reducing abdominal obesity potentially requires a multipronged approach: dietary modification, physical activity, pharmaceutical, endoscopic approaches, and surgical intervention (Fig. 7.10). Endoscopic approaches including intragastric balloons, trans-oral gastric stapling, and gastrojejunal sleeves are currently not FDA approved and will not be discussed further here. Lifestyle changes involve restoring balance between caloric intake (dietary consumption) and expenditure (physical activity and bodily functions). Weight reduction, and consequently abdominal obesity reduction, may necessitate diet modification. While some may advocate specific diets (e.g., Atkins, Zone, Weight Watchers, and others), essentially any diet where calorie intake (consumption) is less than calorie expenditure should result in weight loss. There is a behavioral component to this balance, requiring evaluation of eating habits, for example, a tendency to eat under certain circumstances (emotional or environmental). The second half of the caloric balance pertains to physical activity. Weight reduction may necessitate increase in physical activity. Changes in physical activity should always be evaluated by a physician, in order to prevent injury. Both cardiovascular activity (i.e., running, biking) and resistance training (i.e., activities which increase lean muscle mass) increase energy expenditure and improve the body's natural ability to balance caloric intake and utilization. A pedometer is a simple means by which an individual may monitor one component of physical activity: walking (Fig. 7.11). Lastly, certain genetic factors or illnesses may impact the balance between caloric intake and expenditure. For example, in hypothyroidism, low circulating levels of thyroid hormone lead to a lower basal metabolic rate (less caloric expenditure in body functions at rest), tipping caloric balance towards weight gain.

Pharmaceutical treatment of obesity may be indicated in individuals with BMIs greater than 30 kg/m². These treatment options include drugs such as orlistat, phentermine, or diethylpropion. Any pharmaceutical agent employed for weight loss will carry its own risks and thus should only be administered under a physician's supervision. Prudent evaluation of an individual's risk for metabolic syndrome and its harmful sequelae in comparison with the negative side effects of the proposed drug is necessary before commencing treatment. Phentermine and diethylpropion are sympathomimetic drugs which reduce food intake by creating early satiety in

Fig. 7.11 Illustration of a
pedometer

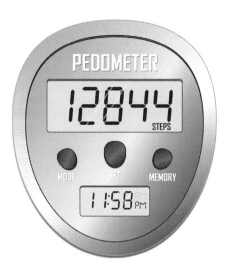

individuals, thus reducing behaviors which lead to excessive caloric intake. Orlistat
is currently the only drug available for long-term treatment of obesity. This pharmaceutical agent alters fat digestion by inhibiting pancreatic lipase and thereby increasing fat excretion by the body. Consequently, caloric intake is reduced, hopefully
creating a favorable caloric balance for weight loss.

For well-informed and motivated adults with a BMI greater than 40 kg/m² who
have unsuccessfully attempted weight loss by nonsurgical approaches (i.e., lifestyle
changes, pharmaceuticals), bariatric surgery may be indicated for stroke risk (and/
or cardiovascular disease) reduction. According to the National Institutes for
Health, the same recommendation may be indicated for adults with a BMI greater
than or equal to 35 kg/m² if other serious comorbidities (i.e., severe diabetes, sleep
apnea, joint disease) exist. Bariatric surgery (weight loss surgery) includes a variety
of procedures including either reducing the size of the stomach with an implanted
medical device (gastric banding), through removal of a portion of stomach, or by
resecting and rerouting the small intestines to a small stomach pouch (gastric bypass
surgery). A prospective, controlled Swedish study comparing obese subjects who
underwent bariatric (gastric) surgery versus obese subjects treated nonsurgically
demonstrated significant risk reduction resulting from the surgery. The bariatric
surgery group showed a 23.4 % decrease in weight after 2 years (versus 0.1 %
increase in nonsurgery group) and a further 16.1 % decrease in weight after 10 years
(versus 1.6 % increase in nonsurgery group). Consequently, the surgery group had
lower 2- and 10-year incidence rates of diabetes and hypertriglyceridemia (serum
triglycerides), which potentially may reduce stroke incidence as well [39]. Bariatric
surgery is largely irreversible and suffers from many negative side effects, most
notably malabsorption. Thus, it should only be considered when the aforementioned criteria are met and the potential disease risk reduction outweighs the negative sequelae.

Conclusion

Weight reduction or management of obesity may require more than one method (lifestyle modification, pharmaceutical, and/or surgical) depending on the etiology and degree of excess adiposity to successfully reduce stroke risk. Careful evaluation of adipose (fat) distribution and quantification (BMI) will assist in stroke risk evaluation and management of other risk factors, such as diabetes, dyslipidemia, and hypertension. It is clear that national programs need to be developed which stress obesity prevention rather than obesity treatment, which has proven so difficult.

References

1. Garabed E. Adolphe Quetelet (1796–1874)—the average man and indices of obesity. Nephrol Dial Transplant. 2008;23:47–51.
2. Clinical Guidelines on the Identification, Evaluation, and Treatment of Overweight and Obesity in Adults—The Evidence Report. National Institutes of Health. Obes Res 1998;6:51S.
3. Overweight and Obesity. National Center for Health Statistics, Health Data Interactive, http://www.cdc.gov/obesity/data/adult.html. Accessed 25 Mar 2012.
4. Biggs ML, Mukamal KJ, Luchsinger JA, Ix JH, Carnethon MR, Newman AB, et al. Association between adiposity in midlife and older age and risk of diabetes in older adults. JAMA. 2010;303:2504–12.
5. Shai I, Jiang R, Manson JE, Stampfer MJ, Willett WC, Colditz GA, et al. Ethinicity, obesity, and risk of type 2 diabetes in women: a 20-year follow-up study. Diabetes Care. 2006;29: 1585–90.
6. Mendell MA, Patel P, Asante M, Ballam L, Morris J, Strachan DP, et al. Relation of serum cytokine concentrations to cardiovascular risk factors and coronary heart disease. Heart. 1997;78:273–7.
7. Mendell MA, Patel P, Ballam L, Strachan D, Northfield TC. C-reactive protein and its relation to cardiovascular risk factors: a population based cross sectional study. BMJ. 1996;312:1061–5.
8. Yudkin JS, Stehouwer CDA, Emeis JJ, Coppack SW. C-reactive protein in healthy subjects: associations with obesity, insulin resistance, and endothelial dysfunction. A potential role for cytokines originating from adipose tissue. Arterioscler Thromb Vasc Biol. 1999;19:972–8.
9. Greenberg AS, Nordan RP, McIntosh J, Calvo JC, Scow RO, Jablons D. Interleukin 6 reduces lipoprotein lipase activity in adipose tissue of mice in vivo and in 3T3-L1 adipocytes: a possible role for interleukin 6 in cancer cachexia. Cancer Res. 1992;52:4113–6.
10. Van Snick J. Interleukin-6: an overview. Annu Rev Immunol. 1990;8:253–78.
11. Kawakami M, Pekala PH, Lane MD, Cerami A. Lipoprotein lipase suppression in 3T3-L1 cells by an endotoxin-induced mediator from exudate cells. Proc Natl Acad Set USA. 1982;82:912–6.
12. Hardardottir I, Grunfeld C, Feingold KR. Effects of endotoxin and cytokines on lipid metabolism. Curr Opin Lipidol. 1994;5:207–15.
13. Hotamisligil GS, Budavari A, Murray DL, Spiegelman BM. Reduced tyrosine kinase activity of the insulin receptor in obesity-diabetes: central role of tumor necrosis factor-α. J Clin Invest. 1994;94:1543–9.
14. Hotamisligil GS, Peraldi P, Budavari A, Ellis R, White MF, Spiegelman BM. IRS-1-mediated inhibition of insulin receptor tyrosine kinase activity in TNF-α and obesity-induced insulin resistance. Science. 1996;271:665–8.
15. Nguyen NT, Magno CP, Lane KT, Hinojosa MW, Lane JS. Association of hypertension, diabetes, dyslipidemia, and metabolic syndrome with obesity: findings from the National Health and Nutrition Examination Survey, 1999 to 2004. J Am Coll Surg. 2008;207:928–34.

16. Howard BV, Ruotolo G, Robbins DC. Obesity and dyslipidemia. Endocrinol Metab Clin North Am. 2003;32:855–67.
17. Wilson PW, D'Agostino RB, Sullivan L, Parise H, Kannel WB. Overweight and obesity as determinants of cardiovascular risk: the Framingham experience. Arch Intern Med. 2002; 162:1867.
18. Huang Z, Willett WC, Manson JE, Rosner B, Stampfer MJ, Speizer FE, et al. Body weight, weight change, and risk for hypertension in women. Ann Intern Med. 1998;128:81–8.
19. Hall JE, Louis K. Dahl memorial lecture: renal and cardiovascular mechanisms of hypertension in obesity. Hypertension. 1994;23:381–94.
20. Ahmed SB, Fisher ND, Stevanovic R, Hollenberg NK. Body mass index and angiotensin-dependent control of renal circulation in healthy humans. Hypertension. 2005;46:1316–20.
21. Ford ES, Giles WH, Dietz WH. Prevalence of the metabolic syndrome among US adults: findings from the third National Health and Nutritional Examination Survey. JAMA. 2002; 287:356–9.
22. Lawlor DA, Smith GD, Ebrahim S. Does the new international diabetes federation definition of the metabolic syndrome predict CHD any more strongly than older definitions? Findings from the British women's heart and health study. Diabetologia. 2006;49:41–8.
23. Meigs JB, Rutter MK, Sullivan LM, Fox CS, D'Agostino Sr RB, Wilson PW. Impact of insulin resistance on risk of type 2 diabetes and cardiovascular disease in people with metabolic syndrome. Diabetes Care. 2007;30:1219–25.
24. Laing SP, Swerdlow AJ, Slater SD, Burden AC, Morris A, Waugh NR, et al. Mortality from heart disease in a cohort of 23,000 patients with insulin-treated diabetes. Diabetologia. 2003;46:760–5.
25. Paterson AD, Rutledge BN, Cleary PA, Lachin JM, Crow RS. The effect of intensive diabetes treatment on resting heart rate in type 1 diabetes control and complications trial/epidemiology of diabetes interventions and complications study. Diabetes Care. 2007;30:2107–12.
26. Hogan P, Dall T, Nikolov P. Economic costs of diabetes in the US in 2002. Diabetes Care. 2003;26:917–32.
27. Beckman JA, Creager MA, Libby P. Diabetes and atherosclerosis: epidemiology, pathophysiology and management. JAMA. 2002;287:2570–81.
28. Duckworth W, Abraira C, Moritz T, Reda D, Emanuele N, Reaven PD, et al. Glucose control and vascular complication in veterans with 2 diabetes. N Engl J Med. 2009;360:129–39.
29. Amarenco P, Labreuche J, Lavallee P, Touboul PJ. Statins in stroke prevention and carotid atherosclerosis: a systematic review and up-to-date +meta-analysis. Stroke. 2004;35:2902–9.
30. Amarenco P. Hypercholesterolemia, lipid lowering agent and the risk of brain infarction. Neurology. 2001;57:S35–44.
31. Hurt-Camejo E, Olsson U, Wiklund O, Bondjers G, Camejo G. Cellular consequences of association of apoB lipoproteins with proteoglycans. Potential contribution to atherogenesis. Arterioscler Thromb Vasc Biol. 1997;17:1011–7.
32. Iuliano L, Mauriello A, Sbarigia E, Spagnoli LG, Violi F. Radiolabeled native low-density lipoprotein injected into patients with carotid stenosis accumulates in macrophages of atherosclerotic plaque: effect of vitamin E supplementation. Circulation. 2000;101:1249–54.
33. Nickenig G, Sachinidis A, Michaelsen F, Böhm M, Seewald S, Vetter H. Upregulation of vascular angiotensin II receptor gene expression by low-density lipoprotein in vascular smooth muscle cells. Circulation. 1997;95:473–8.
34. Uptodate [www.uptodate.com]. Waltham, MA: UptoDate; c1992–2012. Secondary prevention of stroke: Risk factor reduction; 7 Oct 2011 Available from: http://www.uptodate.com/contents/secondary-prevention-of-stroke-risk-factor-reduction?source=search_results&search=hypertension+stroke&selectedTitle=6%7E150. Accessed 25 Mar 2012.
35. Collins R, Peto R, MacMahon S, Hebert P, Fiebach NH, Eberlein KA, et al. Blood pressure, stroke, and coronary heart disease. Part 2, short-term reductions in blood pressure: overview of randomized drug trials in their epidemiological context. Lancet. 1990;335:827–38.
36. Alexander RW. Hypertension and the pathogenesis of atherosclerosis, oxidative stress and the mediation of arterial inflammatory response: a new perspective. Hypertension. 1995;25: 155–61.

37. Grundy SM, Cleeman JI, Daniels SR, Donato KA, Eckel RH, Franklin BA, et al. Diagnosis and management of the metabolic syndrome; an American heart association/national heart, lung, and blood institute scientific statement. Circulation. 2005;112:2735–52.
38. Lee CD, Jacobs Jr DR, Schreiner PJ, Iribarren C, Hankinson A. Abdominal obesity and coronary artery calcification in young adults: the Coronary Artery Risk Development in Young Adults (CARDIA). Am J Clin Nutr. 2007;86:48–54.
39. Sjöström L, Lindroos AK, Peltonen M, Torgerson J, Bouchard C, Carlsson B, et al. Lifestyle, diabetes, and cardiovascular risk factors 10 years after bariatric surgery. N Engl J Med. 2004;351(26):2683–93.

Chapter 8
Pediatric/Adolescent Stroke

Christina DeTallo, Douglas Henry, and Merideth Miller

Key Points

- The evaluation and management of stroke in children is conceptually similar to adult stroke; whereas the basic pathophysiology, residual functional deficits, and rehabilitative strategies share common concepts; however, there are many important details that differ significantly, making the management of pediatric stroke a distinct area of expertise.
- Common causes of childhood stroke include congenital heart disease, clotting disorders, metabolic disorders, mitochondrial disorders, sickle cell disease, and focal arteriopathy.
- In the acute management of stroke, the dietitian's main goal is to ensure optimal nutrition in order to promote healing and prepare the child for physical rehabilitation. Nutritional management in the rehabilitation or chronic phase targets long-term effects of stroke including swallowing problems, immobility, spasticity, limited physical activity, cognitive and behavior changes, limited weight-bearing through the lower extremities, pressure sores, constipation, and gastroesophageal reflux.

C. DeTallo, M.S., R.D., C.S.P., L.D. (✉)
Pediatric Gastroenterology, Cleveland Clinic Children's Hospital, 9500 Euclid Avenue, Cleveland, OH 44195, USA
e-mail: detallc@ccf.org

D. Henry, M.D.
Developmental and Rehabilitative Pediatrics, Cleveland Clinic Children's Hospital for Rehabilitation, 9500 Euclid Avenue, Cleveland, OH 44195, USA
e-mail: henryd@ccf.org

M. Miller, R.D., C.S.P., L.D.
Pediatric Gastroenterology, Cleveland Clinic Children's Hospital, Shaker Campus, 9500 Euclid Avenue, Cleveland, OH 44195, USA
e-mail: millerm5@ccf.org

M.L. Corrigan et al. (eds.), *Handbook of Clinical Nutrition and Stroke*,
Nutrition and Health, DOI 10.1007/978-1-62703-380-0_8,
© Springer Science+Business Media New York 2013

- Nutrition support is typically provided enterally rather than parenterally unless the gastrointestinal tract is compromised. An interdisciplinary approach is the most effective method of evaluation of long-term feeding, nutrient intake, and growth monitoring.
- Obtaining accurate growth parameters can be challenging, especially in children with long-term disability. In children with disabilities, triceps and subscapular skinfolds as well as arm-fat area may be better indicators of undernutrition than the standard weight/length or body mass index (BMI)/age chart. Children's limited food preferences are often one of the biggest challenges for clinicians. Optimal nutritional management of the pediatric stroke patient requires knowledge of childhood-specific nutritional requirements, as well as normal and disease-specific growth and development considerations and cannot be based on adult standards or practices.

Keywords Stroke • Pediatrics • Energy expenditure • Gastrostomy tube

Abbreviations

ADL	Activities of daily living
BEE	Basal energy expenditure
BMI	Body mass index
DRI	Dietary reference intakes
EER	Estimated energy requirement
GER	Gastroesophageal reflux
GI	Gastrointestinal
GT	Gastrostomy tube
MBS	Modified barium swallow
NG	Nasogastric tube
RDA	Recommended dietary allowances
REE	Resting energy expenditure
TEE	Total energy expenditure
TBI	Traumatic brain injury
WHO	World Health Organization

Introduction

The evaluation and management of stroke in children is conceptually similar to adult stroke. The basic pathophysiology (ischemic, embolic, and hemorrhagic), residual functional deficits, and rehabilitative strategies share common concepts in pediatric and adult medicine. However, in each of these domains, there are many important details that differ significantly, making the management of pediatric stroke a distinct area of expertise. For example, it is often difficult to detect stroke in the neonatal period because neurologic deficits are not apparent due to their limited developmental abilities [1]. Additionally, in young children, stroke-related functional deficits may not be apparent for several years, when they reach the developmental age appropriate for those skills. There are also important differences to consider in the nutritional management of pediatric stroke patients. For example, limbs weakened by a stroke during the growing years typically do not achieve their full length at maturity, therefore affecting stature/body mass index (BMI) [2]. The purpose of this chapter is to highlight the nutritional management issues specific to childhood stroke.

Medical Overview

The incidence of ischemic stroke in children varies depending on the study; however, a good estimate comes from the Canadian Ischemic Stroke Registry, which shows an incidence of 3.2 per 100,000 children per year [3]. About 25 % of ischemic strokes occur in the neonatal period [4]. Common causes of childhood stroke include congenital heart disease, clotting disorders (such as protein C deficiency), metabolic disorders (such as homocysteinuria), mitochondrial disorders (such as Kearns–Sayre disease), sickle cell disease, and focal arteriopathy. However, the etiology is not determined in as many as a third of all pediatric strokes [5]. As opposed to adult stroke, atherosclerosis is an extremely rare cause of stroke in children [4]. Multifocal infarcts are also relatively uncommon in children. Recurrent stroke is also unusual, except in specific disorders such as sickle cell disease. Most of the risk factors for pediatric stroke have a genetic basis.

As in adults, the size and location of the stroke determine the long-term functional impact on the individual. This may include weakness, often on one side of the body; vision deficits; swallowing problems; receptive and/or expressive language deficits; and problems with cognition, memory, and behaviors. Any of these effects may be very mild and even resolve, or they may be devastating in nature.

The medications prescribed for some of the conditions causing stroke or its long-term effects may also affect dietary recommendations. Patients may be placed on blood thinners such as aspirin or warfarin. If seizures are present, several different anticonvulsants might be prescribed, which may alter feeding schedules or require folate or vitamin D supplementation. In a child with immobility, vitamin D and calcium supplementation is often recommended. Calcium and vitamin D are particularly important to supplement since more than half of healthy teenagers in the USA have inadequate calcium intake and are vitamin D deficient [1].

Nutritional management in the rehabilitation or chronic phase presents numerous challenges. The long-term effects of the stroke can include swallowing problems, immobility, spasticity, limited physical activity, cognitive and behavior changes, limited weight-bearing through the lower extremities, pressure sores, constipation, and gastroesophageal reflux. All of these problems have nutritional implications. For example, an immobile child who is hypotonic will require fewer calories for his weight, while a similarly immobile child with diffuse spasticity can consume much more than their weight-based caloric needs. Young children may develop an aversive feeding disorder related to the stroke itself, prolonged hospitalization, or intubation. They may avoid certain textures or only eat a small list of specific foods. In the subacute phase children often transition from nasogastric to oral feeds. As they begin to eat more solids, they often do not keep up with their fluid requirements orally. They therefore require extra water as the formula requirement is decreased.

Nutrition Management in the Acute Care Setting

In the acute management of stroke, the dietitian's main goal is to ensure optimal nutrition in order to promote healing and prepare the child for physical rehabilitation. This can be difficult due to frequent interruptions associated with critical care management, procedures, and diagnostic testing which require an empty stomach. During initial nutrition assessment, the clinician should obtain from the guardian a detailed diet history including oral feeding capabilities, route of intake, and supplement or vitamin/mineral intake. This criteria provides the necessary framework for accurate comparison while assessing the appropriateness of alternative means of nutrition support commonly needed in the stroke patient.

Nutrition support is typically provided enterally rather than parenterally unless the gastrointestinal (GI) tract is compromised [1]. Evidence of oral motor feeding difficulties, growth failure, weight status prior to insult, and individual nutrient deficiencies indicates the need for nutrition support. Enteral tube feedings are also required for children who cannot meet their nutritional needs by oral feeding alone. The approach to enteral feeding is dynamic accounting the total nutrient requirement, positioning, oral therapy, behavioral modification, formula selection, route, method of formula administration, feeding intolerance associated with medication interaction, and cultural or ethical concerns [1]. A nasogastric (NG) tube is generally used in the short term to allow for acute nutritional rehabilitation and to ensure the patient will tolerate and/or benefit from enteral feeds. A gastrostomy tube (GT) is placed for long-term feeding needs. When enteral tube feedings are received, nutrition therapy leads to linear growth and weight gain [1]. Short-term nutritional interventions in the acute post stroke phase include optimized health, functional status, and quality of life while maintaining adequate growth and nutritional status during metabolic instability. Treatment options are dependent of the child's age, function, and cognition with drastic differences for those suffering stroke during the neonatal period.

Neonates with stroke are often treated with cooling procedures decreasing metabolic demand warranting close evaluation of glucose and electrolytes [6, 7].

Parenteral nutrition is a common therapy for improved nitrogen balance; however, withholding feeds may have negative consequences including atrophy of intestinal villi [8]. This can predispose the infant to hospital-acquired sepsis leading to increased chances of necrotizing enterocolitis (NEC) [8]. Evidence-based recommendations include initiation of maternal or donor breast milk trophically after 48 h of life with slow volume advancement stimulating bowel function and integrity and preventing bowel atrophy [8].

Seizures are common after stroke and often require anticonvulsant therapy which may compromise vitamin D status. Feeding problems may go unrecognized in the neonatal stroke patient especially when perinatal comorbidities such as failure to thrive and respiratory issues are compromising feeding [1]. A common postneonatal dysfunction documented in the literature is disorganized oral motor skills requiring speech and occupational therapy and diet modification [1].

Growth

An interdisciplinary approach to the long-term care of the child with a brain injury is the most effective method of long-term feeding and nutrition monitoring. These children need the involvement of multiple team members including physicians, dietitians, nurses, occupational therapists, speech language pathologists, social workers, and psychologists. Supporting appropriate nutritional intake may benefit the child in several ways including increased linear growth, health and quality of life improvement, reduction in hospitalizations, decreased irritability and spasticity, improved wound healing and peripheral circulation, decreased incidence of aspiration, increased alertness, and a decrease in the incidence of GER [9].

Weight, height/length, as well as head circumference in infants and children 0–3 years are used to determine adequate growth in typical children. These methods may not be appropriate for children with a brain injury. The weight for height and BMI/age charts may not be reliable for children with lower muscle mass and bone density related to inactivity [10]. These measurements are generally a poor predictor of low fat mass in this population. Weight for height and BMI are monitored much less frequently due to the difficulty in measurement and thus weight is relied on for assessing growth. When compared to healthy children, height for age, weight for age, weight for height, body fat, and arm muscle area are lower in children with neurological impairment. Growth failure can be attributed to the type and severity of neurologic impairment, ambulatory status, cognitive ability, and swallowing function [9].

Obtaining growth parameters, length or height in particular, can be a difficult task due to inability to stand, fixed joint contractures, involuntary muscle spasms, and poor compliance due to cognitive disabilities. Stevenson et al. developed formulas to estimate height utilizing upper arm length, tibial length, and knee height for children with cerebral palsy [10]. These formulas can also be utilized in the stroke population when a reliable height cannot be obtained. Linear growth may be inhibited even when nutritional intake is adequate and thus may not be correctable with nutritional therapy [9]. Parental height is useful to estimate the potential linear growth a child may achieve allowing for a better assessment of current growth than the standard growth charts. The younger the age of the patient when the brain injury occurs, the more likely the linear growth will be effected by the child's nutritional status [9].

Weight should be obtained using the standard infant and standing scales unless there are significant disabilities preventing the child to stand independently. A patient can be weighed in a wheelchair or in the arms of the caregiver, and the weight of the chair or caregiver is then subtracted. Specialized equipment such as a chair or bed scale can be used if available. Fat mass may decrease in the presence of muscle and visceral protein maintenance leading to a lower BMI/age or weight for length. Linear growth can continue to occur while weight gain is lacking due to the body's desire to preserve this parameter. Muscle wasting may occur regardless of nutritional intervention due to decreased or limited mobility [9]. Following neurological insult, children may experience weight loss related to dysphagia and fatigue evidenced by decreased oral intake.

In children with disabilities, triceps and subscapular skinfolds as well as arm-fat area may be a better indicator of under nutrition than the standard weight/length or BMI/age chart. Body fat and mid-arm muscle area can be determined from the mid-arm circumference and triceps skinfold. Standardized equations for these measurements can be used to identify nutritional adequacy. Ninety-six percent of children with depleted fat stores are identified using triceps skinfold compared to 55 % when using weight for height or BMI for age below the 10th percentile [9].

The most effective way to monitor nutritional adequacy is the rate of weight gain. However, in the intensive care setting, it is often difficult to get accurate weights, due to the patient's immobility, intubation, and intravenous lines. In addition, immobile children quickly begin to lose bone and muscle mass [9]. In the first few days of diagnostic assessment and management, children often cannot take nutrition orally. Younger children, especially the neonatal stroke patients, are more likely to have linear growth deficits compared to older children [9]. Tracking weight trends or using body fat measurements may aid in the growth assessments since height measurements can be unreliable. It is important for clinicians to be aware of the pre-stroke growth trends, feeding implications, and daily physical routine to prevent under or over feeding when estimating nutritional needs in neurologically impaired populations, such as children with cerebral palsy, traumatic brain injuries, or hypoxic ischemic encephalopathy.

Estimating Nutrient Needs During Rehabilitation

Energy requirements are disease specific and vary with severity of disability and altered metabolism. Energy can be estimated from Dietary Reference Intake (DRI) standards for basal energy expenditure (BEE), indirect calorimetry, or height

Table 8.1

Equations to estimate energy requirements (EER) for children

Age	EER (kcal/d) = total energy expenditure (TEE) + energy deposition
0–3 months	EER = [89 × weight (kg) – 100] + 175
4–6 months	EER = [89 × weight (kg) – 100] + 56
7–12 months	EER = [89 × weight (kg) – 100] + 22
13–35 months	EER = [89 × weight (kg) – 100] + 20
3–8 years	Boys: EER = 88.5 – (61.9 × age [years]) + PA × (26.7 × weight [kg] + 903 × height [m]) + 20 kcal
	Girls: EER = (135.3 – 30.8 × age [years]) + PA × (10 × weight [kg] + 934 × height [m]) + 20 Kcal
9–18 years	Boys: EER = 88.5 – (61.9 × age [years]) + PA × (26.7 × weight [kg] + 903 × height [m]) + 25 kcal
	Girls: EER = 135.3 – (30.8 × age [years]) + PA × (10 × weight [kg] + 934 × height [m]) + 25 Kcal
Overweight 3–18 years	Boys: TEE = 114 – [50.9 × age (years)] + PA × [19.5 × weight (kg) + 1161.4 × height (m)]
	Girls: TEE = 389 – [41.2 × age (years)] + PA × [15 × weight (kg) + 701.6 × height (m)]

Physical activity coefficient (PA) for determination of energy requirements in children ages 3–18 years

Gender	Sedentary	Low active	Active	Very active
	Typical activities of daily living (ADL) only	ADL + 30–60 min if daily moderate activity (e.g., walking at 5–7 km/h)	ADL + ≥60 min of daily moderate activity	ADL + ≥60 min of daily moderate activity + an additional 60 min of vigorous activity *or* 120 min of moderate activity
Boys	1.0	1.13	1.26	1.42
Girls	1.0	1.16	1.31	1.56

Adapted with permission from Dietary Reference Intakes for Energy, Carbohydrates, Fiber, Fat, Protein, and Amino Acids (Macronutrients), 2005 by the National Academy of Sciences, courtesy of the National Academies Press, Washington, DC

represented as calories per centimeter (calories/cm). The most effective way to monitor nutritional adequacy is rate of weight gain and BMI changes in response to nutrition intervention. Additional supplementation of protein, vitamins, or minerals is essential when energy intake is modified or reduced to obtain desired growth rates. There are no defined evidence-based nutritional allowances for the neurologically impaired child; as a result, it is recommended to calculate nutrient needs derived from the DRIs for protein, vitamins, and minerals commonly used for healthy children [9]. Children walking yield higher energy expenditure resulting in close monitoring and energy adjustment [11]. Nutrient deficiencies in neurologically impaired children are common resulting from metabolic instability and reduced dietary intake. It has been reported that 15–50 % of children are deficient in essential fatty acids, iron, selenium, zinc, and vitamins C, D, and E [9].

Table 8.2
Dietary reference intakes, protein intake

Age	Protein intake (gms/kg/day)
0–6 months	1.52[a]
6–12 months	1.2
12–36 months	1.05
4–13 years	0.95
14–18 years	0.85
>18 years	0.8

Adapted with permission from Dietary Reference Intakes for Energy, Carbohydrates, Fiber, Fat, Protein, and Amino Acids (Macronutrients), 2005 by the National Academy of Sciences, courtesy of the National Academies Press, Washington, DC
[a]This is an adequate intake recommendation; not enough research has been conducted to establish an RDA for this age group

Altered body composition and decreased physical activity can make the task of estimating energy needs difficult. Energy requirements are disease specific and vary based on disability, mobility, feeding difficulties, and altered metabolism. Recommendations are to use the DRI standards for (BEE) when indirect calorimetry is not available. See Table 8.1 for EER equations. Other methods such as calories/cm and the World Health Organization (WHO) Equations may also be useful [12]. Some children with neurologic impairment can grow well receiving calories as low as 61 ± 15 % of the DRI for healthy children; this is believed to be due to their lean body mass and decreased resting energy expenditure (REE) [9]. An REE with a sedentary to low physical activity coefficient (PA) may be adequate for growth. Children who are ambulatory, have spasticity, or movement disorders tend to have a higher REE. Care needs to be taken in assessing changes in medications such as Baclofen which may increase weight gain velocity due to decreased spasticity. The most effective method of promoting optimal growth is monitoring the individual child's overall growth, weight changes, and linear growth and adjusting caloric intake as necessary [9].

Protein needs are based on the DRI for age and gender. The DRIs for protein were determined based on children with normal growth, body composition, and activity level. Protein, essential fatty acids, vitamins, and minerals can be decreased in a diet that is reduced in calories and/or modified in texture. See Table 8.2 for DRI for protein.

Calcium and vitamin D are two of the micronutrients important to bone health. Osteopenia is common in patients who have limited or non-weight-bearing status. Meeting 100 % of the Recommended Dietary Allowances (RDA) for these nutrients is critical in these patients. Decreased sun exposure, decreased intake of calcium and vitamin D in foods and beverages, and chronic use of antiepileptic medications can all be indicators for supplementation. Vitamin D (as 25-hydroxy vitamin D) levels should be monitored at least yearly. Zinc, selenium, and iron have also been noted to be low in patients with decreased oral intake. Standard DRIs for healthy children are recommended for all micronutrients [9, 10].

Diet History During Rehabilitation

An effective means of evaluating dietary intake is to obtain a 3- or 7-day food record including type and volume of foods and beverages consumed. If this is not attainable, a 24 h recall or usual intake can be beneficial in evaluating for nutritional adequacy. From the food records or recall, the dietitian can calculate the macro- and micronutrient intake of the patient and ascertain what supplements may be necessary.

A food record can also be beneficial in observing texture preferences and length of meals. Caregivers tend to overestimate oral intake and underestimate the amount of time spent feeding the child. The longer the meal takes to complete, the more energy the child is expending and allows for possible fatigue leading to increased risk of aspiration. During rehabilitation or hospitalized setting, a structured meal observation offers clinicians accurate oral intake assessment and proactive detection of dysphagia creating an optimal environment to manage nutrition and hydration as it is noninvasive and can be completed quickly [13]. Some children are not able to effectively communicate their hunger, food preferences, or satiety; they must rely on caregivers to regulate for them. This can lead to inappropriate energy intake related to nutrient needs which is the primary cause of under nutrition, growth failure, and overweight in neurologically impaired children [9].

Oral Intake Efficacy

Independent feeding and the efficiency of the feeding process should be evaluated. Children who are able to feed themselves tend to have food loss leading to under nutrition. The dietitian and occupational therapist work together identifying nutrient dense foods to support growth and adaptive utensils and dishes allowing more efficiency during mealtime. Oral motor dysfunction is a major contributing factor of under nutrition. Poor nutritional status and growth typically correlate with the severity of the motor impairment; the more impaired, the higher the level of nutritional insufficiency [9].

The severity of feeding dysfunction correlates with poor nutritional status. Up to 76 % of children with severe traumatic brain injury (TBI) develop acute swallowing difficulties [14]. Dysphagia is a broad term characterized by deficiencies in oral preparation, oral-pharyngeal, and esophageal phases of swallowing [13]. The clinician can pose four questions to families to determine if a referral is warranted for dysphagia evaluation [15]. How long do mealtimes typically take? Are mealtimes stressful? Does the child show any signs of respiratory distress? Has the child not gained weight in the past 2–3 months? A therapist may recommend modified barium swallow (MBS) or videofluroscopic studies for patients who have oral motor impairment offering children varied food and beverage textures in different positions to determine the degree of oral motor dysfunction and aspiration risk, including silent aspiration. These study results aid the occupational or speech therapist in providing guidance for appropriate food textures and therapeutic feeding techniques [9]. Delayed swallow, coughing, gagging, and choking can lead to food accumulation in the mouth increasing risk for aspiration and decreased caloric intake [9]. Treatment of dysphagia focuses on improvement of oro-motor function and reduction of secondary comorbidities and may include adapted eating utensils, texture changes such as puree or mechanical soft foods, treatment of GER, positioning supports, increasing caloric content of foods, addition of supplemental NG or GT feedings, and oral sensorimotor training [13]. GER is common in this population and treatment includes medications, changes in positioning of the head and the body, remaining in an inclined position for at least 30 min after a meal or tube feeding, and smaller, more frequent meals throughout the day. Children with neurological impairment may require a fundoplication to control severe reflux.

Impaired oral motor skills such as inadequate lip closure, drooling, and persistent protrusion of the tongue often result in food loss through spillage decreasing the overall energy intake, but may not be accounted in the reported intake. After a stroke, an NG or GT may be placed to provide adequate nutrition while oral intake is being assessed and trialed or patients are dealing with early satiety. As oral intake improves, the dietitian continues to closely monitor and reevaluate macro- and micronutrient adequacy; adjusting tube feeds to avoid overfeeding and providing vitamin or other nutrient supplement recommendations. Some patients experience hyperresponses such as impulsiveness and the inability to feel satiety [14]. These patients may benefit from a scheduled, structured meal plan to avoid overfeeding and excessive weight gains.

Modified diets should be trialed for infants and children receiving nutrition orally but experiencing inadequate growth. Energy increases for infants are achieved through fortified breast milk and formula concentration. Additives such as butter, powdered milk, cheese, vegetable oil, and heavy whipping cream will increase calories in the diet for those eating solids. Homemade shakes and smoothies can also be utilized to increase calories. Table 8.3 highlights high calorie commercial beverages available. Some children with neurological impairment benefit from a pureed or altered texture diet due to difficulty biting and chewing.

The caregiver should be advised how to puree table foods versus using baby foods. This will allow for increased calories and acceptance of the food offered and can provide more appropriate micronutrients for the older child. Caregivers may benefit from a detailed meal plan including specific quantities and types of food to offer. This provides balance to the diet.

Table 8.3
Pediatric formulas

Infants				
Cow's milk	Soy	Partially hydrolyzed (whey-based)	Protein hydrolysate	Amino acids
Enfamil Premium®	Enfamil Prosobee®	Gerber® Good Start®	Nutramigen®	Elecare Infant®
Similac Advance®	Similac Soy Isomil®	Protect	Pregestimil®	Neocate Infant®
	Gerber Good Start®		Similac Alimentum®	Nutramigen AA®
Nutren Jr®	Bright Beginnings	N/A	Peptamen Jr®	Elecare Jr®
Pediasure®	Soy Pediatric Drink®		Peptamen Jr 1.5®	Neocate Jr®
Pediasure 1.5®			Pediasure Peptide®	EO28 Splash®
Boost Kids Essentials®			Pediasure Peptide 1.5®	Vivonex Pediatric®
Boost Kids Essentials® 1.5				

Adult				
Cow's milk	Soy	Partially hydrolyzed (whey-based)	Protein hydrolysate (whey-based)	Amino acids
Boost®	N/A		Peptamen product line	Vivonex TEN®
Ensure®			Vital product line	Vivonex Plus®
Nutren 1.0®				Vivonex RTF®
Nutren 1.5®				
Osmolyte®				
Promote®				
Replete®				

[17–20]

Pureeing Instructions

- Puree hot foods.
- Remove all liquid from canned fruits and vegetables; these foods contain a significant amount of fluid and may become too thin.
- Add liquid slowly to prevent mixture from becoming too thin.
- Add heavy whipping cream to fruit for calories and taste.
- Steam fresh fruits and vegetables to soften prior to blending.
- Add gravy and/or broth to meats.
- Make batches of foods to save time; use ice cube trays to store pureed foods. Each ice cube from a standard tray is equal to about one ounce.

Difficulty drinking liquids can lead to decreased fluid intake, dehydration, and constipation. Thickened liquids may be recommended allowing children to bypass feeding tube placement for hydration [16]. Thickening agents vary forcing clinicians to pay close attention to product content. Commercial thickeners can increase the caloric content of beverages, while others decrease the concentration through displacement in formulas. Increasing the calories for some patients is beneficial but can cause rapid weight gain that is not warranted in others. Free water is decreased in thickened liquids, and there is not enough data to determine if micronutrients are also bound to the thickener and thus not absorbed in the digestive system [16]. Providing fluid minimums can be beneficial in avoiding constipation and dehydration.

Constipation occurs due to decreased mobility, fluid and fiber intake related to dysphagia, and prescribed medications. Additional medications may still be necessary to alleviate constipation despite fluid and fiber optimization. Some patients are unable to meet fluid requirements or do not pass the MBS safely for oral fluid consumption requiring water boluses via the NG or GT.

It can be difficult for caregivers to agree on feeding tube placement when optimal nutrition cannot be achieved orally. Common misconceptions are children will no longer work toward optimal oral intake or be offered oral if a tube is placed. As long as it is safe, a child can continue to be fed orally and work on oral motor skills. Enteral feedings can reduce the work of the child and the caregiver during feeding times, decrease stress and anxiety surrounding mealtimes, and allow for adequate growth due to decreased energy expenditure required to eat orally. A child may eat typical meals during the day and receive tube feedings overnight or may require daytime boluses if oral intake is significantly below needs. There are a variety of feeding approaches clinicians can utilize, customizing each plan to the individual child for best outcomes. When enteral tube feedings are received, nutrition therapy leads to linear growth and weight gain [9]. Growth should be monitored closely in the beginning to avoid overfeeding and subsequent excessive weight gain [9].

Exclusively tube fed (meaning they have no other nutritional intake, not a group, etc.). Enteral formulas are designed to provide adequate nutrition based on specific volumes. When energy needs are reduced, feeding volume is restricted ultimately decreasing vitamin/mineral intake warranting supplementation. Typical milk-based products can be used if the child does not have allergies. If milk-protein intolerance is a challenge, hydrolysate- or amino acid-based formulas may be beneficial. Please refer to Table 8.3 for common pediatric formulas. Children with decreased activity and energy needs typically require lower volumes compromising micronutrient intake. If energy needs are significantly decreased, protein intake may be inadequate warranting supplementation or formula change to a higher protein containing solution. Decreased formula volume also leads to lower fluid intake requiring free water administration throughout the day. It is critical for clinicians to track and evaluate metrics for long-term nutritional success understanding the balance between the need for frequent changes and/or surveillance to achieve optimal growth velocities.

Conclusion

Optimal nutritional management of the pediatric stroke patient requires knowledge of childhood-specific nutritional requirements, as well as normal and disease-specific growth and development considerations. There are several nutritional challenges surrounding children with disabilities; thus, the nutritional management cannot be based on adult standards or practices. It is a vital part of maximizing a child's recovery from their stroke for optimal patient outcome. Optimal nutrition care plans for pediatric stroke patients are best implemented with an interdisciplinary team experienced in the treatment of children with disabilities. Children's limited food preferences are often one of the biggest challenges for clinician and parent management. Obtaining accurate growth parameters can be difficult, especially in children with long-term disability but a critical step in the evaluation process. Comprehensive medical follow-up is imperative for long-term success.

References

1. Barkat-Masih M, Hamby DK, Ofner S, Golomb MR. Feeding problems in children with neonatal arterial ischemic stroke. J Child Neurol. 2010;25(7):867–72.
2. Stevenson RD, Roberts CD, Vogtle L. The effects of non-nutritional factors on growth in cerebral palsy. Dev Med Child Neurol. 1995;37(2):124–30.
3. deVeber GA, MacGregor D, Curtis R, Supriya M. Neurologic outcome in survivors of childhood arterial ischemic stroke and sinovenous thrombosis. J Child Neurol. 2000;15:316–24.
4. Robinson R. Pediatric stroke: differences from adult symptoms highlighted. Neurol Today. 2010;10(12):22.
5. Friedman N. Pediatric stroke: past, present and future. Adv Pediatr. 2009;56:271–99.
6. Bacani D, Garrin M, Mance M, Yanski A. Therapeutic hypothermia for neonatal hypoxic-ischemic encephalopathy. Nurse Currents. 2011;5(2):1–10.
7. Niklasch D. Induced mild hypothermia and the prevention of neurological injury. J Infus Nurs. 2010;33(4):236–42.
8. Wessel J. Nutrition in hypoxic-ischemic encephalopathy. Nurse Currents. 2011;5(2):12–4.
9. Marchand V, Motil K, NASPGHAN Committee on Nutrition. Nutrition support for neurologically impaired children: a clinical report of the North American Society for Pediatric Gastroenterology, Hepatology and Nutrition. J Pediatr Gastroenterol Nutr. 2006;43:123–5.
10. Kuperminc MN, Stevenson RD. Growth and nutritional disorders in children with cerebral palsy. Dev Disabil Res Rev. 2008;14(2):137–46.
11. Motil KJ. Developmental Delay. In: Corkins MR, Ballint J, Bobo E, Plogsted S, Yaworski JA, Seebeck ND, editors. The A.S.P.E.N. Pediatric Nutrition Support Core Curriculum. 2010;191–203.
12. Ludlow V, Randall R, Burritt E, Rago D. Estimating nutrient needs, pediatric module. ASPEN enteral nutrition practitioner tutorial project; 2010. http://www.nutritioncare.org
13. Calis EA, Veugelers R, Sheppard JJ, Tibboel D, Evenhuis HM, Penning C. Dysphagia in children with severe generalized cerebral palsy and intellectual disability. Dev Med Child Neurol. 2008;50(8):625–30.
14. Morgan AT. Dysphagia in childhood traumatic brain injury: a reflection on the evidence and its implications for practice. Dev Neurorehabil. 2010;13(3):192–203.

15. Prasse JE, Kikano GE. An overview of pediatric dysphagia. Clin Pediatr. 2009;48(3):247–51.
16. Gosa M, Schooling T, Coleman J. Thickened liquids as a treatment for children with dysphagia and associated adverse effects: a systematic review. ICAN Infant Child Adolesc Nutr. 2011;3(6):344–50.
17. Abbott Nutrition. Nutritional products; 2012. http://abbottnutrition.com/Products/Nutritional-Products.aspx
18. Mead Johnson. Nutritional products; 2012. http://www.meadjohnson.com/Brands/Pages/Products-by-Need.aspx
19. Nestle Nutrition. Nutritional products; 2012. http://www.nestle-nutrition.com/products/default.aspx
20. Nutricia North America. Nutritional products; 2012. http://www.nutricia-na.com/pages/products.htm

Chapter 9
Stroke in Younger and Older Adults

Mei Lu

Key Points

- Many of the common stroke risk factors such as obesity, hypertension, hyperlipidemia, diabetes mellitus, physical inactivity, and smoking can occur in all age groups. Incidence and prevalence of metabolic syndrome have been increased among younger adults.
- Predominant causes for stroke differ in different age groups. Atherosclerosis, small vessel disease, and atrial fibrillation are the main causes of stroke in the older adults yet the causes of ischemic stroke in younger adults are diversified.
- Treatment protocol for acute stroke is essentially the same for young and old patients, with a focus on administration of tissue plasminogen activator as a first-line treatment.

Keywords Stroke • Intracranial hemorrhage • Atrial fibrillation • Hypertension • Hyperlipidemia • Diabetic mellitus • Coagulopathy • Dissection • Carotid stenosis • Small vessel disease

Abbreviations

Afib	Atrial fibrillation
AVM	Arterial venous malformation
CADASIL	Cerebral autosomal dominant arteriopathy with subcortical infarcts and leukoencephalopathy

M. Lu, M.D., Ph.D. (✉)
Cerebrovascular Center, Neurological Institute, Cleveland Clinic,
9500 Euclid Avenue/S80, Cleveland, OH 44195, USA
e-mail: lum@ccf.org

M.L. Corrigan et al. (eds.), *Handbook of Clinical Nutrition and Stroke*,
Nutrition and Health, DOI 10.1007/978-1-62703-380-0_9,
© Springer Science+Business Media New York 2013

DM	Diabetes mellitus
FMD	Fibromuscular dysplasia
HTN	Hypertension
MTHFR	Methylenetetrahydrofolate reductase
PFO	Patent foramen ovale
RCVS	Reversible cerebral vasoconstriction syndrome
TPA	Tissue plasminogen activator

Introduction

Stroke is one of the leading causes of morbidity and mortality. The etiology of stroke is diversified and can occur within different age groups; however, the incidence of stroke is more common in elder adults and relatively less in the younger adults. Interestingly, etiologies leading to stroke in younger adults have a wide range of etiologies. Therefore, correctly identifying underlying causes for stroke is essential for the effective treatment of stroke and secondary stroke prevention.

Stroke is one of the most common causes of disabilities in the human society, the fourth most prevalent cause of mortality in the United States, after heart diseases, cancer, and lung disease. The incidence is about 795,000 patients per year to have stroke including new and recurrent stroke. The deaths rate from stroke has declined in the United States [1].

Stroke can be divided into ischemic stroke, due to lack of blood flow of cerebral arterial or venous system, or hemorrhagic stroke, a nontraumatic intracranial hemorrhage. Eighty percent of all stroke cases are due to ischemic stroke [2]. Stroke can occur in all age groups. Stroke is not a disease of a single etiology, but it is quite heterogeneous in its causes. In this chapter, ischemic stroke will be discussed.

Ischemic stroke can also be classified according to vessels affected, including venous, such as venous sinus thrombosis, and arterial strokes. The etiologies of arterial ischemic stroke include large vessel disease, small vessel disease, central embolic (cardioembolic, hypercoagulation), and other etiologies, such as dissection, patent foramen ovale (PFO), or unknown etiologies [3]. The severity of the stroke and subsequent morbidity and mortality depend on the size and location of the lesion, age, and other existing comorbidities. The causes for stroke differ in among differing age groups. Several risk factors for stroke can coexist such as large vessel disease, small vessel disease, and cardioembolic stroke due to similar underlying risk factors. Therefore, it is important to thoroughly evaluate the patient with stroke, for effective secondary prevention.

Pathological processes leading to an ischemic stroke can be classified as vascular atherosclerosis of large artery, non-atherosclerotic vasculopathy, usually associated with genetic defects and commonly causes carotid or vertebral arterial dissections, such as fibromuscular dysplasia (FMD), infection, inflammatory, or drug-induced vasculitis. Small artery disease includes hypertension, diabetes mellitus, hyperlipidemia, cerebral autosomal dominant arteriopathy with subcortical infarcts and leukoencephalopathy (CADASIL), and Fabry disease. Central embolic stroke includes cardiogenic embolism from atrial fibrillation (afib), valvular disease, and ventricular thrombosis from low cardiac ejection fraction and aortic arch atheroma. Many hematological disorders can produce hypercoagulable states and high viscosity disorder, causing embolic stroke as well. Other etiology includes mitochondrial disorder such as mitochondrial encephalomyopathy, lactic acidosis, and stroke-like episodes (MELAS). Stroke of unknown etiologies accounts for about 30 % of cases which also includes probable unidentified metabolic and genetic causes [4].

Predominant causes for stroke differ in different age groups. Atherosclerosis, small vessel disease, and atrial fibrillation are the main causes of stroke in the older adults. However the causes of ischemic stroke in younger adult are diversified. Despite the fact that cardiogenic embolisms are common in older adults with stroke due to afib. It is also common among younger patients with stroke and accounts for about 20 % of all strokes but with differing etiologies, mostly caused by valvular disease, PFO, cardiomyopathy, endocarditis, and cardiac mass [5]. Several of stroke mechanisms, such as small vessel disease, large vessel atherosclerosis, and atrial fibrillation could coexist, since the pathologies shares the common risk factors. Therefore, it is important to thoroughly analyze the patient with stroke and identify its causes for a better secondary prevention and treatment.

Ischemic Stroke in Old Patients

The incidence of stroke is highest among older adults, as over 80 % of strokes occur in the people 65 years of age or more [1]. Hypertension, diabetes mellitus, hyperlipidemia, obesity, inactivity, and age are the most common risk factors for stroke in this population. The outcome after the stroke is highly influenced by age. The increased vulnerability of elderly people to ischemic stroke is associated with changes that occur in the aged brain. In addition, presence of obstructive sleep apnea also plays a role in older patients with stroke.

The common stroke mechanisms in older patient include embolic stroke from arterial to arterial embolization and hypoperfusion from large vessel atherosclerotic changes (such as carotid stenosis and/or occlusion, vertebral stenosis, or intracranial vascular stenosis/occlusion), small vessel disease due to HTN, DM, hyperlipidemia, smoking, and cardioembolic stroke from afib and aortic arch atheroma or hypercoagulation state. Infections such as gout, urinary tract infections, or pneumonia are common in older patient, which can cause the worsening the atherosclerotic plaque, increasing inflammation and prothrombotic triggering events that could lead to the occurrence of ischemic stroke.

Statistically, with increased age above 80s, the cardioembolic stroke risk tends to increase dramatically due to atrial fibrillation [6]. Anticoagulation is the most effective secondary prevention for stroke caused by atrial fibrillation. Advanced age by itself is not a contraindication for anticoagulation [7]. In addition to atrial fibrillation, atheroma formation in the aortic arch and ascending aorta, cardiomyopathy with low ejection fraction of ischemic nature, subclinical myocardial infarction, and valvular degenerative changes are also central embolic sources for stroke in this group of patients.

Hypercoagulable states are increased in the elderly patient populations. Increased age is an independent risk factor for risk for hypercoagulation. Further, with increased age, the incidence and prevalence of malignancy are increased. It is well-known that acquired hypercoagulated states have been associated with certain malignancy, including leukemia and adenocarcinomas.

Since atherosclerosis is the major contributing risk factor for acute stroke, primary and secondary prevention for risk factor modification has been proven itself to be cost-effective. Effective stroke prevention and treatment requires combination of efforts from physicians and patients to modify the risk factors, including healthy diet and exercise.

Ischemic Stroke in Young Patient

Current data shows stroke is more common in young patients than previously thought. In recent years, there is a trend of an increase in stroke rate among younger adults. The rate of premature atherosclerosis has been increased with the rise in HTN, DM, obesity, physical inactivity, and metabolic syndrome among younger patients [1]. Although less common than in elderly patients with stroke, the risk factors such as hyperlipidemia, hypertension, and smoking are becoming the common risk factors for stroke in younger patient [5].

Nonartherosclerotic large vessel angiopathy is another common cause for ischemic stroke in younger patient. Cervicocephalic arterial dissection (10–25 %), carotid, and/or vertebral dissection are the most common causes among others. Possible etiologies for dissection include trauma and connective tissue disease (such as Ehlers-Danlos syndrome, Marfan's syndrome, Pseudoxanthoma elasticum, fibromuscular dysplasia). Inflammatory vasculitis, such as Takayasu's disease, in contrast to temporal arteritis in older adult, is relatively more common [8].

Congenital heart disease such as PFO and potential right to left shunt heart or vascular disease such as pulmonary arterial venous malformation (AVM) are important factors causing paradoxical embolic stroke for younger adult.

It is well-known that the genetic disorders such as homocysteinuria, Fabry's, MELAS, and CADASIL syndrome can cause stroke in younger patients. Homocysteinuria is a cause for premature atherosclerosis in younger patient, in addition to common risk factors (such as smoking, hypertension, diabetes mellitus, hyperlipidemia). This condition may respond to folic acid, pyridoxine, vitamin B12, and dietary therapy, but current data for the efficacy of treatment is controversial (see Chap. 7).

Illicit drugs such as cocaine, heroin and phencyclidine, and estrogen hormone therapy are contributors to stroke in the young adult group. After excluding the previous contributors, moyamoya, primary CNS vasculitis, and reversible cerebral vasoconstriction syndrome (RCVS) are other possible etiologies.

Migraine is believed as an important cause of ischemic stroke by some investigators in younger population even though they can be a prodrome of an embolic event from PFO or arterial dissections. Its contribution varied from 4 to 20 % based on literature. Stroke risk is higher among younger patients with migraine [9]. The direct association between migraine and stroke is still in search.

Hypercoagulable state including acquired and congential condition, such as disseminated intravascular coagulation, thrombocytosis, polycythemia vera, and thrombotic thrombocytopenic purpura and sickle-cell disease, homocysteinemia, deficiency of antithromin III, protien C or S, increased factor VIII, factor V leiden, factor II and MTHFR Mutations, is risk factor for stroke, In addition, hypercoagulation can be due to immunomediated process, such as antiphospholipid syndrome.

Stroke from venous occlusion is less commonly seen in clinical practice comparing to arterial stroke. Their causes include dehydration, para-meningeal infection, meningitis, neoplasm, birth control medication use, polycythemia, leukemia, inflammatory bowel diseases. Among the genetic cause, factor V Leiden mutation; G20210A is the most common cause for venous stroke. Sickle-cell disease should be considered in young African descendents. Malignancy such as leukemia and adenocarcinoma is also commonly presented as stroke as their first presentation. Certain malignancies are associated with positive lupus anticoagulants which can cause hypercoagulative states.

Clinical Presentation

Stroke often presents with sudden onset of neurological deficits. The signs and symptoms are depending on the area and anatomic location being affected. There is no significant difference in the neurological changes in younger patients compared to older patients. However, with the same location, degree of brain damage, and collateral flow, the initial deficit could be worse and less localized with associated encephalopathy in older patient due to decreased brain function reserve (previous insults, atrophy) and brain functional decompensation. Since stroke has variety etiologies, it is important to get specific information from history and physical examination to help to elucidate the underlying etiology.

It is important to investigate the common risk factors including HTN, DM, hyperlipidemia, obesity, smoking, physical inactivity, and excessive alcohol use. Evaluation for peripheral vascular disease, carotid disease, coronary artery disease, heart failure with low ejection fraction, cardiac arrhythmia (particularly atrial fibrillation), and history of blood clot formation (deep vein thrombosis) is essential. These findings are important for young and older stroke patients with possible etiologies from large vessel atherosclerosis, small vessel disease, and central and cardioembolic stroke. Particularly, thorough evaluation is important for possible paroxysmal atrial fibrillation in elderly patient, since the efficacy of secondary prevention with anticoagulation versus antiplatelet therapy differs significantly.

In younger patients, additional information is crucial, since there is a wide range of possible etiologies for stroke. Patients with history of migraine, headache, neck pain, recent neck injury, or manipulation are important clues to consider migraine-related stroke, dissection (especially with Horner's syndrome), intracranial hemorrhage, and even possible subarachnoid hemorrhage. Family history of connective tissue diseases, hyperextensible skin and hyperflexible joint, and dislocation of lens on the examination are suggestive of connective tissue disease such as Ehlers-Danlos syndrome and Marfan's syndrome. History of birth control medication use or hormone replacement is important for female patient with both arterial and venous ischemic stroke. Skin rash, ocular abnormality, joint problem, and other organ involvement are suggestive of possible autoimmune connective tissue diseases. Bruit from large vessels, asymmetry in blood pressure, and decreased pulse are indicative of vascular abnormality. History of African descent, anemia, and bleeding tendency are clues for stroke (ischemic, seen in patient with sickle-cell disease, or hemorrhagic intracranial hemorrhage). Stroke related to endocarditis is suspected in patients with history of fever and/or intravenous drug use. In patients with lobar hemorrhage, history of dementia is important, since amyloid angiopathy is associated with Alzheimer's disease. If a patient has a history or family history of multisystem involvement such as myopathy (muscle pain/weakness) and/or small fiber neuropathy (autonomic dysfunction/disturbance of skin sensation), then metabolic causes, including mitochondrial disorder or Fabry disease, should be considered. It is crucial to have a complete history and physical examination performed related to signs and symptoms caused by stroke.

Evaluation

If infection is suspected for younger patients with embolic stroke from drug use or endocarditis, blood cultures with endocarditis protocol are mandatory. Normally for younger patients with evidence of embolic stroke and negative intravenous drug use history, laboratory work up for hypercoagulation and rheumatological work up are strongly indicated. Serial cardiac enzymes are indicated if having history of chest pain, acute heart failure, arrhythmia, and EKG changes to evaluate for possible myocardial infarction-related stroke.

Imaging studies of brain and cerebral blood vessels are mandatory for acute stroke patients. Computerized topography (CT) of brain is usually the initial imaging study to evaluate subarachnoid, intracranial, and intraventricular hemorrhage. If MRI of brain is not readily available, CT study can be used to evaluate venous sinus thrombosis because it usually presented as hemorrhagic ischemic stroke. CT is fast, easily available, less expensive, and very sensitive to hemorrhagic changes, but not sensitive enough for early ischemic changes when comparing to MRI.

MRI of the brain can provide more detailed information regarding acute ischemic stroke, especially small stroke or an old stroke. MRI is very important for detecting embolic stroke, involving multiple vascular territories for early detection of stroke (in minutes). In addition, MRI of the brain can provide information regarding microbleeding, which could be from hypertension, or a sign of amyloid angiopathy. MRI of brain can provide important information regarding possible etiologies according to the size, shape, and pattern of the infarction area. For example, a small lacunar infarction in the pons is likely due to small vessel disease, related to hypertension, diabetes mellitus, hyperlipidemia, and smoking. However, a stroke in the watershed zone on one side of the brain is likely due to large vessel atherosclerosis, such as carotid stenosis, or dissection due to impaired flow.

It is crucial to evaluate the status of aortic, cervical, and intracranial arteries for stroke diagnosis and treatment as well as secondary stroke prevention. In addition, carotid ultrasound, transcranial Doppler, CT angiogram, and MR angiogram are very important to identify involved vascular lesions. The conventional angiogram is the gold standard but has become optional. The provider can select between CT angiogram or MR angiogram depending on the cost, complications, sensitivity and false-positive rate, patient's clinical conditions, and comorbidities. Sometime, more than one modality is required to obtain an accurate assessment for stroke patients. For example, CTA can overestimate the degree of stenosis when there is significant calcification, which can be confirmed by other modality, such as MRA, or carotid ultrasound or angiogram. Transcranial Doppler is an excellent tool to evaluate suspected embolic event with emboli monitoring, right to left shunt with bubble study (PFO or pulmonary AVM), and cerebral vascular reserve with breath-holding test.

Cardiac evaluation for acute stroke is necessary. Routine EKG is necessary to evaluate for possible left ventricular hypertrophy, arrhythmia, and ischemic changes. In addition, cardiac monitoring, including long-term monitoring as outpatient are important especially in older adult suspicious for paroxymal atrial fibrillation or flutter and sick sinus syndrome. Transthoracic echocardiogram will be helpful to evaluate left ventricular function, cardiac valvular diseases, and possible PFO with contrast. Transesophageal echocardiogram is more sensitive for atrial thrombus detection, vegetation on the valve, and atheroma detection of aortic arch, which are also possible sources of central embolic stroke. In elderly patients with embolic stroke, but without obvious cardioembolic etiologies, hypercoagulable states, or malignancy need to be evaluated in patients with family history of clot formation, malignancy, history of recurrent venous thrombosis, unexplained weight loss, and profound venous or arterial thrombosis.

Treatment

Treatment protocol for acute stroke is basically the same for younger patients as well as older patients. The first-line treatment is intravenous thrombolysis with tissue plasminogen activator (TPA) within 3 h window of onset of initial stroke symptoms [10]. Currently, the studies suggest the benefit of TPA could extend up to 4.5 h in selected patients. In the trial, the patient's age is limited to under 80 years old, since the hemorrhagic rate may be higher in older patient [11]. For patients who are not candidates for TPA, or patient with large vessel stenosis/occlusion which could not be recanalized by TPA, endovascular recanalization may be beneficial. In additional to recanalization, medical treatment is important to correct underlying medical problems such as fever, uncontrolled hypertension, hypotension, hypo/hyperglycemia, and underlying infections. For symptomatic carotid stenosis (>70 %), it is recommend to have surgery done as soon as possible normally within 2 weeks for secondary stroke prevention [12]. In addition, it is important to prevent and treat early for stroke complications, including dysphagia, aspiration pneumonia, deep vein thrombosis, pressure ulcer, orthostatic hypotension, and major depression.

For secondary ischemic stroke prevention, in addition to risk factors, control antiplatelet treatment is advised for atherosclerotic etiology, and anticoagulation is indicated for central embolic stroke such as atrial fibrillation [13] and hypercoagulation state. For young patients with uncommon etiologies, specific treatment is needed. For example, blood transfusion is beneficial for stroke related to sickle-cell disease. Enzyme replacement may be beneficial for the patient with Fabry disease. The effect of vitamin supplements remains controversial in treatment of patients with hyperhomocysteinemia (see Chap. 6). Immunosuppression therapy is essential for patient with underlying vasculitis and related autoimmune diseases. There is no proven benefit for PFO closure over medical treatment at this time for secondary stroke prevention [14].

Conclusion

Stroke is a syndrome, with diverse etiologies, It can occur in patient from all age group. However, the likelihood of etiology for stroke is different in patient from different age group. Correction diagnosis of underlying etiology of stroke is crucial for the effective treatment and secondary prevention.

References

1. Roger VL, Go AS, Lloyd-Jones DM, Benjamin EJ, Berry JD, Borden WB, et al. American Heart Association Statistics Committee and Stroke Statistics Subcommittee. Executive summary: heart disease and stroke statistics-2012 update: a report from the American Heart Association. Circulation. 2012;125(1):188–97.
2. Donnan GA, Fisher M, Macleod M, Davis SM. Stroke. Lancet. 2008;371(9624):1612–23.
3. Adams Jr HP, Bendixen BH, Kappelle LJ, Biller J, Love BB, Gordon DL, et al. Classification of subtype of acute ischemic stroke. Definitions for use in a multicenter clinical trial. TOAST. Trial of Org 10172 in Acute Stroke Treatment. Stroke. 1993;24:35–41.

4. Cotter PE, Belham M, Martin PJ. Towards understanding the cause of stroke in young adults utilising a new stroke classification system (A-S-C-O). Cerebrovasc Dis. 2012;33(2):123–7.
5. Putaala J, Metso AJ, Metso TM, Konkola N, Kraemer Y, Haapaniemi E, et al. Analysis of 1008 consecutive patients aged 15 to 49 with first-ever ischemic stroke: the Helsinki young stroke registry. Stroke. 2009;40(4):1195–203.
6. Riley AB, Manning WJ. Atrial fibrillation: an epidemic in the elderly. Expert Rev Cardiovasc Ther. 2011;9(8):1081–90.
7. Marinigh R, Lip GY, Fiotti N, Giansante C, Lane DA. Age as a risk factor for stroke in atrial fibrillation patients implications for thromboprophylaxis: Implications for thromboprophylaxis. J Am Coll Cardiol. 2010;56(11):827–37.
8. Camilo O, Goldstein LB. Non-atherosclerotic vascular disease in the young. J Thromb Thrombolysis. 2005;20(2):93–103.
9. Bousser MG, Welch KM. Relation between migraine and stroke. Lancet Neurol. 2005;4(9): 533–42.
10. Tissue plasminogen activator for acute ischemic stroke. The National Institute of Neurological Disorders and Stroke rt-PA Stroke Study Group. N Engl J Med. 1995;333(24):1581–7.
11. Hacke W, Kaste M, Bluhmki E, Brozman M, Dávalos A, Guidetti D, et al. ECASS Investigators. Thrombolysis with alteplase 3 to 4.5 hours after acute ischemic stroke. N Engl J Med. 2008;359(13):1317–29.
12. Rothwell PM, Eliasziw M, Gutnikov SA, Warlow CP, Barnett HJ. Endarterectomy for symptomatic carotid stenosis in relation to clinical subgroups and timing of surgery. Carotid Endarterectomy Trialists Collaboration. Lancet. 2004;363(9413):915–24.
13. Saxena R, Koudstaal P. Anticoagulants versus antiplatelet therapy for preventing stroke in patients with nonrheumatic atrial fibrillation and a history of stroke or transient ischemic attack. Cochrane Database Syst Rev. 2004 (4):CD000187.
14. Kutty S, Sengupta PP, Khandheria BK. Patent foramen ovale: the known and the to be known. J Am Coll Cardiol. 2012;59(19):1665–71.

Part III
Medical Management of Stroke

Chapter 10
Medical Management of Stroke

William S. Tierney and J. Javier Provencio

Key Points

- The acute management of stroke involves understanding both the location and the underlying cause of the stroke to effectively treat the patient.
- Early recognition and treatment of acute ischemic stroke with tissue plasminogen activator is the most effective treatment available to the majority of patients.
- Hemorrhagic stroke types are less common than ischemic stroke, but their treatments are completely different and mistakes in diagnosis are potentially catastrophic.
- The delivery of appropriate substrates to the brain as soon after injury is critical to maximize the potential for recovery.

Keywords Stroke • Medical management • Intracerebral hemorrhage • Subarachnoid hemorrhage • Substrate delivery

Abbreviations

CT   Non-Contrast Computed Tomography
DCI   Delayed Cerebral Ischemia
DCV   Delayed Cerebral Vasospasm

W.S. Tierney, M.S. (✉)
Cleveland Clinic Foundation, Cleveland Clinic Lerner College of Medicine,
Cleveland, OH, USA
e-mail: tiernew@ccf.org

J.J. Provencio, M.D., F.C.C.M.
Cerebrovascular Center and Neuroscience, Neurologic Institute, Cleveland Clinic,
Cleveland Clinic Lerner College of Medicine, Cleveland, OH, USA
e-mail: provenj@ccf.org

M.L. Corrigan et al. (eds.), *Handbook of Clinical Nutrition and Stroke*,   139
Nutrition and Health, DOI 10.1007/978-1-62703-380-0_10,
© Springer Science+Business Media New York 2013

DDAV   Delayed Deterioration Associated with Vasospasm
ICH   Intracerebral Hemorrhage
NIHSS   NIH Stroke Scale
rt-PA   Recombinant Tissue Plasminogen Activator

Introduction

Stroke is defined as an acute neurologic deficit ascribable to a vascular territory. Today we understand stroke as either an acute ischemic event from occlusion of a cerebral artery, subarachnoid hemorrhage usually from the rupture of an aneurysm or trauma, intracerebral hemorrhage from the rupture of a small intracerebral artery, or cerebral vein thrombosis. We will discuss the first three in this chapter.

Ischemic Stroke

Ischemic stroke is the most common stroke subtype and can be traced to several different etiologies: thrombosis within the cerebral arteries, the lodging of an embolism within one of these arteries, and hypoperfusion insults caused by lowering of the blood pressure. The pathophysiology of ischemic stroke stems from decreased or eliminated blood flow in a cerebral artery, and symptoms are specific to the vessels affected. The region of brain tissue affected by a stroke has two parts: a core that is comprised of dead brain tissue and a rim around the core that has injured, but not dead, brain cells referred to as the "ischemic penumbra." Within minutes of the initial ischemic event, the affected areas, core and penumbra, cease to show activity. If some blood flow remains in the penumbra, the silenced neurons may have the potential to recover. However, after blood flow falls below a threshold, the neurons within the ischemic penumbra quickly become irreparably damaged [1]. The distribution of pathology and symptoms is determined by which blood vessels are affected, the existence of collateral blood vessels which may provide nutrients to the affected tissue, and the function of the specific brain region in question. Medical management aims to maximize the amount of brain tissue which survives and to limit secondary damage caused by the body's response to the stroke.

An understanding of the circulation serving the brain allows the astute clinician to anticipate the effects of a stroke, predict and avoid secondary complications, and prepare for rehabilitation. The brain is supplied via three major arterial sources: the bilateral internal carotid arteries and the posterior basilar artery. These three sources are connected via the circle of Willis. This arterial circle allows the major arteries of the brain to provide assistance to one another if one becomes occluded. While this collateral flow is protective against some cerebrovascular pathologies, sudden events (hemorrhage, thrombus formation, or embolism) usually result in ischemic damage because the arteries of the circle cannot respond with increased collateral flow quickly enough to maintain perfusion. Of course, ischemic events which occur distal to the circle of Willis will cause damage if other collateral blood vessels cannot assist. To approach the treatment of ischemic strokes, it is best to break the progression into three phases: the acute phase, the secondary phase, and the rehabilitation phase.

Diagnosis

During the acute phase, the clinician's primary goal is to restore cerebral blood flow and thereby minimize ischemic damage to the brain. This phase begins with stroke onset and persists until the edema, which often accompanies stroke, has subsided. Because the longer the period of ischemia the worse the outcome, reaching a correct diagnosis quickly is important. There are several clinical tools used to aid the prehospital responder (EMTs and ambulance personnel) in the recognition and diagnosis of stroke. Is the Recognition of Stroke in the Emergency Rooms (ROSIER) Scale [2] which attributes one point to the acute onset of each (1) asymmetric facial weakness, (2) asymmetric arm weakness, (3) asymmetric leg weakness, (4) speech disturbance, and (5) visual field defects, and then subtracts one point if a loss of consciousness/syncope has occurred, or if the patient demonstrates seizure activity. If the total, which falls within the range of -2 and 5, is greater than 0 AND in the absence of hypoglycemia, a diagnosis of stroke or transient ischemic attack is made. A simplified version of this test is the Fast Arm Speech Test (FAST) [3]. Using this method, the clinician suspects stroke if any of three factors is present: facial asymmetry, arm/leg weakness, and speech disturbance. The ROSIER Scale predicts stroke with a sensitivity of 82 % and a specificity of 42 %, while the FAST Scale has a sensitivity of 82 % and a specificity of 37 %. Diagnoses based on initial impression of clinical staff maintain a sensitivity of 77 % and a specificity of 58 % [4]. Other comparable tools exist with similar sensitivities and specificities.

The NIH Stroke Scale (NIHSS) is the most widely used and accepted tool for analyzing the severity of stroke by clinicians. This test can be administered as soon as the patient is suspected of having a stroke and its results predict outcome after stroke with good specificity and sensitivity [5]. The NIHSS uses 11 questions to assess symptoms of cerebrovascular disease and is comprehensive without requiring a lengthy neurological examination. The final result of the test, which can be administered by a trained professional in 11 min, is a score between 0 and 42. A score of 0 represents a non-symptomatic patient, while a score of 18 or greater represents a patient with severe stroke.

Imaging is a crucial step in determining therapy options for stroke patients and the acquisition of clinically useful imaging must therefore be pursued as soon as stroke is suspected. Non-contrast computed tomography (CT) is the most widely used imaging modality and is especially important in separating hemorrhagic from ischemic stroke. Because the treatment of these two diseases is quite different, it is crucial that this distinction be made early and before clot-dissolving treatment. CT has its shortcomings in that its resolution is limited immediately after stroke. Contrast angiographic CT (CTA) and CT perfusion (CTP) are becoming more widely used in some centers because of their ability to define regions of insufficient perfusion. At present, magnetic resonance imaging (MRI) is the optimal imaging technique for the definitive diagnosis of stroke. In a study [6], noncontrast CT has only 26 % sensitivity for the detection of early ischemia, while MRI has a sensitivity of 83 %. Additionally, MRI is effective in the detection of hemorrhagic versus ischemic stroke and therefore should be a part of each workup after a patient is admitted to a stroke service. It should be noted however that in many hospitals expedient MRI imaging may be impossible. Imaging of the extracranial carotid arteries is also recommended to rule out occlusive carotid disease or basilar occlusion.

The First Three (Four-and-a-Half) Hours

The immediate clinical goal after a diagnosis of ischemic stroke is to achieve reperfusion of the occluded vasculature. The only drug approved for this purpose is recombinant tissue plasminogen activator (rt-PA), a potent clot-dissolving (thrombolytic) agent. The intravenous administration of rt-PA is approved by the FDA within 3 h of ischemic stroke, but the American Stroke Association suggests administration up to 4.5 h after the ischemic event in appropriate patients based on clinical findings of clinical trials [7]. After stroke, transportation to a hospital, triage, imaging, and diagnosis, even this 4.5 h window becomes a challenging standard to meet in all but the most efficient modern hospital systems. As a thrombolytic agent, rt-PA should only be used to treat ischemic strokes because it will promote catastrophic bleeding into the brain parenchyma of the hemorrhagic stroke patient, so attention to diagnostic detail during this brief treatment window is of paramount importance. Therefore, as soon as a diagnosis of acute ischemic stroke has been reached, rt-PA should be administered to reestablish blood flow to the affected area. Earlier administration is associated with better clinical outcome [8]. The odds ratio of a favorable outcome after rt-PA treatment of ischemic stroke is 2.55 if the rt-PA is administered within 90 min of stroke, 1.64 if administered 91–180 min after stroke, 1.34 if administered 181–270 min after stroke, and 1.22 if administered 271–360 min after stroke [8].

Managing Secondary Damage of Ischemic Stroke

During the secondary phase, the clinical team aims to limit secondary damages of ischemic stroke. The most dangerous complication of using rt-PA is the development of post-thrombolysis intracranial hemorrhage. While the action of rt-PA as a "clot-buster" makes it the modern standard for medical treatment of ischemic stroke, it also decreases the capacity of the blood to generate clots in response to hemorrhage. It should be made clear that the benefit of rt-PA administration justifies the relatively minor risk of intracerebral hemorrhage following intravenous thrombolytic therapy. About 6 % of individuals who receive intravenous rt-PA for ischemic stroke suffer a subsequent intracerebral hemorrhage, usually with poor prognosis. Clinical trials have shown that rt-PA administration improve clinical outcomes without changing mortality rates [9].

The mechanism of this increased chance for hemorrhage is due to damage to the blood vessels of the brain which lie within the ischemic penumbra. The ischemic conditions cause these vessels to lose some or all of their autoregulatory capacity, and reestablishment of blood flow into these damaged vascular beds is accompanied by increased likelihood that the compromised vessels will rupture. Certain clinical and laboratory factors have been found to increase the rate of intracerebral hemorrhage following rt-PA administration. These include thrombocytopenia, hyperfibrinogenemia, low plasminogen activator inhibitor levels, low-density lipoprotein-bound cholesterol, baseline serum glucose, and/or history of diabetes mellitus [10]. However, based on current medical standards, these factors do not necessarily preclude rt-PA administration and clinical judgment based on the size and location of the stroke, the expected prognosis without thrombolytic therapy, and patient and/or patient family preference. It is worth reiterating that, on the whole, ischemic stroke patients who qualify benefit from rt-PA administration despite the increased risk of hemorrhage.

In the event of an intracerebral hemorrhage following thrombolytic treatment of ischemic stroke, treatment strategies generally aim to restore clotting function in an attempt to limit hemorrhage. Studies of these therapies are lacking in the literature because of the rare instance of post-thrombolysis intracerebral hemorrhage and because of the severity of the condition. Accepted therapies include the administration of procoagulants often used to treat intracerebral hemorrhage, aminocaproic acid, fresh frozen plasma/cryoprecipitate, and the infusion of platelets. Furthermore, thrombolytic therapy should be discontinued and blood pressure should be maintained within normal physiological ranges. In patients who express symptoms of intracerebral hemorrhage, clot evacuation is recommended and has been show to improve outcomes after peripheral thrombolysis [8].

Hemorrhage: Intracerebral Hemorrhage and Subarachnoid Hemorrhage

Intracranial hemorrhage is caused by a bleed rather than a blockage of a blood vessel. Hemorrhages can be divided based on the location of blood into two broad subgroups: subarachnoid hemorrhage and intracerebral hemorrhage. Subarachnoid hemorrhages occur in the subarachnoid space (see Fig. 10.1; meningeal compartments with stroke locations), while intracerebral hemorrhages occur in small vessels which branch directly into the brain parenchyma.

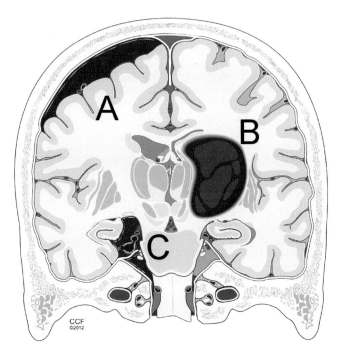

Fig. 10.1 The three types of stroke discussed in this chapter are ischemic stroke, intracerebral hemorrhage, and subarachnoid hemorrhage. (**a**) Hematomas, such as the subdural hematoma shown here, represent another class of intracranial bleeds. Ischemic stroke is caused by the blockage of a cerebral vessel either by an embolic event or a thrombotic event inside the vessel. The damage is primarily due to the loss of blood flow to the territory blocked off by the clot. (**b**) An intracerebral hemorrhage occurs when a small vessel branching into the brain ruptures and a blood clot forms in the brain. ICH causes its primary damage through the rapid accumulation of blood within the brain and the resulting compression of the surrounding tissue. (**c**) Subarachnoid hemorrhage occurs when a cerebral aneurysm bursts in the subarachnoid space surrounding the brain. Blood quickly fills the cerebrospinal fluid space near the bleeding vessel and causes increased intracranial pressure, which results in pressure-related brain damage (reprinted with permission, Cleveland Clinic Center for Medical Art & Photography © 2012. All Rights Reserved)

Diagnosis of hemorrhage is a key component of appropriate stroke treatment. Because the rt-PA treatment of ischemic stroke can significantly increase bleeding, incorrect diagnoses of a hemorrhage poses an additional threat to patient well-being. Unlike ischemic stroke, hemorrhages often lead to headache. The hallmark symptom of subarachnoid hemorrhage is the development of an intense headache which patients will usually describe as the worst they have ever experienced [11]. Additional symptoms typically include loss of consciousness, nausea, vomiting, retinal hemorrhage, focal neurological signs, and meningismus [12]. Primary hemorrhages may be more difficult to differentiate from ischemic stroke as they often present with hemiparesis, headache, and no other symptoms. Atypical presentations are relatively common and misdiagnoses can lead to worsening of patient condition;

non-contrast computed tomography (CT) scans are relied upon heavily in patients with suspected hemorrhage. CT scan has a sensitivity to detect hemorrhage of 90–100 % [13] when the scans are high quality, obtained using state-of-the-art equipment, and are read by a skilled technician.

Secondary measures to specifically diagnose SAH include obtaining a lumbar puncture to check for the presence of bilirubin in the CSF, a condition called xanthochromia. It can take as long as 12 h for xanthochromia to present and it persists as a clinical sign for 2 weeks following ictal event. Outside of this time frame, cerebral angiography supplies a definitive diagnosis of cerebral aneurysms if hemorrhagic lesion is observed. Nontraumatic subarachnoid hemorrhage is the result of a ruptured berry aneurysm in about 80 % of cases and the result of a non-aneurismal hemorrhagic event in the other 20 %.

Primary Intracerebral Hemorrhage Treatment

Intracerebral hemorrhage is usually the result of an arterial rupture in the small perforating arteries branching directly off of larger cerebrovascular arteries. Once a diagnosis of intracerebral hemorrhage (ICH) has been reached, primary treatment aims to minimize the involvement of the tissue surrounding the infarct. The initial intracerebral hemorrhage usually causes a rapid irreversible damage to the area immediately surrounding the bleed as the pressure of trapped blood within the cerebral parenchyma increases. Preventing rebleeding of the hemorrhage and taking measures to reduce the intracranial pressure are the primary goals of the physician in the acute phase of ICH. Critical care physicians should work to stabilize the mean arterial pressure below 125 mmHg [14] (or 160 mmHg systolic as recommended in the 2010 American Heart Association Guidelines [15]) for the first 6 h following hemorrhage to minimize hemorrhage expansion.

If imaging studies indicate that the hemorrhagic mass is large or if the patient begins to demonstrate signs of intracranial pressure (decreased alertness, oculomotor deficits, hemiparesis, nausea or vomiting, or decreases in vital signs), they should have an intracranial pressure monitoring device placed immediately. The most common intracranial pressure measurement device is an intraventricular catheter inserted through a hole in the skull, through the brain, and into one of the cerebral ventricles. Direct measurement of CSF pressure, a good indicator of global intracerebral pressure, can be acquired using this device, and it also acts as a shunt to drain off CSF and reduce ICP. Another option is an intraparenchymal pressure monitoring device. These devices measure pressure directly in the parenchyma of the brain and are less invasive than intraventricular catheterization, but they do not offer the therapeutic advantage of CSF drainage.

Measures to lower intracranial pressure should include keeping the patient sitting at an approximately 45° angle to maximize venous drainage through the jugular veins. CSF drainage, the mainstay of ICP control has been the use of osmotically active agents to increase the osmotic gradient between the blood and brain and therefore remove water from the cerebral interstitial space. In addition, increased plasma osmolarity causes a diuresis which further increases the gradient. There is considerable debate about whether osmotic agents work in the area of ischemia where the blood–brain barrier (the functional barrier that restricts solutes from entering and leaving the brain) function is disrupted. Mannitol is the most commonly used osmotic diuretic. The use of mannitol in intracerebral hemorrhage is well characterized and conceptually based on decreasing the amount of water in the brain parenchyma to reduce the intracranial pressure. Data for the use of mannitol in the treatment of intracerebral hemorrhage are mixed with no clear conclusions as to its efficacy across the entire population of ICH patients [16]. However, mannitol has been shown to improve markers of parenchymal metabolic function in patients with intracerebral hemorrhage [17] and investigation of its merits as a clinical treatment is still under way. Intravenous hypertonic saline solution has become more commonly administered to quickly draw water from the brain parenchyma and reduce intracerebral pressure in the same way as mannitol. It is an effective therapy for reducing intracranial pressure [18] but its use is still unsupported by large clinical trials. However, data seem to indicate that saline helps to improve brain metabolic and cerebrovascular function after ICH [19] and further research will help us fully understand the use of this injection in the ICH patient. Both treatments have significant side effects including pulmonary edema and volume overload which limit their use in patients with poor heart function.

A final treatment option for the ICH patient is surgical intervention. A few options exist. Craniectomy is the removal of a piece of the skull to allow the brain to expand beyond the constraints of the calvarium and therefore reduce the pressure caused by the confining skull [20]. This intervention has not been studied in a prospective trial. Alternately, surgical evacuation of the hemorrhage has been tested in the multinational STICH trial which showed no benefit versus surgery. Because of the results of this trial, evacuation is not recommended universally although considerable interest remains in looking for subsets of patients who may respond to evacuation, particularly if it is less invasive than open craniotomy [21]. A trial is underway to determine if stereotactically placed external catheters into the hemorrhage bed followed by administration of tPa may be beneficial in the treatment of ICH.

Subarachnoid Hemorrhage Treatment

Subarachnoid hemorrhage from aneurysm rupture represents only 3 % of strokes but accounts for a disproportionate 25 % of lost life-years due to stroke. Other causes of SAH include trauma, arterial dissections, drug use, and various minor causes. Patients with SAH must be stabilized before treatment can be attempted. Many aneurysms result in the depression of respiration and other vital automatic functions. The first goal of the team must therefore be to stabilize these vital functions before directed treatment can begin.

The first goal of SAH treatment aims to decrease the likelihood that the aneurysm will rebleed and cause further damage. Rebleeding occurs in 15 % of patients within the first day after admission for SAH if the aneurysm is not secured [22] and the risk remains high for the 6 months following the ictal event. There are two strategies employed to reduce rebleeding risk. To temper the immediate risk, medical therapies take the stress from the damaged aneurysm. For a more permanent fix, surgical therapies obliterate the aneurysm. Medical management of SAH consists of lowering systemic blood pressure to decrease the sheer stress on the aneurysm. In addition, antiepileptic medications are often prescribed to decrease the risk of aneurysm re-rupture during the autonomic changes associated with seizures although there is considerable debate about whether this is a worthwhile treatment option.

Antifibrinolytic drugs, medications that promote clotting of blood in the aneurysm, have been used in some institutions but are not widely used throughout the United States. A number of trials [23, 24] have shown that while antifibrinolytic treatments successfully prevent rebleeding, they come at the cost of new blood clots resulting in ischemic strokes, heart attacks, or pulmonary emboli. Therefore, antifibrinolytic therapy is not recommended as a standard at this time.

Surgical intervention to prevent rebleeding after SAH has been the standard of care for post-SAH patients since such treatments became readily available in the 1950s. Microsurgical clipping of the ruptured aneurysm consists of opening the skull and placing a small clip around the most proximal part of the aneurysm (called the "neck"). Intravascular intervention is a relatively new technique for treating SAH [25]. The technique involves the insertion of a platinum coil coated in a procoagulant into the site of rupture to decrease rebleeding risk and promote vascular recovery. The technique is usually successful in closing the ruptured vessel and has low complication rates. The durability of coiling is still not as well understood as that of clipping the aneurysm.

Because intravascular technique success is impacted by the anatomy of the aneurysm (thick-necked aneurysms are difficult to coil) and the surgical technique is limited by vascular anatomy as well as posthemorrhage swelling, the choice to either coil or clip is not an easy one. A neurosurgeon, with or without a trained interventionalist, must make this determination case by case. Regardless of the method employed, early occlusion of a ruptured aneurysm is the most efficacious method of prevention of rebleeding. The standard in the United States is quickly becoming that aneurysm ablation should be accomplished before the second day in most cases.

Delayed Deterioration Associated with Vasospasm After SAH

There is a curious syndrome that occurs almost exclusively in patients with aneurismal SAH and accounts for a great deal of morbidity. Approximately one-third of SAH patients develop a syndrome of delayed deterioration associated with cerebral vasospasm. Interestingly, non-aneurismal SAH etiologies seem to be relatively free from this complication [26]. While the etiology of delayed cerebral deterioration remains unknown, strategies for treatment have shown to be marginally effective. Standard of care measures are based on clinical precedent rather than basic science concepts.

Over the years, this syndrome has had many names associated with it including cerebral vasospasm, delayed cerebral ischemia (DCI), and delayed cerebral vasospasm. We have chosen to call it delayed deterioration associated with vasospasm (DDAV) to indicate that we do not understand the cause.

Blood pressure management is the standard therapeutic option for the treatment of DDAV. Initially, prior to aneurysm clipping or coiling, blood pressure is kept very low to mitigate sheer forces and prevent rebleeding. In patients who develop DDAV, augmentation of blood pressure is thought to be beneficial. The theoretical basis of this treatment is that higher blood pressure will increase blood flow through spastic cerebral arteries ensuring blood flow to the areas of the brain they serve. There has not been a good scientific test of this theory. In an associated therapy, blood volume management is focused on increasing blood volume to ischemic areas of the brain. While no definitive guidelines exist, it is common practice to administer saline to ensure euvolemia and maintain blood pressure in the above normal range [27] to best promote cerebral perfusion. In many institutions, supplemental albumin is administered to augment blood volume. The administration of albumin is currently being tested in a clinical trial.

Blood glucose control is an evolving area of interest with conflicting results. Hyperglycemia has been shown to significantly worsen outcomes after SAH [28]. However, even moderate hypoglycemia is also associated with vasospasm and increased disability after SAH [29]. More shockingly, some patients with relatively normal blood glucose levels have been found to have severely decreased brain interstitial fluid glucose levels calling into question whether blood testing is the appropriate monitoring technique [30]. However, brain interstitial fluid testing still not part of common practice. It is recommended that normoglycemia be maintained throughout the SAH patient's hospital stay [31] to avoid negative impacts of both hypoglycemia and hyperglycemia. No optimal blood-glucose range has been agreed upon to date, and this is a clinical target for SAH research. In our institution, as of the writing of this book, we use a goal of 100–150 mg/dl of glucose in the blood to prevent both severe hyperglycemia and severe hypoglycemia.

A number of pharmacologic therapies for DDAV have been employed or tested. The most commonly used is oral nimodipine, a calcium channel blocker. Interestingly, nimodipine does not prevent the associated vasospasm (vascular constriction) but improves outcome in patients who experience delayed deterioration. This drug was originally tested based on the theory that it would reduce cerebral vasospasm through interaction with vascular wall, but current understanding is that it exerts a neuroprotective effect independent of its vasoactive properties. In addition, HMG Co-A reductase inhibitors (statins) have been tested in small studies of patients with the theory that they are anti-inflammatory. Results are mixed, and they are used sporadically around the United States. Magnesium sulfate has also been tested in part because of its ability to block calcium channels but resulting trials have been disappointing.

Finally, a series of trials in humans to test increasingly potent vasodilators to counteract the cerebral vasospasm have all shown similar findings; cerebral vasospasm can be ameliorated but this does not improve patient outcome. This opens the possibility that the major injury from DDAV may not be ischemic. Recently, inflammation in the brain has been studied and promising preclinical data may support human trials in the near future.

The Role of Nutrition in ICU Therapies for Stroke

Interesting Historical SAH Treatments

In the 1970s through the 1990s, it was common practice in SAH to manage patients with a set of "SAH orders" based on loosely held theories and assumptions. The orders were based in two fundamental tenants: (1) that fluids administered to patients with cerebral edema leads to increased cerebral edema and (2) that the SAH patient is unable to effectively metabolize food. These lead to treatment algorithms that included minimal intravenous and oral fluids for up to 2 weeks and no food for up to a week. It is now known that both of these tenants are incorrect and, in fact, this strategy was likely detrimental to both cerebral edema prevention and patient outcome.

Modern Substrate Delivery in Stroke Care

The critical care management of patients with stroke aims to maintain regular homeostasis and prevent further neurological damage. Central to the issue of prevention of damage is the prevention of ischemia. Reduced oxygen and nutrient delivery to the tissues affected by the hemorrhage or ischemic stroke will increase the risk to damaged but recoverable brain cells. This concept is clinically applied by increasing cerebral substrate delivery through increasing perfusion pressure and blood volume [27]. It has been shown that in the setting of local hypoxia and interstitial glucose levels found in the brain's white matter correlate strongly with patient outcome in subarachnoid hemorrhage and traumatic brain injury [32, 33]. These data have led to the clinical definition of a neurological "metabolic crisis" as interstitial levels of glucose below 0.7 mmol/l and ratio of lactate/pyruvate of $\leq$40 [34]. Metabolic crisis is therefore an indicator or poor nutrient delivery to the brain as well as decreased aerobic metabolism. Metabolic crisis in the neurocritical patient has been shown to be a strong predictor of negative outcome [33]. In addition to supporting clinical practice regarding glycemic control and blood pressure management, the correlation of cerebral metabolic distress with decreased patient outcomes suggests that maintaining nutrient and oxygen levels carefully should be the clinical

Table 10.1
Characterization and treatment strategies for stroke

	Acute treatment	Chronic treatment	Rehabilitation
Acute Ischemic Stroke (AIS)	Open blocked vessel	Rescue the cells of the ischemic penumbra	Aggressive early rehabilitation.
Intracerebral Hemorrhage (ICH)	Normalize blood pressure	Manage increased cerebral pressure from edema	Depending on patient condition:
Subarachnoid Hemorrhage (SAH)	Lower blood pressure Secure the aneurysm	Manage delayed cerebral deterioration associated with vasospasm	• Cognitive rehabilitation • Motor rehabilitation • Occupational (fine motor) rehabilitation

standard of care for at least subarachnoid hemorrhage and probably all forms of stroke. For example, excessive shivering in the setting of fever has been shown to place a significant metabolic burden on the patient [35]. While intracranial catheters to measure metabolic data are currently not available widely for clinical management, research using these techniques has been enlightening thus far. More importantly, these techniques are challenging our assumptions of the optimal delivery of nutrients and oxygen to the brain. It is expected that advances in the near future may significantly change our understanding in nutrient delivery and our clinical practice.

Conclusion

In conclusion, the medical management of acute ischemic stroke, intracerebral hemorrhage, and subarachnoid hemorrhage is dependent on a rapid recognition of the correct diagnosis, rapid action to protect the brain, and a clear understanding of neuroanatomy to understand the ramifications of the resultant injury (see Table 10.1). Advances in care are continually being tested and evaluated for efficacy. It is very likely that in the near future, there will be new treatments for the different types of stroke. The real improvements may be in preventative measures, which are outside the scope of this chapter.

References

1. Bradley W. Neurology in clinical practice. 5th ed. Boston [u.a.], MA: Butterworth-Heinemann; 2008.
2. Nor AM, Davis J, Sen B, Shipsey D, Louw SJ, Dyker AG, et al. The Recognition of Stroke in the Emergency Room (ROSIER) scale: development and validation of a stroke recognition instrument. Lancet Neurol. 2005;4(11):727–34.

3. Nor AM, McAllister C, Louw SJ, Dyker AG, Davis M, Jenkinson D, et al. Agreement between ambulance paramedic- and physician-recorded neurological signs with Face Arm Speech Test (FAST) in acute stroke patients. Stroke. 2004;35(6):1355–9.
4. McArthur KS, Quinn TJ, Dawson J, Walters MR. Diagnosis and management of transient ischaemic attack and ischaemic stroke in the acute phase. BMJ. 2011;342((mar31 2)): d1938–8.
5. Adams Jr HP, Davis PH, Leira EC, Chang KC, Bendixen BH, Clarke WR, et al. Baseline NIH stroke scale score strongly predicts outcome after stroke: a report of the trial of Org 10172 in acute stroke treatment (TOAST). Neurology. 1999;53(1):126–31.
6. Chalela JA, Kidwell CS, Nentwich LM, Luby M, Butman JA, Demchuk AM, et al. Magnetic resonance imaging and computed tomography in emergency assessment of patients with suspected acute stroke: a prospective comparison. Lancet. 2007;369(9558):293–8.
7. Lansberg MG, Bluhmki E, Thijs VN. Efficacy and safety of tissue plasminogen activator 3 to 4.5 hours after acute ischemic stroke. Stroke. 2009;40(7):2438–41.
8. Lees KR, Bluhmki E, von Kummer R, Brott TG, Toni D, Grotta JC, et al. Time to treatment with intravenous alteplase and outcome in stroke: an updated pooled analysis of ECASS, ATLANTIS, NINDS, and EPITHET trials. Lancet. 2010;375(9727):1695–703.
9. Wahlgren N, Ahmed N, Dávalos A, Ford GA, Grond M, Hacke W, et al. Thrombolysis with alteplase for acute ischaemic stroke in the Safe Implementation of Thrombolysis in Stroke-Monitoring Study (SITS-MOST): an observational study. Lancet. 2007;369(9558): 275–82.
10. Sandercock PAG, Counsell C, Gubitz GJ, Tseng M-C. Antiplatelet therapy for acute ischaemic stroke. Cochrane Database Syst Rev. 2008;(3):CD000029.
11. Davenport R. Acute headache in the emergency department. J Neurol Neurosurg Psychiatry. 2002;72 suppl 2:ii33–7.
12. Edlow JA, Caplan LR. Avoiding pitfalls in the diagnosis of subarachnoid hemorrhage. N Engl J Med. 2000;342(1):29–36.
13. Manno EM. Subarachnoid hemorrhage. NeurolClin. 2004;22(2):347–66.
14. Owens WB. Blood pressure control in acute cerebrovascular disease. J Clin Hypertens. 2011;13(3):205–11.
15. Morgenstern LB, Hemphill 3rd JC, Anderson C, Becker K, Broderick JP, Connolly Jr ES, et al. Guidelines for the management of spontaneous intracerebral hemorrhage: a guideline for healthcare professionals from the American Heart Association/American Stroke Association. Stroke. 2010;41(9):2108–29.
16. Bereczki D, Fekete I, Prado GF, Liu M. Mannitol for acute stroke. Cochrane Database Syst Rev. 2007;(3):CD001153.
17. Helbok R, Kurtz P, Schmidt JM, Stuart RM, Fernandez L, Malhotra R, et al. Effect of mannitol on brain metabolism and tissue oxygenation in severe haemorrhagic stroke. J Neurol Neurosurg Psychiatr. 2011;82(4):378–83.
18. Qureshi AI, Suri MFK, Ringer AJ, Guterman LR, Hopkins LN. Regional intraparenchymal pressure differences in experimental intracerebral hemorrhage: effect of hypertonic saline. Crit Care Med. 2002;30(2):435–41.
19. Al-Rawi PG, Tseng M-Y, Richards HK, Nortje J, Timofeev I, Matta BF, et al. Hypertonic saline in patients with poor-grade subarachnoid hemorrhage improves cerebral blood flow, brain tissue oxygen, and pH. Stroke. 2010;41(1):122–8.
20. Chibbaro S, Di Rocco F, Mirone G, Fricia M, Makiese O, Di Emidio P, et al. Decompressive craniectomy and early cranioplasty for the management of severe head injury: a prospective multicenter study on 147 patients. World Neurosurg. 2011;75(3–4):558–62.
21. Siddique MS, Mendelow AD. Surgical treatment of intracerebral haemorrhage. Br Med Bull. 2000;56(2):444–56.
22. Hijdra A, Braakman R, van Gijn J, Vermeulen M, van Crevel H. Aneurysmal subarachnoid hemorrhage. Complications and outcome in a hospital population. Stroke. 1987;18(6): 1061–7.

23. Vermeulen M, Lindsay KW, Murray GD, Cheah F, Hijdra A, Muizelaar JP, et al. Antifibrinolytic treatment in subarachnoid hemorrhage. N Engl J Med. 1984;311(7):432–7.
24. Roos Y. Antifibrinolytic treatment in subarachnoid hemorrhage: a randomized placebo-controlled trial. STAR Study Group. Neurology. 2000;54(1):77–82.
25. Guglielmi G, Viñuela F, Duckwiler G, Dion J, Lylyk P, Berenstein A, et al. Endovascular treatment of posterior circulation aneurysms by electrothrombosis using electrically detachable coils. J Neurosurg. 1992;77(4):515–24.
26. van Gijn J, Rinkel GJ. Subarachnoid haemorrhage: diagnosis, causes and management. Brain. 2001;124(Pt 2):249–78.
27. Muench E, Horn P, Bauhuf C, Roth H, Philipps M, Hermann P, et al. Effects of hypervolemia and hypertension on regional cerebral blood flow, intracranial pressure, and brain tissue oxygenation after subarachnoid hemorrhage. Crit Care Med. 2007;35(8):1844–51.
28. Lanzino G, Kassell NF, Germanson T, Truskowski L, Alves W. Plasma glucose levels and outcome after aneurysmal subarachnoid hemorrhage. J Neurosurg. 1993;79(6):885–91.
29. Naidech AM, Levasseur K, Liebling S, Garg RK, Shapiro M, Ault ML, et al. Moderate Hypoglycemia is associated with vasospasm, cerebral infarction, and 3-month disability after subarachnoid hemorrhage. Neurocrit Care. 2010;12(2):181–7.
30. Oddo M, Schmidt JM, Carrera E, et al. Impact of tight glycemic control on cerebral glucose metabolism after severe brain injury: a microdialysis study. Crit Care Med. 2008;36(12): 3233–8.
31. Schmutzhard E, Rabinstein AA. The Participants in the International Multi-Disciplinary Consensus Conference on the Critical care Management of Subarachnoid Hemorrhage, Spontaneous subarachnoid hemorrhage and glucose management. Neurocrit Care. 2011; 15(2):281–6.
32. Bellander B-M, Cantais E, Enblad P, Hutchinson P, Nordström C-H, Robertson C, et al. Consensus meeting on microdialysis in neurointensive care. Intensive Care Med. 2004; 30(12):2166–9.
33. Sarrafzadeh A, Haux D, Küchler I, Lanksch WR, Unterberg AW. Poor-grade aneurysmal subarachnoid hemorrhage: relationship of cerebral metabolism to outcome. J Neurosurg. 2004; 100(3):400–6.
34. Helbok R, Schmidt JM, Kurtz P, Hanafy KA, Fernandez L, Stuart RM, et al. Systemic glucose and brain energy metabolism after subarachnoid hemorrhage. Neurocrit Care. 2010;12(3): 317–23.
35. Badjatia N, Strongilis E, Gordon E, Prescutti M, Fernandez L, Fernandez A, et al. Metabolic impact of shivering during therapeutic temperature modulation: the bedside shivering assessment scale. Stroke. 2008;39(12):3242–7.

Chapter 11
Malnutrition in Stroke

Janis Dale, Christine Kijak, and Norine Foley

Key Points

- The published estimates of the prevalence of malnutrition associated with stroke range from 6 to 62 %.
- There are very few previously validated tools available with which to assess nutritional status; none have been evaluated for their application in stroke.
- Following stroke, patients may be at increased risk for the development of malnutrition, due to a variety of factors that affect their willingness or ability to self-feed including dysphagia, depression, cognitive deficits, visual neglect, and upper-extremity paresis. The overly restrictive use of therapeutic diets may also contribute.
- Although there is limited evidence, patients do not appear to be hypermetabolic in the first few weeks following stroke. Elevations of peripheral plasma markers of inflammation have been well described in the acute phase of stroke, but their clinical significance is unknown.

Keywords Nutritional status • Malnutrition • Stroke • Risk factors • Nutritional assessment • Validity

J. Dale, R.D. C.D.E.
Stroke and Neurological Rehabilitation Program, Neurotrauma Rehabilitation Program, St. Joseph's Health Care, Parkwood Hospital, 801 Commissioners Road East, London, ON, Canada N6C 5J1

C. Kijak, R.D.
Stroke and Neurological Rehabilitation Program, Amputee Rehabilitation Program, St. Joseph's Health Care, Parkwood Hospital, 801 Commissioners Road East, London, ON, Canada N6C 5J1

N. Foley, M.Sc., R.D. (✉)
Aging, Rehabilitation and Geriatric Care Program, Lawson Health Research Institute, Parkwood Hospital, 801 Commissioners Road East, London, ON, Canada N6C 5J1
e-mail: norine.foley@sjhc.london.on.ca

M.L. Corrigan et al. (eds.), *Handbook of Clinical Nutrition and Stroke*,
Nutrition and Health, DOI 10.1007/978-1-62703-380-0_11,
© Springer Science+Business Media New York 2013

Abbreviations

ASPEN American Society for Parenteral and Enteral Nutrition
SGA Subjective global assessment
MNA Mini nutritional assessment
BMI Body mass index
FM Fat mass
TSF Triceps skinfold
NOD Neurogenic oropharyngeal dysphagia
REE Resting energy expenditure

Definitions of Malnutrition

There is no standardized, validated, or universally accepted definition of the term "malnutrition." Debate and confusion continue to this day over the appropriate use of the term. This lack of consensus is problematic and can limit our ability to correctly identify a malnourished person and evaluate the benefit of nutritional interventions. The American Society for Parenteral and Enteral Nutrition (ASPEN) describes malnutrition as a "subacute or chronic state of nutrition, in which a combination of varying degrees of overnutrition or undernutrition and inflammatory activity has led to a change in body composition and diminished function" [1]. The authors also noted that this is an interim definition pending the development of a consensus with ASPEN collaborators. A new approach which recognizes the contribution of cytokine-mediated inflammation on the development of malnutrition has recently been proposed. This system distinguishes between the effects of uncomplicated, chronic starvation and acute or chronic diseases with superimposed inflammation [2, 3]. Hoffer has suggested that the use of the term is too vague to be meaningful and discourages its use [4]. In the hospitalized patient, malnutrition can be difficult to identify as it is associated with muscle wasting, due to age, immobility, or inflammatory processes [2, 4].

To date, efforts to achieve a consensus definition of malnutrition have been unsuccessful. During a recent Delphi process, while 22 experts could agree that deficiency of energy and protein and a decrease in fat-free mass were all relevant to the construct of malnutrition, they could not agree which element was most important [5]. There was agreement that the operational definition should include measures of involuntary weight loss, nutritional intake, and body mass index (BMI); however, there was no consensus on cutoff levels that would indicate the presence of malnutrition.

Prevalence of Malnutrition in the Stroke Population

Determining the prevalence of malnutrition following stroke is difficult since no nutritional assessment tools have been developed and validated for this population. Further, no existing, previously developed, disease-specific assessment tools have been validated for use in stroke. As a result, a variety of methods have been used, yielding widely differing estimates, none of which may be valid [6–9]. A systematic review identified 18 studies in which the nutritional status of patients was assessed after inpatient admission for stroke [10]. The reported frequency of malnutrition ranged from 6 to 62 %. The authors suggested that a substantial proportion of the variation was attributed to the heterogeneity of nutritional assessment methods. Among the 18 trials reviewed, 17 different assessment methods were used. The frequency of malnutrition tended to be lower, ranging from 7.8 to 26.3 % in the four included studies [9, 11–13] that used validated assessment methods. Other factors such as comorbidities, complications from stroke, stroke type, and patient characteristics would have influenced the variability of reported estimates of malnutrition but were not examined in this review.

Timing of assessment may also affect the reported prevalence of malnutrition. To date, 10 studies have assessed nutritional status within 7 days of stroke onset [9, 11–20]. The prevalence of malnutrition ranged from 7.8 to 32 %; however, in two of these studies [13, 17], "at-risk" patients were identified as malnourished, likely inflating the estimate. Although unclear if these were incident (new) or prevalent (existing) cases of malnutrition, the results may suggest that malnutrition may not be as widespread immediately following stroke as previously thought. This finding may not be surprising considering that stroke, in the developed world, is an "event" associated with conditions of overnutrition including obesity, hyperlipidemia, and diabetes mellitus, notwithstanding the proportion of patients who may be malnourished at the time of stroke onset or those who may be particularly vulnerable due to medical comorbidities or complications.

In studies where nutritional assessment was conducted using a traditional approach, using biochemical and anthropometric data, the estimates of malnutrition vary greatly. Foley et al. [10] demonstrated how the choice of cutoff values and the number of indicators required to elicit a diagnosis of malnutrition affected the estimates of malnutrition. For example, when albumin was used by itself to indicate malnutrition, 6.1–22 % of stroke patients were identified as malnourished based on cutoffs of 40 g/L and 25 g/L, respectively. When investigators increased the number of abnormal markers required to diagnose malnutrition, the prevalence of malnutrition decreased. Seventy-three percent of subjects were diagnosed as malnourished if one abnormal measurement was required, compared with only 2 % if four abnormal markers were considered indicative of malnutrition. Joosten et al. [21] aptly demonstrated how the application of differing diagnostic criteria affected the estimates of malnutrition in a sample of 151 elderly patients admitted to an acute geriatric ward. In this study, malnutrition was identified using the methods from six previously published reports in which the nutritional status of hospitalized patients had been assessed using a traditional approach. The prevalence of malnutrition varied from 6.5 to 85 % depending on which criteria were applied.

Nutritional Assessment

To the best of our knowledge, there are only two nutritional assessment tools that have been developed with evidence of validity and reliability. Subjective Global Assessment (SGA) was designed to predict complication risk in preoperative, gastrointestinal surgical patients. It was intended to be used as prognostic, rather than a diagnostic tool. As a result, SGA is not meant to diagnose malnutrition but rather to predict the risk of patients developing nutrition-associated complications [22]. The developers of the tool reasoned that in the absence of a diagnostic gold standard and the difficulties in differentiating malnutrition from the disease process, this approach was preferred. SGA categorizes patients as well nourished, moderately malnourished (or suspected of being malnourished), or severely malnourished based on weight history, food intake, gastrointestinal symptoms, functional status, and the metabolic demands of the disease state [23]. A physical examination evaluates the presence of edema, muscle wasting, and subcutaneous fat loss. There is no standardized way to conduct SGA nor method to weight information from all the assessment items to arrive at a final score (category). In the original study, interrater reliability was quite good. Two physicians each examined 59 patients and agreed that they belonged in the same category in 48 cases [23]. The corresponding chance-corrected Kappa statistic was 0.72. Other reliability estimates have not been as good. When used to assess the nutritional status of 90 patients admitted to a geriatric unit agreement between a clinician and a researcher was 77.8 % (Kappa=0.56) [24]. Agreement between a medical resident and a specialist in clinical nutrition was 79 % (Kappa=0.66) when assessing 175 general surgical patients [25]. In the years since SGA was introduced, it has been adapted for use in a wide range of disease states. In the published literature, it has been used to assess the nutritional status of stroke patients in only a single study [9], although an adaptation of SGA developed for use in cancer patients, the patient-generated SGA [26], was used in two stroke studies [18, 27].

Mini nutritional assessment (MNA) was developed as tool to identify geriatric patients at risk for malnutrition and encompasses anthropometric measurements, mobility, medication, lifestyle, and dietary history [28]. The tool includes items that are indicative of both actual nutritional states (e.g., BMI) as well as items which indicate risk for the development of malnutrition (e.g., takes more than 3 prescription drugs/day). MNA is comprised of two sections: one for screening (MNA-short form) and one for assessment. The screening portion consists of six questions. Scores of less than 12 are indicative of either malnutrition or risk of malnutrition and are a signal to continue with the assessment portion of the tool. In terms of applicability to stroke, two of the screening items may not be suitable since they can be related to the effect of stroke and not nutritional state per se. Impaired mobility is a typical consequence of stroke; reflecting its severity and neuropsychological status (depression) may be difficult to assess if a patient is aphasic. The full MNA will also be difficult to complete if patients have cognitive or language deficits secondary to stroke. When the full MNA was used to assess nutritional risk among small groups of hospitalized elderly patients, its reliability among nurses was good (Kappa = 0.78) [29]. In a study that included patients recovering from stroke, reliability among nurses was also good (Kappa = 0.67) [30]. The tool was less reliable when conducted by two clinicians (Kappa = 0.41) [31].

In the absence of a validated tool, a traditional approach is often used, both clinically and for research purposes. The strengths and limitations of some of the more commonly used measurements are discussed below.

Biochemical Measurements

Albumin is a hepatic protein marker which has been commonly used to evaluate nutritional status. In earlier studies in the stroke literature, a strong emphasis was placed on its value in diagnosing malnutrition, without considering that its production is downregulated during acute illness [32]. During acute illness, serum albumin may fall and remain depressed in spite of adequate nutritional support, until the underlying inflammatory process improves or resolves. Albumin does have prognostic value as an indicator of morbidity and mortality because it reflects underlying disease burden and inflammatory condition or injury [2]. Patients' serum albumin was associated with poorer functional mobility, increased complications, and lower self-care scores in a group of geriatric stroke patients [33]. Gariballa et al. [34] demonstrated that stroke patients with hypoalbuminemia had a greater risk of infective complications. Serum albumin concentration was a strong and independent risk factor of mortality 3 months after acute stroke, and the lower the serum albumin concentration, the more likely a patient would need institutional care after discharge from hospital.

It has been suggested that albumin may be more appropriate for detection of malnutrition in the rehabilitation setting because of its longer half-life; however, its serum levels may be affected by mild to moderate inflammation characteristic of chronic disease. Therefore, its use may also be limited in this setting. Sarcopenic obesity and congestive heart failure are two examples of chronic disease conditions characterized by inflammation, which are relatively common in the stroke population [2, 35]. A normal albumin level can also mask malnutrition, because in the absence of inflammation, it can remain in the normal range in spite of chronic profound weight loss [36].

Prealbumin has a shorter half-life (2.5 days) and smaller body pool than albumin [37]. Although it is used in the clinical setting for nutrition support monitoring, it is also decreased during periods of acute illness in the presence of inflammation and is not specific to nutritional status [2, 38]. In fact, no correlation between change in prealbumin levels and percent of calorie or protein needs delivered was found in a group of 154 patients receiving enteral nutrition. Only C-reactive protein, a positive acute-phase protein, correlated significantly (inversely) with change in serum prealbumin [39]. Dennis et al. [40] reported a similar pattern. Daily protein intake accounted for only 6 % of the variability in a model examining change in serum prealbumin among 111 men admitted to a veterans' hospital for recuperative and rehabilitative care. The results of these studies suggest that prealbumin may also be a better marker for inflammation than nutritional status. In clinical practice, C-reactive protein is often ordered with prealbumin, helping to confirm the presence of inflammation.

Anthropometrics

Examples of anthropometric measurements include body weight, mid-arm muscle circumference, and skinfold thickness, which can be measured using skinfold calipers and a measuring tape. With a traditional approach, the identification of malnutrition is usually inferred, based on a single value or multiple values falling outside population reference ranges or below a given percentile within these ranges. Anthropometric measurements can be difficult to obtain in a hospital setting. Even a basic measurement such as a standing height can be difficult to get. Since self-reported heights can be inaccurate [11], knee height and demispan are two of examples of alternate methods available to estimate height in individuals not able to stand safely [41]. Ethnic-specific equations for demispan and knee height are available [42].

Some ethnic groups have more fat mass (FM) per unit BMI and therefore can have lower cutoff values for health risk [43]. In patients over 60, the reported lower BMI cutoffs associated with the lowest risk for underweight, reduced physical function, and mortality range markedly from 20 kg/M^2 [41] to 24 kg/M^2 [44]. The Canadian Best Practice Recommendations for Stroke Care recommends that persons at risk for stroke or who have had a stroke should maintain a BMI of 18.5–24.9 kg/m^2 or a waist circumference of <80 cm for women and <94 cm for men [45]. However, age and premorbid nutritional status should also be considered. For example, the BMI cutoff point for a frail 85-year-old ought to be higher than that for a healthy 65-year-old. Elderly obese patients with waist circumferences greater than target may still be at significant risk for accelerated lean body mass depletion due to inflammation-associated illness or injury and immobility post-stroke.

Subcutaneous fat scores may also be measured indirectly. Common measurement sites include triceps, biceps, subscapular, and suprailiac. Ideally, the measurements from four sites should be summed and then compared with population norms of healthy individuals of similar age and sex. A single measurement of triceps skinfold (TSF) may underestimate overall adiposity, as there is a redistribution of fat from extremities to the trunk associated with aging [46]. TSF measurements are often difficult to perform, particularly in obese, bedridden patients, while most equations were developed for younger, normal-weight individuals [42]. Inherent flaws with skinfold measurements include insensitivity to change and intra-observer and inter-observer variability [32]. In routine clinical practice, skinfold measurement is not used frequently.

Malnutrition and Poor Outcome

Malnutrition is a potentially modifiable risk factor which has negative consequences for the individual with stroke. Using different assessment techniques, premorbid undernutrition was found to be an independent predictor of mortality at 30 days [9, 16] and 6 months [47] following stroke and was associated with increased dependency or poor outcome, after controlling for age, stroke severity, pre-stroke function, and living arrangements [9, 11, 12, 47]. Malnutrition after the first week of stroke was also associated with a greater incidence of infections and pressure sores, and longer lengths of hospital stays, although it ceased to be an independent predictor of poor outcome 1 month post-stroke, after controlling for swallowing impairment and stroke severity [16].

The Effectiveness of Nutritional Interventions

Among stroke patients with preexisting malnutrition, it may be reasonable to predict that some form of nutritional supplementation will improve their nutritional status, which in turn will help to improve outcomes. The literature is limited on the subject. Gariballa et al. [34] randomized non-dysphagic "malnourished" stroke patients to receive a protein and energy supplement in addition to a regular hospital diet or oral diet exclusively for 4 weeks or until death or discharge. Despite significantly increased intake of protein and energy among patients in the supplemented group over the study period, no significant differences in weight were evident at follow-up. Patients receiving supplements experienced smaller declines in serum albumin compared to patients in the control group (−1.5 vs. to 4.4, $p = 0.025$). In terms of non-nutritional secondary outcome measures, including a scale assessing activities of daily living, infective complications, and length of hospital stay, no differences were observed between the groups.

In two smaller studies that recruited patients who were either malnourished or at risk for malnutrition following stroke, patients were randomized to receive oral protein and energy supplements or either to control [48] or routine care [20] groups. In both studies, better outcomes were associated with patients who received supplements. Significant improvements in total Functional Independence Measure™ scores, and its motor subscore, as well as 2 and 6 min timed walk tests were found with the "intensive group" versus the standard group [48]. Patients receiving individual nutritional intervention compared with patients with no individualized treatment had fewer problems with mobility and self-care and significantly improved muscle grip strength [20]. Energy intakes were also higher and weight loss significantly less among patients in the treatment group.

If the metabolic sequelae of stroke put all patients at risk for the development of malnutrition regardless of their initial nutritional state, then perhaps it would be advantageous to provide supplemental nutrition universally soon after hospitalization.

However, evidence from the Feed or Ordinary Diet (FOOD) trial suggests that routine supplement may not affect global outcome. The FOOD trial allocated 4,023 non-dysphagic patients to receive either a routine hospital diet alone or oral sip feedings in addition to the regular hospital diet to establish whether oral protein energy supplementation would improve the outcomes of stroke patients [12]. In this trial, both malnourished (8 %) and non-malnourished patients were randomized to the same two diets. The nutritional intake of individuals was not measured due to the difficulty of obtaining and evaluating food intake records from such a large sample size. The results at 6 months demonstrated no significant differences between the two groups in mortality rate, functional outcome, or quality of life. The results from two smaller studies, which also included non-dysphagic patients, indicated that protein and energy supplementation may help to cognitive function following stroke [48, 49]. The authors hypothesized that among other mechanisms, the additional supply of amino acids could help to reactivate the synthesis of neural proteins, thereby increasing neuron energy and neurotransmitter function.

Risk Factors for the Development of Malnutrition Following Stroke

Premorbid risk factors associated with the development of malnutrition following stroke include a history of smoking [53], advanced age [10], female sex [13], and residential care [10]. The consequences of stroke can further increase a patient's risk for poor energy and protein intake and subsequent nutritional decline post-stroke. Fatigue, depression, and anxiety may result in decreased appetite and intake [49]. Patients who are unable to communicate food preferences due to aphasia may also be at risk for decreased intake [50]. Decreased or inability to self-feed related to upper paresis, apraxia, or visual deficits may result in an inability to open containers at meals and reluctance to ask staff for help. Lack of access to between-meal snacks placed within easy reach may also contribute to inadequate intake. Half of patients surveyed in acute care hospitals in London, UK, identified barriers outside of the food itself such as organizational (meal timing and lack of assistance), physical (inappropriate eating utensils and seating), and environmental (unpleasant smells, interruptions) as impacting negatively on food intake [51]. Visual field losses such as homonymous hemianopsia (the loss of half the field of view on the same side in both eyes) may prevent a patient from seeing food on one side of the plate and potentially reduce intake unless the patient is cued to scan the affected side.

Dysphagia

Stroke is the most frequent cause of neurogenic oropharyngeal dysphagia (NOD). In the acute phase of stroke, the frequency of NOD varies depending on the size and location of stroke and the timing and method of assessment but is reported to be between 29 and 78 % [52]. It is estimated that up to half of patients will return to good swallowing function within 14 days, while the other half will develop chronic dysphagia [53]. Dysphagia can lead to the development of malnutrition through a number of mechanisms. Patients who are able to eat orally may fear eating and/or choking, be unwilling, or lack a desire to eat, partly due to the decreased palatability of texture-modified diets [53]. Implementing strict therapeutic diets in combination with texture-modified diets can lead to reduced menu options, poor variety, patient dissatisfaction with meals, and inadequate intake. Dysphagic patients who also require pureed diets and thickened fluids can be particularly challenging. In these cases, insulin or oral hypoglycemic agents should be adjusted as opposed to further diet restriction to minimize the risk of malnutrition and optimize glycemic control. Dysphagic patients requiring enteral feeding may be at decreased risk for the development of malnutrition unless intolerance to the feeding formula develops or there are preexisting medical conditions, such as malignancies or organ failure.

There are limited and conflicting reports of the adequacy of energy and protein intakes of patients consuming texture-modified dysphagia diets during hospitalization [54, 55]. The results from one study, which was stroke specific, indicated that previously well-nourished patients received an average of 80–90 % of their protein and energy requirements, regardless of diet type during the first 21 days of hospitalization [55]. Average energy intake was 19.4–22.3 kcal/kg/day over five observation points representing 80.3–90.0 % of measured requirements. Average protein intake ranged met 81–90 % of requirements. Patients receiving enteral nutrition had higher energy and protein intakes than those on regular or dysphagia diets, but there were nonsignificant differences in the average energy and protein intakes of patients receiving dysphagia versus regular diets. The authors suggested that dysphagia diets were higher in calories due to thickening agents and that patients received additional assistance at meals, increasing intake. There were several limitations associated with this study. The sample size was relatively small, diets could have been upgraded during the study period, and only well-nourished patients were included.

In patients without swallowing difficulties, Gariballa et al. [56] reported that the average 2-week energy intake of stroke patients who consumed a regular hospital diet was 1,338 kcal representing 74 % of their predicted requirement. This level of adequacy was not significantly different from 42 age- and sex-matched nonstroke patients who consumed 1,317 kcal, or 73 % of requirement, suggesting that the intakes of stroke patients were similar to those of other non-intensive care unit, hospitalized patients.

Effects of Therapeutic Diets on Intake

Post-stroke patients may be placed on specific diets to treat obesity, diabetes, hyperlipidemia, and hypertension. These diets should be implemented with care since dietary restrictions can lead to decreased food intake, especially in the elderly (>65 years) and the oldest old (>80 years) [57]. Diet regimes for patients with these conditions should be individualized according to patient goals. Patients capable of making an informed decision or their substitute decision maker should be made aware of the potential risks and benefits of therapeutic diets prior to implementation. Initiating weight loss diets for patients over 75 years is controversial as the restrictions may promote sarcopenia and loss of bone mass. In these cases, moderate calorie restriction in combination with exercise may be considered to help minimize loss of muscle mass [57]. Similarly, sodium-restricted diets are often less palatable, lack variety, and may result in decreased intake. They may be of less value on in normotensive patients. A liberalized approach (i.e., 3 g sodium/day vs. no added salt vs. no restriction) based on individual need and use of clinical judgement may work best to promote adequate nutritional intake and minimize the risk of unintentional weight loss [57, 58]. For example, a frail, elderly individual unable to prepare meals and relying on frozen prepared meals would be educated on a no-added-salt diet. In terms of diets to help control hypercholesterolemia, there is no evidence to date that supports the use of low-cholesterol diets in older individuals. Instead, the emphasis should be placed on a well-balanced diet focusing on the intake of healthy fats and oils, in moderation [57].

Hypermetabolism and Catabolism

Patients do not appear to be hypermetabolic following uncomplicated stroke, although the data are limited. Only two studies have been conducted to measure the resting energy expenditure of patients following stroke; evidence from these suggests that stroke patients are not at an increased risk for the development of malnutrition due to the effects of hypermetabolism. Finestone et al. [50] measured the resting energy expenditure (REE) of 91 stroke patients using indirect calorimetry on several occasions immediately following stroke and at 3 months and compared the results with 10 healthy elderly subjects. The average REE of stroke patients was 1,521–1,663 kcal/day which represented 107–114 % of the predicted estimated REE using the Harris Benedict equation, which was similar to control subjects. They also reported that there was no difference on resting energy expenditure when comparing stroke location, stroke size, or stroke severity. The authors concluded that resting energy expenditure of stroke patients was not different from that of controls, and for clinical purposes, a "stress factor" was not required when calculating energy requirements. A smaller study completed by Weekes et al. [59] measured the REE of 15 patients 24–72 h post-stroke and again 10–14 days later ($n = 11$) and reported that REE was 107 % of predicted value. These authors also concluded that stroke patients do not have elevated energy needs.

Patients may also be catabolic following trauma, infection, or injury as a result of an acute-phase response, mediated through the effects of cytokines and counter-regulatory hormones [60]. Activated macrophages and other leukocytes release pro-inflammatory cytokines, such as tumor necrosis factor-alpha, and Interleukin-1 (IL-1), which stimulate the production of interleukin-6 (IL-6) [60]. Cytokines in turn stimulate hepatocytes to synthesize and secrete acute-phase proteins, which promote inflammation and fever, activate the complement cascade, and stimulate chemotaxis of phagocytes [61]. The production of acute-phase proteins may be increased or decreased in response to acute illness. The hepatic production of albumin, prealbumin, and transferrin is known to be downregulated during periods of acute illness [60, 62]. While a classic acute-phase response is most commonly associated with systemic insults, tissue infarction, which occurs following ischemic stroke, can also elicit this response. General agreement exists that a systemic acute-phase response occurs following stroke although the exact mechanism, timing, and magnitude of the response remain uncertain. Elevations of peripheral plasma markers of inflammation have been well described following stroke [63–68], although their clinical significance is unclear. It is possible that prolonged elevations of these cytokines lead to a cascade of events that result in rapid muscle wasting and weight loss. However, the acute-phase response, as its name suggests, is usually short lived. Although malnutrition can impair cell-mediated immunity, it is more likely that the inflammatory response mimics malnutrition by influencing the production of proteins used as markers of nutritional status.

Conclusions

There is evidence of an association between stroke and the development of malnutrition. Patients who are malnourished at the time of stroke or those with significant complications or comorbidities likely will experience further declines in nutritional status as a result of poor intake; however, it is less obvious how previously well-nourished patients become malnourished. Results from several studies suggest that patients are not hypermetabolic in the acute-phase post-stroke, protein and energy intakes are marginally adequate, and absorption of nutrients is unimpaired, but the body of relevant literature is small and findings may not be generalizable. In addition, there are no nutrition assessment tools that have been validated for use with individuals who have experienced stroke. In the published literature, a variety of assessment techniques have been used, yielding a wide variety of estimates for the prevalence of malnutrition following stroke, suggesting that the current means employed to identify malnutrition may be unreliable or invalid. To overcome this uncertainty, there is an urgent need for a consensus process to develop both a definition and an operational definition of malnutrition, which can then be used to guide the development of standardized assessment tools suitable for use in the stroke population.

References

1. American Society for Parenteral and Enteral Nutrition (A.S.P.E.N.) Board of Directors and Clinical Practice Committee. Definition of terms, style and conventions used in A.S.P.E.N. Board of Directors-approved documents. American Society for Parenteral and Enteral Nutrition. 2009.
2. Jensen GL, Bistrian B, Roubenoff R, Heimburger DC. Malnutrition syndromes: a conundrum vs continuum. J Parenter Enteral Nutr. 2009;33(6):710–6.

3. Jensen GL, Mirtallo J, Compher C, Dhaliwal R, Forbes A, Grijalba RF, et al. Adult starvation and disease-related malnutrition: a proposal for etiology-based diagnosis in the clinical practice setting from the International Consensus Guideline Committee. J Parenter Enteral Nutr. 2010;34(2):156–9.

4. Hoffer LJ. The need for consistent criteria for identifying malnutrition. Nestle Nutr Workshop Ser Clin Perform Programme. 2009;12:41–52.

5. Meijers JM, van Bokhorst-de van der Schueren MA, Schols JM, Soeters PB, Halfens RJ. Defining malnutrition: mission or mission impossible? Nutrition. 2010;26(4):432–40.

6. DePippo KL, Holas MA, Reding MJ, Mandel FS, Lesser ML. Dysphagia therapy following stroke: a controlled trial. Neurology. 1994;44(9):1655–60.

7. Finestone HM, Greene-Finestone LS, Wilson ES, Teasell RW. Malnutrition in stroke patients on the rehabilitation service and at follow-up: prevalence and predictors. Arch Phys Med Rehabil. 1995;76(4):310–6.

8. Choi-Kwon S, Yang YH, Kim EK, Jeon MY, Kim JS. Nutritional status in acute stroke: undernutrition versus overnutrition in different stroke subtypes. Acta Neurol Scand. 1998;98(3): 187–92.

9. Davis JP, Wong AA, Schluter PJ, Henderson RD, O'Sullivan JD, Read SJ. Impact of premorbid undernutrition on outcome in stroke patients. Stroke. 2004;35(8):1930–4.

10. Foley NC, Salter KL, Robertson J, Teasell RW, Woodbury MG. Which reported estimate of the prevalence of malnutrition after stroke is valid? Stroke. 2009;40(3):e66–74.

11. Dennis MS, Lewis SC, Warlow C. Effect of timing and method of enteral tube feeding for dysphagic stroke patients (FOOD): a multicentre randomised controlled trial. Lancet. 2005;365(9461):764–72.

12. Dennis MS, Lewis SC, Warlow C. Routine oral nutritional supplementation for stroke patients in hospital (FOOD): a multicentre randomised controlled trial. Lancet. 2005;365(9461): 755–63.

13. Crary MA, Carnaby-Mann GD, Miller L, Antonios N, Silliman S. Dysphagia and nutritional status at the time of hospital admission for ischemic stroke. J Stroke Cerebrovasc Dis. 2006;15(4):164–71.

14. Axelsson K, Asplund K, Norberg A, Alafuzoff I. Nutritional status in patients with acute stroke. Acta Med Scand. 1988;224(3):217–24.

15. Unosson M, Ek AC, Bjurulf P, von Schenck H, Larsson J. Feeding dependence and nutritional status after acute stroke. Stroke. 1994;25(2):366–71.

16. Davalos A, Ricart W, Gonzalez-Huix F, Soler S, Marrugat J, Molins A, et al. Effect of malnutrition after acute stroke on clinical outcome. Stroke. 1996;27(6):1028–32.

17. Westergren A, Karlsson S, Andersson P, Ohlsson O, Hallberg IR. Eating difficulties, need for assisted eating, nutritional status and pressure ulcers in patients admitted for stroke rehabilitation. J Clin Nurs. 2001;10(2):257–69.

18. Martineau J, Bauer JD, Isenring E, Cohen S. Malnutrition determined by the patient-generated subjective global assessment is associated with poor outcomes in acute stroke patients. Clin Nutr. 2005;24(6):1073–7.

19. Yoo SH, Kim JS, Kwon SU, Yun SC, Koh JY, Kang DW. Undernutrition as a predictor of poor clinical outcomes in acute ischemic stroke patients. Arch Neurol. 2008;65(1):39–43.

20. Ha L, Hauge T, Spenning AB, Iversen PO. Individual, nutritional support prevents undernutrition, increases muscle strength and improves QoL among elderly at nutritional risk hospitalized for acute stroke: a randomized, controlled trial. Clin Nutr. 2010;29(5):567–73.

21. Joosten E, Vanderelst B, Pelemans W. The effect of different diagnostic criteria on the prevalence of malnutrition in a hospitalized geriatric population. Aging (Milano). 1999;11(6): 390–4.

22. Detsky AS, Baker JP, Mendelson RA, Wolman SL, Wesson DE, Jeejeebhoy KN. Evaluating the accuracy of nutritional assessment techniques applied to hospitalized patients: methodology and comparisons. J Parenter Enteral Nutr. 1984;8(2):153–9.

23. Baker JP, Detsky AS, Wesson DE, Wolman SL, Stewart S, Whitewell J, et al. Nutritional assessment: a comparison of clinical judgement and objective measurements. N Engl J Med. 1982;306(16):969–72.

24. Ek AC, Unosson M, Larsson J, Ganowiak W, Bjurulf P. Interrater variability and validity in subjective nutritional assessment of elderly patients. Scand J Caring Sci. 1996;10(3):163–8.
25. Hirsch S, de Obaldia N, Petermann M, Rojo P, Barrientos C, Iturriaga H, et al. Subjective global assessment of nutritional status: further validation. Nutrition. 1991;7(1):35–7.
26. Ottery FD. Definition of standardized nutritional assessment and interventional pathways in oncology. Nutrition. 1996;12(1 Suppl):S15–9.
27. Lim HJ, Choue R. Nutritional status assessed by the Patient-Generated Subjective Global Assessment (PG-SGA) is associated with qualities of diet and life in Korean cerebral infarction patients. Nutrition. 2010;26(7–8):766–71.
28. Guigoz Y, Vellas B, Garry P. The mini nutritional assessment: a practical assessment tool for grading the nutritional state of elderly patients. Facts Res Gerontol. 1994;4(Suppl):15–59.
29. Bleda MJ, Bolibar I, Pares R, Salva A. Reliability of the mini nutritional assessment (MNA) in institutionalized elderly people. J Nutr Health Aging. 2002;6(2):134–7.
30. Baath C, Hall-Lord ML, Idvall E, Wiberg-Hedman K, Wilde LB. Interrater reliability using modified norton scale, pressure ulcer card, short form-mini nutritional assessment by registered and enrolled nurses in clinical practice. J Clin Nurs. 2008;17(5):618–26.
31. Gazzotti C, Pepinster A, Petermans J, Albert A. Interobserver agreement on MNA nutritional scale of hospitalized elderly patients. J Nutr Health Aging. 1997;1(1):23–7.
32. Corrigan ML, Escuro AA, Celestin J, Kirby DF. Nutrition in the stroke patient. Nutr Clin Pract. 2011;26(3):242–52.
33. Aptaker RL, Roth EJ, Reichhardt G, Duerden ME, Levy CE. Serum albumin level as a predictor of geriatric stroke rehabilitation outcome. Arch Phys Med Rehabil. 1994;75(1):80–4.
34. Gariballa SE, Parker SG, Taub N, Castleden CM. Influence of nutritional status on clinical outcome after acute stroke. Am J Clin Nutr. 1998;68(2):275–81.
35. Stenholm S, Harris TB, Rantanen T, Visser M, Kritchevsky SB, Ferrucci L. Sarcopenic obesity: definition, cause and consequences. Curr Opin Clin Nutr Metab Care. 2008;11(6):693–700.
36. Narayanan V, Gaudiani JL, Mehler PS. Serum albumin levels may not correlate with weight status in severe anorexia nervosa. Eat Disord. 2009;17(4):322–6.
37. Gibson R. Nutritional assessment. 2nd ed. New York: Oxford University Press; 2005.
38. Fuhrman MP, Charney P, Mueller CM. Hepatic proteins and nutrition assessment. J Am Diet Assoc. 2004;104(8):1258–64.
39. Davis CJ, Sowa D, Keim KS, Kinnare K, Peterson S. The Use of prealbumin and C-reactive protein for monitoring nutrition support in adult patients receiving enteral nutrition in an urban medical center. J Parenter Enteral Nutr. 2012;36(2):197–204.
40. Dennis RA, Johnson LE, Roberson PK, Heif M, Bopp MM, Cook J, et al. Changes in prealbumin, nutrient intake, and systemic inflammation in elderly recuperative care patients. J Am Geriatr Soc. 2008;56(7):1270–5.
41. Hirani V, Mindell J. A comparison of measured height and demi-span equivalent height in the assessment of body mass index among people aged 65 years and over in England. Age Ageing. 2008;37(3):311–7.
42. Dart A, Keller H. Review of anthropometric measures for older adults. http://www.drheatherkeller.com/pdf/Anthropometry%20Review-%20Final%202009.pdf. Accessed Feb 15,2012.
43. Deurenberg-Yap M, Chew SK, Deurenberg P. Elevated body fat percentage and cardiovascular risks at low body mass index levels among Singaporean Chinese, Malays and Indians. Obes Rev. 2002;3(3):209–15.
44. Implications for reducing chronic disease risk. Washington, DC: Food and Nutrition Board, Committee on Diet and Health, National Research Council, National Academies Press; 1989.
45. Lindsay P, Gubitz G, Bayley M, Hill M, Davies-Schinkel C, Singh S, et al. Canadian best practice recommendations for stroke care (updated 2010). ON, Canada: Canadian Stroke Strategy Best Practices and Standards Writing Group; 2010. p. 2010.
46. Shatenstein B, Kergoat MJ, Nadon S. Anthropometric changes over 5 years in elderly Canadians by age, gender, and cognitive status. J Gerontol A Biol Sci Med Sci. 2001;56(8):M483–8.

47. FOOD Trial Collaboration. Poor nutritional status on admission predicts poor outcomes after stroke: observational data from the FOOD trial. Stroke. 2003;34(6):1450–6.
48. Rabadi MH, Coar PL, Lukin M, Lesser M, Blass JP. Intensive nutritional supplements can improve outcomes in stroke rehabilitation. Neurology. 2008;71(23):1856–61.
49. Finestone HM, Greene-Finestone LS. Rehabilitation medicine: 2. Diagnosis of dysphagia and its nutritional management for stroke patients. CMAJ. 2003;169(10):1041–4.
50. Finestone HM, Greene-Finestone LS, Foley NC, Woodbury MG. Measuring longitudinally the metabolic demands of stroke patients: resting energy expenditure is not elevated. Stroke. 2003;34(2):502–7.
51. Naithani S, Whelan K, Thomas J, Gulliford MC, Morgan M. Hospital inpatients' experiences of access to food: a qualitative interview and observational study. Health Expect. 2008;11(3):294–303.
52. Martino R, Foley N, Bhogal S, Diamant N, Speechley M, Teasell R. Dysphagia after stroke: incidence, diagnosis, and pulmonary complications. Stroke. 2005;36(12):2756–63.
53. Ickenstein GW, Hohlig C, Prosiegel M, Koch H, Dziewas R, Bodechtel U, et al. Prediction of outcome in neurogenic oropharyngeal dysphagia within 72 hours of acute stroke. J Stroke Cerebrovasc Dis. 2012;21(7):569–76.
54. Wright L, Cotter D, Hickson M, Frost G. Comparison of energy and protein intakes of older people consuming a texture modified diet with a normal hospital diet. J Hum Nutr Diet. 2005;18(3):213–9.
55. Foley N, Finestone H, Woodbury MG, Teasell R, Greene FL. Energy and protein intakes of acute stroke patients. J Nutr Health Aging. 2006;10(3):171–5.
56. Gariballa SE. Malnutrition in hospitalized elderly patients: when does it matter? Clin Nutr. 2001;20(6):487–91.
57. Darmon P, Kaiser MJ, Bauer JM, Sieber CC, Pichard C. Restrictive diets in the elderly: never say never again? Clin Nutr. 2010;29(2):170–4.
58. Zeanandin G, Molato O, Le DF, Guerin O, Hebuterne X, Schneider SM. Impact of restrictive diets on the risk of undernutrition in a free-living elderly population. Clin Nutr. 2012;31(1):69–73.
59. Weekes E, Elia M. Resting energy expenditure and body composition following cerebrovascular accident. Clin Nutr. 1992;11(1):18–22.
60. Gabay C, Kushner I. Acute-phase proteins and other systemic responses to inflammation. N Engl J Med. 1999;340(6):448–54.
61. Moshage H. Cytokines and the hepatic acute phase response. J Pathol. 1997;181(3):257–66.
62. Fleck A. Clinical and nutritional aspects of changes in acute-phase proteins during inflammation. Proc Nutr Soc. 1989;48(3):347–54.
63. Beamer NB, Coull BM, Clark WM, Hazel JS, Silberger JR. Interleukin-6 and interleukin-1 receptor antagonist in acute stroke. Ann Neurol. 1995;37(6):800–5.
64. Muir KW, Weir CJ, Alwan W, Squire IB, Lees KR. C-reactive protein and outcome after ischemic stroke. Stroke. 1999;30(5):981–5.
65. Fassbender K, Rossol S, Kammer T, Daffertshofer M, Wirth S, Dollman M, et al. Proinflammatory cytokines in serum of patients with acute cerebral ischemia: kinetics of secretion and relation to the extent of brain damage and outcome of disease. J Neurol Sci. 1994;122(2):135–9.
66. Ferrarese C, Mascarucci P, Zoia C, Cavarretta R, Frigo M, Begni B, et al. Increased cytokine release from peripheral blood cells after acute stroke. J Cereb Blood Flow Metab. 1999;19(9):1004–9.
67. Syrjanen J, Teppo AM, Valtonen VV, Iivanainen M, Maury CP. Acute phase response in cerebral infarction. J Clin Pathol. 1989;42(1):63–8.
68. Smith CJ, Emsley HC, Gavin CM, Georgiou RF, Vail A, Barberan EM, et al. Peak plasma interleukin-6 and other peripheral markers of inflammation in the first week of ischaemic stroke correlate with brain infarct volume, stroke severity and long-term outcome. BMC Neurol. 2004;4:2.

Chapter 12
Fluid and Electrolyte Management

Melissa Ellis and Tina S. Resser

Key Points

- Hyponatremia is divided into subcategories according to tonicity, classified as isotonic, hypotonic, and hypertonic.
- SIADH and CSW are two forms of hypotonic hyponatremia commonly seen with CNS disease. While the clinical presentation overlaps, it is critical to distinguish the diagnosis as therapies differ significantly.
- Hypernatremia commonly results from an altered thirst mechanism and/or lack of water intake; however, its ability to cause cellular dehydration in brain tissue is often induced in certain neurologic populations.
- Hypokalemia has been associated with both an increase in stroke incidence and a poor outcome at 3 months.
- Hyperglycemia increases risk for the incidence of all stroke subtypes, hemorrhagic conversion of ischemic stroke, expanded hematoma volume in hemorrhagic stroke, and worse outcome after a stroke occurs.
- Stroke patients commonly experience acid–base disorders which may be a result of their injury or due to medications which can cause metabolic acidosis.

Keywords Sodium • Potassium • Stroke • Electrolyte • Glucose

Abbreviations

ADH Antidiuretic Hormone
CDI Central Diabetes Insipidus

M. Ellis, M.S.N., A.C.N.P.-B.C. • T.S. Resser, M.S.N., A.C.N.P.-B.C., C.N.R.N. (✉)
Neurological Intensive Care Unit, Cleveland Clinic, 9500 Euclid Avenue, Unit H22,
Cleveland, OH, USA
e-mail: ressert@ccf.org

M.L. Corrigan et al. (eds.), *Handbook of Clinical Nutrition and Stroke*,
Nutrition and Health, DOI 10.1007/978-1-62703-380-0_12,
© Springer Science+Business Media New York 2013

CSW	Cerebral Salt Wasting
DI	Diabetes Insipidus
dDAVP	Desmopressin
NDI	Nephrogenic Diabetes Insipidus
SIADH	Syndrome of Inappropriate Antiduiretic Hormone
tPA	tissue Plasminogen Activator

Introduction

Electrolyte disturbances in stroke patients are a common phenomenon. While many of these derangements occur during the acute hospital stay, research demonstrates that some electrolyte disturbances may increase the risk for stroke, stroke complications, and even mortality. This chapter will review the most common electrolyte disorders encountered in stroke care, as well as reviewing common issues relating to fluid management in acute stroke.

Disorders of Sodium Concentration

Normal plasma sodium concentration is between 135 and 145 milliequivalents per liter (mEq/L). Sodium influences osmotic equilibrium, blood volume, and blood pressure and plays a major role in acid–base balance. The concentration of plasma sodium depends on its dilution with water. Normal sodium concentration is achieved through an integration of thirst and secretion of vasopressin (antidiuretic hormone), aldosterone, and natriuretic peptides, which directly or indirectly influence the reabsorption and excretion of sodium [1].

In healthy patients water balance is maintained by thirst and antidiuretic hormone (ADH). ADH is secreted to prevent water loss in the kidneys, restoring normal plasma osmolality and reducing sodium concentrations. The primary stimulus for ADH release is an increase in serum osmolality [2]. The change in serum osmolality is sensed by osmoreceptors in the hypothalamus that further induce or depress thirst and ADH release form the posterior pituitary.

Hyponatremia

Hyponatremia is common among neurological patients with etiology and associated risks of morbidity widely varying [3, 4]. Anderson et al. found hyponatremia to be associated with a 60-fold increase in mortality, usually due to associated medical problems such as heart, lung, liver, brain, or kidney disease [5–7]. Hyponatremia is defined as a plasma sodium concentration less than 135 mEq/L and generally refers to inappropriate or excessive supply of free water [8].

Table 12.1

Causes of hypotonic hyponatremia based on volume status [11]

Hypovolemia	Euvolemia	Hypervolemia
Cerebral salt wasting	SIADH	SIADH
Remote diuresis, especially thiazides	Cortisol deficiency	Heart failure
Extrarenal losses: vomiting, diarrhea, excessive sweating	Hypothyroidism	Renal failure/severe nephrotic syndrome
Iatrogenic (hypotonic solutions, insufficient volume replacement)	Iatrogenic (hypotonic solutions)	Hepatic failure/cirrhosis
	Medications causing an increase in ADH secretion	Iatrogenic (hypotonic solutions, excessive volume)
	Water intoxication	

Hyponatremia can be divided into subcategories according to tonicity, classified as isotonic, hypertonic, or hypotonic. Isotonic hyponatremia (serum osmolality 280–295) is commonly seen in patients following transurethral resection of the prostate or hysterectomy. It is less commonly seen as a laboratory artifact in those with extreme hyperlipidemia and hyperproteinemia, also known as "pseudohyponatremia." Hypertonic hyponatremia (serum osmolality >295) occurs from the accumulation of non-osmotically active particles, such as urea, ethanol, and glucose, which produce transcellular fluid shifts, diluting plasma sodium concentration [9]. This occurs with severe hyperglycemia where the serum sodium concentration falls by 1.6 mmol/L for each 100 mg/dL rise in glucose concentration [10]. Mannitol is another common solute producing osmotic shifts. Hyponatremia that results from hypertonic or isotonic states does not result in neuronal cellular swelling and is usually of little clinical significance. However, hypotonic hyponatremic patients warrant treatment. Hypotonic hyponatremia is caused by excessive water intake or water retention and is further divided according to volume status (Table 12.1).

The diagnostic approach to differentiating hyponatremia includes a detailed history and physical examination with appropriate lab testing. Laboratory tests such as basic chemistry panel, lipid panel, plasma osmolality, urine osmolality, and urine sodium concentration provide valuable information in the differential diagnosis of hyponatremia [8].

Neurological dysfunction is the principle manifestation of hyponatremia [11]. The resulting encephalopathy is related to an osmotic water shift leading to increased cellular volume, specifically cerebral edema. Severity is dependent upon onset and absolute decrease in plasma concentrations. Although neurologic abnormalities may be present, typically patients with sodium concentrations >125 mmol/L remain asymptomatic. Patients with sodium concentrations between 115 and 125 mmol/L may experience symptoms that include headache, malaise, nausea, emesis, muscle cramps, depressed reflexes, lethargy, and confusion [12, 13]. In extreme hyponatremia (<115 mEq/L) or with acute onset, complications include seizures, coma, respiratory arrest, permanent brain damage, brainstem herniation, and death [12, 13].

Table 12.2
Clinical features of SIADH and CSW [14]

	SIADH	CSW
Volume status	Euvolemia	Hypovolemia
Plasma BUN/creatinine	Normal	Increased
Hematocrit	Normal	Increased
Plasma uric acid	Decreased	Normal or decreased

While multiple factors contribute to hypotonic hyponatremia (Table 12.1), syndrome of inappropriate antidiuretic hormone (SIADH) and cerebral salt wasting (CSW) are two common causes in the setting of central nervous system (CNS) disease. There is considerable overlap in the clinical presentation and it is often difficult to distinguish between these two conditions (Table 12.2). Appropriate diagnosis is crucial as therapies not only differ but may result in negative clinical consequences if treated inappropriately [14].

Syndrome of Inappropriate Antidiuretic Hormone

The primary mechanism underlying SIADH is excessive release of ADH, resulting in renal water reabsorption and volume retention [14]. This non-osmotic release of vasopressin usually occurs from the posterior pituitary or an ectopic source. As water intake is improperly excreted, the resultant water retention leads to hyponatremia. Inappropriate antidiuresis commonly occurs with central nervous system disturbances. Any CNS disorder, including cerebrovascular accident, head trauma, hemorrhage, meningitis, encephalitis, and acute psychosis may enhance the release of ADH. Other common causes include pulmonary diseases (pneumonia, tuberculosis), malignant tumors (most commonly small cell carcinoma of the lung), and physical/emotional stressors [15].

SIADH is a diagnosis of exclusion. This syndrome should be suspected in any patient experiencing hyponatremia in the setting of an inappropriately elevated urine osmolality (>100 mOsm/kg) in the setting of hypotonicity. Further diagnostic criteria are as follows [8, 16]:

1. Elevated urine sodium concentration (usually above 40 mEq/L)
2. Absence of extracellular volume depletion
3. Low blood urea nitrogen and serum uric acid concentration
4. Relatively normal acid–base and potassium balance
5. Normal adrenal and thyroid function
6. Normal cardiac and hepatic function

Prior to making the diagnosis of SIADH, there must be no stimuli that could potentially stimulate the non-osmotic release of ADH (Table 12.3), and pharmacologic agents that enhance ADH must be withdrawn (Table 12.4).

Table 12.3
Stimuli that may stimulate
ADH release [21]

Hypovolemia
Hypotension
Positive-pressure ventilation
Pain
Stress
Nausea
Medications

Table 12.4
Pharmacologic agents that enhance ADH action [26]

Stimulate ADH release	Potentiate ADH action	ADH analogs
Nicotine	Chlorpropamide	Oxytocin
Carbamazepine	Methylxanthines	Desmopressin acetate
Antidepressants	NSAIDS	
Narcotics		
Antipsychotics		
Certain antineoplastic drugs		

Cerebral Salt Wasting

CSW is characterized by hyponatremia and volume depletion due to inappropriate sodium wasting in the urine [17]. The mechanism by which cerebral disease leads to renal salt wasting is poorly understood with controversy among clinicians over its existence. The most probable process involves decreased neuronal input to the kidneys and/or the release of one or more natriuretic factors [18, 19]. Decreased sympathetic input to the kidney may alter renal tubular sodium reabsorption, whereas intracranial disease may stimulate release of natriuretic peptides, which in turn suppresses aldosterone secretion and alter kidney function [18, 20].

The clinical characteristics of CSW are similar to SIADH. In CSW, ADH secretion is appropriately stimulated leading to elevated levels that meet criteria for SIADH, often leading to incorrect diagnosis [21]. The primary distinction lies in the volume status of the patient. SIADH is characterized by a volume-expanded state with patients presenting euvolemic to hypervolemic. Oppositely, CSW is characterized by a volume-depleted state, resulting in hypovolemia [22].

Hyponatremia resulting from CSW is the most common electrolyte disorder after aneurysmal subarachnoid hemorrhage [2]. Serum sodium levels tend to decline between the second and tenth day following the hemorrhage, paralleling cerebral vasospasm [23]. Other common causes of cerebral salt wasting include traumatic brain injury, intracranial and metastatic neoplasm, meningitis, encephalitis, and CNS surgeries [24].

Management

When treating SIADH or CSW, the goal of therapy aims at treating the underlying disease and implementing therapies to raise and maintain serum sodium concentrations. When correcting hyponatremia, the therapeutic plan varies with the presence and severity of symptoms.

Symptomatic hyponatremia, particularly when symptoms suggest seizures, coma, and respiratory and cardiac disturbances, requires treatment with hypertonic saline. Symptoms occur with an acute drop in the serum sodium to 120 mEq/L in less than 48 h. Acute hyponatremia promotes cerebral edema which may be fatal in patients already suffering a neurological insult [3]. Cautious administration of hypertonic saline solutions will raise serum sodium concentrations and improve neurological manifestations. Hypertonic therapies should aim to raise the serum sodium concentration by 1.5–2 mEq/L/h for 3–4 h [25]. Subsequent replacement should be adjusted so the total rise over 24 h not exceeds 12 mEq/L with frequent serum sodium monitoring.

Asymptomatic hyponatremia, with mild to moderate symptoms, warrants less aggressive treatment. Patients who experience confusion or lethargy may benefit from hypertonic therapies but usually only require fluid restriction. If hypertonic saline is used, the initial rate of correction should only raise the serum sodium level by 0.5 mEq/L in the first 3–4 h. The maximum rate of correction should not exceed 12 mEq/L in 24 h [25]. Adaptive mechanisms to defend cell volume occur with hyponatremia lasting more than 2 days. Strict sodium replacement and slower correction is advised to avoid precipitating *central pontine myelinolysis* (CPM). This demyelinating disorder is characterized by flaccid paralysis, dysarthria, and dysphagia [26].

While free water restriction (less than 800 mL/day) is the mainstay therapy in most patients with SIADH-associated hyponatremia, treatment often requires the administration of sodium chloride, either intravenous or oral [27]. When choosing intravenous fluids, the replacement osmolality must exceed the osmolality of the urine, failure to will further lower serum sodium concentrations and worsen the hyponatremia. Oral salt tablets and administration of a loop diuretic aid in the reduction of urine osmolality, increasing urinary water excretion. Excessive ADH release may also be corrected with vasopressin receptor antagonist therapies such as vaptans or tetracyclines.

As CSW is a volume-depleted state, it should be treated with the administration of intravenous saline. Depending on severity of symptoms, either isotonic or hypertonic saline is used to correct volume depletion and maintain a positive fluid balance. Salt tablets combined with intravenous saline and use of fludrocortisones, a potent mineralocorticoid, has been shown to achieve sodium balance more frequently [28, 29]. Once euvolemic, therapy is aimed at maintaining a positive salt balance and preventing volume depletion by matching urinary output with volume repletion [24].

Hypernatremia

Hypernatremia is defined as plasma sodium concentration greater than 145 mEq/L. It is a state of sodium excess relative to extracellular volume [30]. It commonly occurs from an altered thirst mechanism and/or lack in water intake. Symptoms are nonspecific and relate to cellular dehydration, especially in the brain [16]. As water leaves the intracellular compartment and cells begin to shrink, CNS manifestations such as irritability, restlessness, lethargy, muscle twitching, spasticity, and hyper-reflexia occur [31]. If cellular brain shrinkage continues to occur, traction is placed on surrounding vessels and may result in cerebral hemorrhage [32].

Urine osmolality, urine sodium, urinary output, and overall volume status are essential in the differential diagnosis of hypernatremia. Basic chemistry panel and plasma renin level will exclude electrolyte abnormalities, renal impairment, or primary aldosteronism. Assessment should also include age, mobility, and access to water. History of diarrhea, recent vomiting, prolonged exposure to heat, exercise or sweating, recent burns, or traumatic brain injury should be assessed. The primary mechanism by which hypernatremia occurs may be divided into two categories based upon functioning or impaired renal water-conserving ability.

Hypernatremia with Intact Renal Water-Conserving Ability

Urine osmolality >400 mOsm/kg indicates proper renal water-conserving ability. It can further be divided as nonrenal losses, renal losses, and primary sodium gain.

Nonrenal Losses: Insensible and Sensible Losses

Hypernatremia is commonly caused by inadequate fluid intake and inadequate replacement of fluid losses. Inadequate intake is usually related to lack of or inability to access water. Increased fluid losses are often attributed to gastrointestinal losses, diuretic therapy, and both insensible and sensible losses. Unreplaced loss of hypotonic fluids promotes cellular dehydration, leading to *hypernatremic encephalopathy*, which can be accompanied by seizures, coma, and other neurological deficits [33].

Primary hypodipsia results from a defect of thirst, usually associated with the destruction of the hypothalamic thirst or osmoreceptor function [16]. This disorder is often the result of primary and metastatic hypothalamic tumors, less commonly granulomatous disease, vascular abnormalities, and trauma [34].

Renal Losses: Osmotic Diuresis

Nonelectrolyte solutes, such as glucose, mannitol, and urea, increase urine output with a sodium concentration below plasma, resulting in increased serum osmolality and serum sodium [35]. Osmotic diuresis reduces brain volume by removing free water from brain tissue and eliminating it from circulation through renal excretion [36, 37]. Mannitol is the mainstay of hyperosmolar therapy, used to treat neurological emergencies such as cerebral edema or increased intracranial pressure [38]. This cause of hypernatremia is often confused for diabetes insipidus (DI). It too presents with inappropriately low urine osmolarity that can be distinguished by measuring the osmoles excreted in the urine per day. Osmotic diuresis will present with >400 mOsm/day, whereas DI will be <300 mOsm/day [26].

Primary Sodium Gain

Primary sodium gain is induced by the administration of hypertonic therapies or, less commonly, salt poisoning. Hypervolemic hypernatremia is seen with aggressive administration of hypertonic saline or bicarbonate-containing solutions. While mannitol remains the mainstay for hyperosmolar therapy, hypertonic solutions are an alternative for the treatment for cerebral edema [38]. Bolus dosing and continuous infusions are commonly used in patients with cerebrovascular disease. Hypertonic therapies act as osmotic agents by dehydrating brain tissue and have been shown to decrease intracranial pressure and enhance cerebral perfusion and may prevent herniation or cerebral death [39]. CNS disorders produce cerebral edema and secondary injury related to mass effect, such conditions warrant the use of hypertonic therapies. They include large cerebrovascular infarcts, traumatic brain injury, and intracranial hypertension.

Hypernatremia with Impaired Renal Water-Conserving Ability

Urine osmolality <300 indicates impaired renal water-conserving ability. Urine osmolality less than 300 mmol/L in the setting of hypernatremia and polyuria is diagnostic of DI [40].

Diabetes Insipidus

DI results from an insufficient production or lack of appropriate renal response to ADH. Clinical manifestations include polydipsia and polyuria with the excretion of large amounts of hypotonic dilute urine. The defect may be central (vasopressin deficient) or nephrogenic (vasopressin resistant). Both conditions may be inherited or acquired. Polyuria is usually evident within 24 h of the primary insult [41].

Absence of ADH release from the posterior pituitary is characteristic of central DI. It often results from damage to the hypothalamo-neurohypophyseal axis, commonly from neurosurgery, traumatic brain injury, neoplasms, vascular accidents, anoxic encephalopathy, or infections [26]. Insensitive or defective renal responsiveness to ADH is characteristic of nephrogenic DI. This condition results in defective renal concentrating abilities, commonly as a result of intrinsic renal diseases, drugs, radiocontrast dyes, sickle cell anemia, and electrolyte disorders [26].

To differentiate between central DI (CDI) and nephrogenic DI (NDI), patients are challenged with a synthetic replacement for vasopressin, commonly desmopressin (dDAVP). If the urine osmolality is at least two times greater than baseline after 1–2 h, the patient is likely to have CDI. If the response to dDAVP is less, the patient is likely to have NDI [40].

Management

When correcting hypernatremia, the therapeutic plan varies with onset, symptoms, and if the hypernatremia is induced, as often may be the case in the neurocritical patient. As with hyponatremia, brain adaptation occurs with hypernatremia, and if treatment is warranted, correction should be calculated based on symptoms and onset. The primary treatment of hypernatremia is the administration of water to correct existing water deficits and ongoing losses. Water may be replaced enterally with pure water or intravenously with isotonic, hypotonic, or dextrose solutions [16] and can be calculated as

$$\text{Free water deficit} = [0.6 \times \text{body weight (kg)}] \times [(\text{plasma sodium} / 140) - 1].$$

Acute hypernatremia (<24 h) may be replaced rapidly [16]. Chronic hypernatremia (>24 to 48 h) should be calculated and replaced slowly. Therapy is often aimed at correcting serum sodium of approximately 1–2 mEq/L/h until symptoms resolve, typically with 50 % of the calculated free water deficit replaced in the first 12–24 h. The remainder is corrected over the next 24–48 h [42]. If a decline in neurologic status occurs during free water replacement, it may indicate cerebral edema and therapy must be temporarily discontinued with reevaluation of plan. In hypovolemic patients, initial therapy is aimed at restoring intravascular volume, then at correcting the water deficit. In hypervolemic patients, a loop diuretic may be administered, and in some circumstances dialysis may be indicated [16].

When managing DI, the overall goal is to decrease polydipsia and polyuria, allowing one to maintain a normal lifestyle. As central DI is a result of deficient secretion of ADH, it is treated with hormone replacement. The drug of choice is dDAVP, a synthetic analogue of vasopressin. Other water-retaining agents include L-arginine vasopressin. Hormone replacement is ineffective in nephrogenic DI. Therapy is aimed at reducing symptomatic polyuria through diuretics and dietary salt restriction [43]. If drug-induced NDI is suspected, any precipitating medications must be removed as soon as possible (Table 12.5).

Table 12.5

Drug-induced NDI [26]

Lithium
Demeclocycline
Methoxyflurane
Amphotericin B
Phenytoin
Aminoglycosides
Several cancer treatment drugs

Disturbances in Potassium

Potassium is a basic need for the brain and essential for neuronal cell health, function, and cerebral circulation [45]. Disturbances in potassium are common in stroke patients throughout the stroke spectrum. Understanding the etiology for a patient's potassium disturbance and correcting this common condition improves patient outcome. Symptoms of potassium derangements and suggestions for treatment are included in Tables 12.6 and 12.7.

Numerous studies have demonstrated that hypokalemia defined as a serum potassium less than 3.4 mg/dL increases risk for stroke incidence and mortality [44–46, 49, 55]. One study by Ascherio et al. [47] supported a reduced reduction of all stroke subtypes in subjects with an increased dietary potassium intake, particularly in hypertensive men. Multiple theories for potassium's benefit have been proposed, including its lowering effect on blood pressure, as well as inhibition of free radical formation, vascular smooth muscle proliferation, and arterial thrombosis [47]. While dietary potassium intake and stroke risk has more often been studied, Landmark proposed that the blood pressure-reducing benefit of thiazide and loop diuretics may be challenged by their subsequent potassium depletion [48]. Hypokalemia in stroke patients has been correlated with an independent risk for poor outcome at 3 months, irrespective of stroke severity, admission hypertension, or smoking [49].

Hypokalemia is a common finding among patients acutely hospitalized for stroke. The cause for this is multifold: medications, delays in nutrition, and exaggerated renal and gastrointestinal potassium losses may all impact serum potassium levels. Approximately 20 % of adult stroke patients can present to the hospital hypokalemic, independent of diuretic use [49]. Finestone et al. [50] found that nearly half of the patients admitted for acute stroke presented malnourished, again raising the argument for dietary potassium intake and stroke risk. Exaggerating the risk for malnutrition is a delay in feeding start once a stroke patient is hospitalized [51]. Dysphagia, delays for enteral access, and holding of nutrition for studies and procedures in the stroke patient can increase hypokalemia risk. A study by Oh and Seo [52] noted more stroke patients became hypokalemic after enteral feeds were initiated, although the mechanism was not clearly discussed.

Table 12.6
Symptoms of hypokalemia and hyperkalemia [80]

Hypokalemia ($K<3.5$ mmol/L)	Hyperkalemia ($K>5.0$ mmol/L)
Muscle weakness	Confusion or irritability
Anorexia	Listlessness
Vomiting	Paresthesias arms and legs
Hypotension	Flaccid paralysis
Weak pulse	Bradycardia
ECG changes: flattened ST segment and T wave, U wave elevation, dysrhythmias	ECG changes: peaked T waves, dysrhythmias

Table 12.7
Tips for potassium replacement [80]

1. Consider oral replacement when patient is asymptomatic and K <3.8 mmol/L
2. Correct magnesium first if also low
3. Oral replacement can average 40–100 mEq/day divided into 2–4 doses
4. If combining oral and intravenous replacement, do not administer more than 120 mEq in 6 h. Recheck potassium before further intervention
5. Potassium chloride can never be administered intramuscularly or by intravenous push
6. Intravenous replacement must always be administered on programmable pump
7. The maximum concentration for peripheral intravenous K replacement 10 mEq/100 mL
8. The maximum concentration for central intravenous K replacement 20 mEq/50 mL
9. The *preferred* concentration for central intravenous K replacement 20 mEq/100 mL
10. Central infusion potassium should be administered at 20 mEq/h

Potassium losses through the gut or kidney can potentiate hypokalemia. Due to stroke-related dysphagia, many patients require liquid forms of medications. One of the common additives to these liquid forms, sorbitol, can worsen diarrhea and gastrointestinal potassium losses [51]. Hypokalemia is also a common occurrence after the administration of mannitol, commonly prescribed to lower intracranial pressure in patients suffering from stroke-related intracranial hypertension. Of note, hyperkalemia can occur if mannitol is administered to a patient with renal failure [53, 54, 56]. Clinical thoughtfulness such as monitoring potassium following mannitol administration and crushing pills and potassium (rather than prescribing liquid forms) are important measures to maintain more normal serum potassium levels.

Disturbances in Chloride

Virtually all patients admitted for any stroke type will receive fluid resuscitation with 0.9 % sodium chloride at some time during their acute hospitalization. Normal saline is the most common crystalloid of choice for stroke patients. Hypotonic solutions are generally avoided for their potential to raise intracerebral edema [68].

However, it is important to note that aggressive resuscitation with saline is associated with the development of hyperchloremic metabolic acidosis [68].

Saline infusion indications in the acute stroke patient are widespread. Many stroke patients arrive volume depleted and are resuscitated with normal saline on arrival to the emergency department. Since many stroke patients have dysphagia or are nil per os status for tests and procedures, most will receive saline infusion during their hospital stay to prevent dehydration. Subarachnoid hemorrhage patients experiencing vasospasm or cerebral salt wasting will often require aggressive fluid administration with crystalloid (most often normal saline) [67]. Finally, stroke patients with cerebral edema may require hypertonic saline for their management.

Despite the usefulness and necessity of saline fluid resuscitation, large volume resuscitations can be associated with hyperchloremic metabolic acidosis. Morgan described that the pathology of this metabolic acidosis is due to saline's reduction of plasma and extracellular strong ion difference, a driving force in acid–base balance. The result is a normal to reduced anion gap metabolic acidosis [69].

The effects of hyperchloremic metabolic acidosis in stroke patients are not well studied. In the intensive care unit setting, Gunnerson et al. found that there were no differences in mortality among critically ill patients who had hyperchloremic acidosis versus those who did not [68]. Other studies among surgical patients have found several potential side effects, including decreased gastric perfusion, renal vasoconstriction, and elevated GFR, and the higher frequency of sodium bicarbonate infusions and blood products [68, 69].

Disturbances in Glucose

Disturbances in glucose and stroke risk, management, and outcome have long been studied. Hyperglycemia (diabetic and nondiabetic) as well as hypoglycemia are common findings in stroke patients which have important implications for the patient and practitioner. Anticipation of these disturbances is key to their appropriate management.

Diabetes mellitus doubles ones risk for acute hemorrhagic or ischemic stroke [57, 76]. This risk is associated with different types of ischemic stroke, including large-vessel occlusion, lacunar, and thromboembolic strokes. Moreover, patients who are diabetic and/or are hyperglycemic and receive tissue plasminogen activator (tPA) in the acute stroke setting are at an increased risk for intracranial hemorrhage after tPA administration. This risk increases with severity of the glucose elevation [58–60].

Hyperglycemia is a complex problem relating to hemorrhagic stroke. While diabetes is associated with an increased risk for intracerebral hemorrhage (ICH), hyperglycemia after the development of ICH may increase hematoma expansion, worsen outcome, and increase risk of death [77, 78]. Acute hyperglycemia in hospitalized patients is common among all stroke subtypes, even among nondiabetics. This has been described to be due to a catecholamine surge and physiologic stress response in severe neurological injury [61, 62]. Chronic hyperglycemia, whether in the diabetic or nondiabetic patient admitted for all stroke types, increases risk for death, severe disability, and lessens functional independence long term [61, 63]. The ideal glucose control for stroke patients has not yet been defined, as Oddo et al. [64] demonstrated that tight glucose control (defined 80–120 mg/dL) in severely brain injured patients may worsen outcome.

Disturbances in Magnesium

Magnesium is an important electrolyte and may have properties which protect the brain by acting as a glutamate receptor antagonist and calcium channel blocker [70]. The normal serum range for magnesium is 1.7–2.7 mg/dL [80]. Hypomagnesemia is associated with vasoconstriction, vascular endothelial injury, and progression of atherosclerosis [70]. In patients with symptomatic peripheral arterial disease, low serum magnesium levels are associated with an increase in neurologic events [47, 70].

Hypomagnesemia is the most common electrolyte disturbance among all critically ill patients. Its occurrence after aneurysmal subarachnoid hemorrhage (SAH) is common, occurring in over a third of patients [65, 66]. Correcting magnesium levels in SAH patients is important as its deficiency may propagate delayed cerebral ischemia [66]. Symptoms of hypomagnesemia may include irritability, confusion, arrhythmias, weakness, muscle fasciculations, nystagmus, and seizures [80]. While hypermagnesemia in SAH has not proven beneficial, achieving normal magnesium levels in all stroke patients is recommended. While hypomagnesemia has been linked to stroke development, there is ongoing research evaluating the neuroprotective effects of early magnesium administration in stroke patients to improve long-term outcomes [71]. Suggestions for magnesium replacement are noted in Table 12.8.

Table 12.8
Suggestions for magnesium replacement [80]

1. Consider oral replacement when Mg >1.2 mg/dL. Oral absorption varies between 15 and 50 %
2. Intramuscular injection can be considered. Maximum dose 1 g magnesium sulfate per injection site
3. Intravenous replacement preferred when Mg <1.2 mg/dL, patient is symptomatic, or patient cannot take oral dosing
4. Intravenous infusion magnesium sulfate should not exceed 1 g over 7 min

*use of magnesium oxide may cause increased stooling due to a laxative effect which should not be mistaken for enteral nutrition intolerance

Disturbances in Phosphorus

Stroke patients are at risk for developing hypophosphatemia. Normal serum phosphorus levels range between 2.4 and 4.5 mg/dL (0.8–1.5 mmol/L) [80]. A review of factors associated with hypophosphatemia in stroke is noted in Table 12.9 [41]. Strokes attributed to malignancy or severe dehydration may present with concurrent hypophosphatemia. Careful monitoring of phosphorus levels should be assessed for any patient deemed at risk for hypophosphatemia or refeeding syndrome. Refeeding syndrome is a complex syndrome which can cause a multitude of cardiovascular, neurologic, and other systemic side effects if encountered [79]. While hypophosphatemia is the most common sign of refeeding syndrome (RFS), a patient may also present with hypomagnesemia, thiamine deficiency, sodium and fluid retention, and changes in energy metabolism [79]. If untreated, hypophosphatemia can have an impact on cardiac output, hemolysis, oxyhemoglobin dissociation, and muscle weakness [41]. Information regarding phosphorus replacement is reviewed in Table 12.10.

Hyperphosphatemia is not independently associated with stroke although may be encountered in the stroke patient with concurrent renal disease.

Table 12.9
Risk factors for developing hypophosphatemia [41]

1. Preexisting condition of malnutrition, alcoholism, or debilitation while admitted for stroke
2. Nausea and vomiting secondary to increased intracranial pressure or posterior fossa lesions
3. Dysphagia with poor oral intake/nutrition
4. Altered mental status with secondary poor oral intake/nutrition
5. Poor appetite with secondary poor oral intake/nutrition
6. Prolonged "NPO" status for diagnostic tests and/or interventions
7. Prolonged respiratory alkalosis

Table 12.10 Phosphorus replacement key points [80]

1. Multiply calcium and phosphorus before choosing to replace. If product exceeds 60, note there is risk of calcium phosphate precipitation systemically
2. Antacids containing magnesium, calcium, or aluminum may contribute to low phosphorus levels
3. Oral phosphorus replacements should be divided into TID dosing and should be diluted into 75 mL water when administered enterally
4. Phosphorus less than 1 mg/dL should be replaced intravenously
5. Intravenous replacement phosphorus dose for acute drop 0.25 mmol/kg ideal body weight (IBW)
6. Intravenous replacement phosphorus dose for chronic drop 0.5 mmol/kg IBW
7. With intravenous replacement, phosphorus level will increase by an average of 1.2 mg/dL at dose 0.25 mmol/kg
8. Reduce dose by half if patient has concomitant renal insufficiency
9. Intravenous phosphorus replacement is traditionally infused over 4–6 h due to reported risks of hypocalcemia, hypotension, metastatic calcification, and renal failure

Table 12.11
Replacing calcium [80]

1. Multiply calcium and phosphorus before choosing to replace. If product exceeds 60, note there is risk of calcium phosphate precipitation systemically
2. Correct magnesium if also low. Normal serum magnesium levels will aid in calcium replacement measures
3. Oral dosing should be in divided doses
4. Choose intravenous replacement when corrected calcium <7.7 mg/dL or patient is at high risk for hypocalcemia
5. Total calcium is raised an average of 0.5 mg/dL for every 1 g intravenous calcium gluconate

Disturbances in Calcium

Normal serum calcium is defined as either total calcium: 8.4–10.2 mg/dL (2.1–2.6 mmol/L) or ionized calcium: 3.8–5.3 mg/dL (0.95–1.35 mmol/L) [80]. Ionized hypocalcemia is a common finding in general intensive care units, although epidemiologic studies measuring the frequency in acute stroke patients has not been reported. Common causes among critically ill patients may include hypomagnesemia, renal failure, sepsis, and blood transfusions [41]. Severe hypocalcemia may have neurologic manifestations such as hyperreflexia, paresthesias, or tetany [41]. Suggestions for replacement are noted in Table 12.11. Hypocalcemia should be defined using ionized calcium measurements as serum calcium is protein bound and may provide a spurious result [72].

Corrected calcium is measured as $(4 - [\text{plasma albumin}] \times 0.8 + [\text{serum calcium}])$ [80].

Hypercalcemia due to primary hyperparathyroidism has been reported as a very rare cause of cerebrovascular occlusion and stroke in both adults and children. Its cause is postulated to be due to calcium-mediated vasoconstriction and renal insufficiency [72]. Differential diagnosis of hypercalcemia should be included for any patient who is admitted with acute ischemic stroke of unknown cause and concomitant elevated serum calcium.

Disturbances in Bicarbonate

Normally, bicarbonate (HCO_3) and carbon dioxide (CO_2) work together to maintain the body's acid–base balance. Stable carbon dioxide requires the brain and lungs working together to provide normal ventilation. However, acute stroke can cause a number of disturbances with secondary or iatrogenic disturbances in this delicate balance.

Respiratory Disturbances

Control of breathing is found in the central nervous system [74]. Acute ischemic stroke may directly involve respiratory pathways or may alter ventilation due to secondary insult such as cerebral edema or aspiration. Any number of respiratory abnormalities may be found in acute stroke patients, including Cheyne–Stoke, ataxic, cluster, apneustic, or central neurogenic hyperventilation [73]. One study found over half of stroke patients tachypneic and experiencing Cheyne–Stroke respirations. Special attention should be made to monitor HCO_3 and CO_2 for any stroke patient suspected to be at risk for acid–base disorder.

Metabolic Disturbances

Metabolic acidosis is a common finding in stroke and may be due to either renal losses of bicarbonate or accumulation of organic acids. Mannitol and hypertonic saline are associated with renal losses of bicarbonate through their osmotic diuretic effect. Excessive isotonic saline administration may also cause a normal anion gap metabolic acidosis.

Excessive lactic acid may be found in the stroke patient who is severely dehydrated, seizing, or suffering from mitochondrial encephalomyopathy, lactic acidosis, and stroke-like episodes [75]. Therapy should be directed at correcting the primary disorder.

Conclusion

Electrolyte anomalies are discovered throughout the stroke spectrum. Whether encountered as part of stroke prevention care, during acute stroke management, or monitored in the rehabilitation of stroke rehabilitation, understanding the implications of electrolyte derangements and appreciating the importance of prevention, diagnosis, and treatment are key factors to patient safety.

References

1. Singer GG, Brenner BM. Fluid and electrolyte disturbances. Harrisons principles of internal medicine. 17th ed. New York: McGraw Hill; 2008. p. 274–85.
2. Dunn FL, Brennan TJ, Nelson AE, Roberton GL. The role of blood osmolality and volume in regulating vasopressin secretion in the rat. J Clin Invest. 1973;52:3212.
3. Arieff AI. Hyponatremia, convulsions, respiratory arrest, and permanent brain damage after receiving elective surgery in healthy women. N Engl J Med. 1986;314:1529–35.

4. Chung HM, Kluge R, Schrier RW, Anderson RJ. Postoperative hyponatremia. A prospective study. Arch Intern Med. 1986;146:333–6.
5. Anderson RJ, Chung H-M, Kluge R, Schrier RW. Hyponatremia: a prospective analysis of its epidemiology and the pathogenetic role of vasopressin. Ann Intern Med. 1985;102:164–8.
6. Kennedy PGE, Mitchell DM, Hoffbrand BL. Severe hyponatremia in hospital patients. Br Med J. 1978;2:1251–3.
7. Baran D, Hutchinson TA. The outcome of hyponatremia in a general hospital population. Clin Nephrol. 1984;22:72–6.
8. Rose BD, Post TW. Clinical physiology of acid-base and electrolyte disorders. 5th ed. New York: McGraw-Hill; 2001. p. 703–61.
9. Feig PU, McCurdy DK. The hypotonic state. N Engl J Med. 1977;297:1444.
10. Katz MA. Hyperglycemia-induced hyponatremia-calculation of expected serum sodium depression. N Engl J Med. 1973;289:843.
11. Cole CD, Gottfried ON, Liu JK, et al. Hyponatremia in the neurosurgical patient: diagnosis and management. Neurosurg Focus. 2004;16(4):E9.
12. Adrogue HJ, Madias NE. Hyponatremia. N Engl J Med. 2000;342:1581–9.
13. Arieff AI, Llach F, Massry SG. Neurological manifestations and morbidity of hyponatremia: correlation with brain water and electrolytes. Medicine. 1976;55:121–9.
14. Biff PF. Hyponatremia in patients with central nervous system disease: SIADH versus CSW. Trends Endocrinol Metab. 2003;14(4):182–7.
15. Robertson GL. Disorders if the neurohypophysis. Harrison's principles of internal medicine. 17th ed. New York: McGraw Hill; 2008. p. 2217–23.
16. Fried LF, Palevsky PM. Hyponatremia and hypernatremia. Med Clin North Am. 1997;81:585–609.
17. Gutierrez OM, Lin HY. Refractory hyponatremia. Kidney Int. 2007;71:79–82.
18. Berendes E, Walter M, Cullen P, Prien T, Van Aken H, Horsthemke J, Schulte M, et al. Secretion of brain natriuretic peptide in patients with aneurysmal subarachnoid hemorrhage. Lancet. 1997;349:245–9.
19. Berger TM, Kistler W, Berendes E, Raufhake C, Walter M. Hyponatremia in a pediatric stroke patient: syndrome of inappropriate antidiuretic hormone secretion or cerebral salt wasting. Crit Care Med. 2002;30:792–5.
20. Harrigan MR. Cerebral salt wasting syndrome. Crit Care Clin. 2001;17:125–38.
21. Rabinstein AA, Wijdicks EF. Hyponatremia in critically ill neurological patients. Neurologist. 2003;9:290–300.
22. Maesaka JK, Gupta S, Fishbane S. Cerebral-salt wasting syndrome: does it exist. Nephron. 1999;82:100–9.
23. Wijdicks EF, Vermeulen M, Hijdra A, Van Gijn J. Hyponatremia and cerebral infarction in patients with ruptured intracranial aneurysms: is fluid restriction harmful. Ann Neurol. 1985;17:137–40.
24. Momi J, Tang CM, Abcar AC, et al. Hyponatremia—what is cerebral salt wasting. Perm J. 2010;14(2):62–5.
25. Rose BD, Post TW. Hypoosmolal states-hyponatremia. Clinical physiology of acid-base and electrolyte disorders. 5th ed. New York: McGraw-Hill; 2001. p. 696–745.
26. Sambandam KK. Electrolyte abnormalities. The Washington manual of critical care medicine. Philadelphia, PA: Lippincott Williams & Wilkins; 2008. p. 153–60.
27. Verbalis JG, Goldsmith S, Greenberg A, Schrier R, Sterns RH. Hyponatremia treatment guidelines 2007: expert panel recommendations. Am J Med. 2007;120:S1.
28. Hasan D, Lindsay KW, Wijdicks EF, Murray GD, Brouwers PJ, Bakker WH, et al. Effect of fludrocortisone acetate in patients with subarachnoid hemorrhage. Stroke. 1989;20(9):1156–61.
29. Mori T, Katayama Y, Kawamata T, Hirayama T. Improved efficiency of hypervolemic therapy with the inhibition of natriuresis by fludrocortisone in patients with aneurysmal subarachnoid hemorrhage. J Neurosurg. 1999;91(6):947–52.

30. Adrogue HJ, Madias NE. Hypernatremia. N Engl J Med. 2000;342:1493–9.
31. Arieff AI, Guisado R. Effect on the central nervous system of hypernatremic and hyponatremic states. Kidney Int. 1976;10:116.
32. Kugler JP, Hudstead T. Hyponatremia and hypernatremia in the elderly. Am Fam Physician. 2000;61(12):3623–30.
33. Arieff AI, Ayus JC. Strategies for diagnosing and managing hypernatremic encephalopathy. J Crit Illn. 1996;11:720–7.
34. Robertson GL, Aycinena P, Zerbe RL. Neurologic disorders of osmoregulation. Am J Med. 1982;72:339.
35. Gipstein RM, Boyle JD. Hypernatremia complicating prolonged mannitol diuresis. N Engl J Med. 1965;272:1116.
36. Nath F, Galbraith S. The effect of mannitol on cerebral white matter water content. J Neurosurg. 1986;65:41.
37. Paczynski RP. Osmotherapy. Basic concepts and controversies. Crit Care Clin. 1997;13:105.
38. Hauer EM, Stark D, Staykov D, Stiegleder T, Schwab S, Bardutzky J. Early continuous hypertonic saline infusion in patients with severe cerebrovascular disease. Crit Care Med. 2001;39(7):1766–72.
39. Zornow MH. Hypertonic saline as a safe and efficacious treatment of intracranial hypertension. J Neurosurg Anesthesiol. 1996;8:175–7.
40. Ozer K, Balasubramanyam A. Diabetes insipidus in Bope and Kellerman: Conn's current therapy 2012. 1st ed. Philadelphia, PA: Elsevier Saunders; 2012. p. 690–3.
41. Marino PL. Hypertonic and hypotonic conditions. The ICU book of facts and formulas. Philadelphia, PA: Lippincott Williams & Wilkins; 2009. p. 409–26.
42. Beck LH. Changes in renal function with aging. Clin Geriatr Med. 1998;14:199–209.
43. Robinson A, Verbalis JG. Williams textbook of endocrinology. 11th ed. Philadelphia, PA: Elsevier Saunders; 2008. p. 291–323.
44. Green DM, Ropper AH, Kronmal RA, Psaty BM, Burke GL. Serum potassium level and dietary potassium intake as risk factors for stroke. Neurology. 2002;59:314–20.
45. Khaw KT, Barrett-Conner E. Dietary potassium and stroke-associated mortality. N Engl J Med. 1987;316(5):235–40.
46. Smith NL, Lemaitre RN, Heckbert SR, Kaplan RC, Tirschwell DL, Longstreth WT, Psaty BM. Serum potassium and stroke risk among treated hypertensive adults. Am J Hypertens. 2003;16(10):806–13.
47. Ascherio A, Rimm EB, Hernán MA, Giovannucci EL, Kawachi I, Stampfer MJ, Willett WC. Intake of potassium, magnesium, calcium, and fiber and risk of stroke among US men. Circulation. 1998;98:1198–204.
48. Landmark K. Hypokalemia can accelerate the development of cerebrovascular and cardiovascular disease. Tidsskr Nor Laegeforen. 2002;122(5):499–501.
49. Gariball SE, Robinson TG, Fotherby MD. Hypokalemia and potassium excretion in stroke patients. J Am Geriatr Soc. 1997;45(12):1454–8.
50. Finestone HL, Greene-Finestone LS, Wilson ES, Teasell RW. Malnutrition in stroke patients on the rehabilitation service and at follow-up: prevalence and predictors. Arch Phys Med Rehabil. 1995;76:310–6.
51. Corrigan ML, Escuro AA, Celestin J, Kirby DF. Nutrition in the stroke patient. Nutr Clin Pract. 2011;26(3):242–52.
52. Oh H, Seo W. Alterations in fluid, electrolytes, and other serum chemistry values and their relations with enteral tube feeding in acute brain infarction patients. J Clin Nurs. 2007;16:298–307.
53. Davis M, Lucatorto M. Mannitol revisited. J Neurosci Nurs. 1994;26(3):170–4.
54. Cottrell JE, Robustelli A, Post K, Turndorf H. Furosemide and mannitol induced changes in intracranial pressure and serum osmolality and electrolytes. Anesthesiology. 1977;47:28–30.
55. Fang J, Madhavan S, Alderman MH. Dietary potassium intake and stroke mortality. Stroke. 2000;31:1532–7.

56. Forsyth LL, Liu-DeRyke X, Parker D, Rhoney DH. Role of hypertonic saline for the management of intracranial hypertension after stroke and traumatic brain injury. Pharmacotherapy. 2008;28(4):469–84.
57. The Emerging Risk Factors Collaboration. Diabetes mellitus, fasting blood glucose concentration, and risk of vascular disease: a collaborative meta-analysis of 102 prospective studies. Lancet. 2010;375:2215–22.
58. Lansberg MG, Albers GW, Wijman CA. Symptomatic intracerebral hemorrhage following thrombolytic therapy for acute ischemic stroke: a review of the risk factors. Cerebrovasc Disord. 2007;24:1–10.
59. Demchuk AM, Morganstern LB, Krieger DW, Chi TL, Hu W, Wein T, et al. Serum glucose level and diabetes predict tissue plasminogen activator-related intracerebral hemorrhage in acute ischemic strokes. Stroke. 1999;30:34–9.
60. Bruno A, Levine SR, Frankel MR, Brott TG, Lin Y, Tilley BC, et al. Admission glucose level and clinical outcomes in the NINDS rt-PA stroke trial. Neurology. 2002;59:669–74.
61. Capes SE, Hunt D, Malberg K, Pathak P, Gerstein HC. Stress hyperglycemia and prognosis of stroke in nondiabetic and diabetic patients: a systematic review. Stroke. 2001;32:2426–32.
62. Allport LE, Bucher KS, Baird TA, MacGregor L, Desmond PM, Tress BM, et al. Insular cortical ischemia is independently associated with acute stress hyperglycemia. Stroke. 2004;35:1886–91.
63. Frontera JA, Fernandez A, Claasen J, Schmidt M, Schumacher HC, Wartenberg K, et al. Hyperglycemia after SAH: predictors, associated complications, and impact on outcomes. Stroke. 2006;37:199–203.
64. Oddo M, Schmidt M, Carrera E, Badjatia N, Connolly ES, Presciutti M, et al. Impact of tight glycemic control on cerebral glucose metabolism after severe brain injury: a microdialysis study. Crit Care Med. 2008;36(12):3233–8.
65. Winn HR. Youman's neurological surgery. 6th ed. Amsterdam: Elsevier; 2011.
66. Saleh AAE, Megahed MMAE, Ibrahim KH. Hypomagnesaemia, hyponatremia and hypercholesterolemia on admission as prognostic predictors for patients with subarachnoid haemorrhage. Internet J Interv Med. 2010;1(1). doi: 10.5580/3e2. http://archive.ispub.com/journal/the-internet-journal-of-interventional-medicine/volume-1-number-1/hypomagnesemia-hyponatremia-and-hypercholesterolemia-on-admission-as-prognostic-predictors-for-patients-with-subarachinoid-haemorrhage-1.html#sthash.n9MG9ZZC.dpbs.
67. Darby BT. Intensive care in neurosurgery. Rolling Meadows, IL: Thieme; 2003.
68. Gunnerson KJ, Saul M, Kellum JA. Lactic nonlactic metabolic acidosis: a retrospective outcome evaluation of critically ill patients. Crit Care. 2006;10(1):R22.
69. Morgan TJ. Clinical review: the meaning of acid–base abnormalities in the intensive care unit—effects of fluid administration. Crit Care. 2005;9(2):204–11.
70. Ohira T, Peacock JM, Iso H, Chambless LE, Rosamond WD, Folsom AR. Serum and dietary magnesium and risk of ischemic stroke; The atherosclerosis risk in communities study. Am J Epidemiol. 2009;169(2):1437–44.
71. Saver JL, Kidwell C, Eckstein M. FAST-MAG Trial Investigators. Prehospital neuroprotective therapy for acute stroke: results of the field administration of stroke therapy magnesium (FAST-MAG) pilot trial. Stroke. 2004;35:e106–8.
72. Mitre N, Mack K, Babovic-Vuksanovic D, Thompason G, Kumar S. Ischemic stroke as the presenting symptom of primary hyperparathyroidism due to multiple endocrine neoplasia type 1. J Pediatr. 2008;153(4):582–5.
73. Lee MC, Klassen AC, Resch JA. Respiratory pattern disturbances in ischemic cerebral vascular disease. Stroke. 1974;5:612–6.
74. Guz A. Brain, breathing, and breathlessness. Respir Physiol. 1997;109:197–204.
75. Hirano M, Pavlakis SG. Mitochondrial myopathy, encephalopathy, lactic acidosis, and stroke like episodes (MELAS): current concepts. J Child Neurol. 1994;9(1):4–13.
76. Feldman E, Broderick JP, Kernan WN, Viscoli CM, Brass LM, Brott T, et al. Major risk factors for intracerebral hemorrhage in the young are modifiable. Stroke. 2005;36:1881–5.

77. Kimura K, Iguchi Y, Inoue T, Shibazaki K, Matsumoto N, Kobayashi K, et al. Hyperglycemia independently increases the risk of early death in acute spontaneous intracerebral hemorrhage. J Neurol Sci. 2007;255(1):90–4.
78. Qureshi AI, Palesch YY, Martin R, Novitzke J, Cruz-Flores S, Ehtisham A, et al. Association of serum glucose concentrations during acute hospitalization with hematoma expansion, peri-hematomal edema, and three month outcome among patients with intracerebral hemorrhage. Neurocrit Care. 2011;15(3):428–35.
79. Mehanna HM, Moledina J, Travis J. Refeeding syndrome: what it is, and how to prevent it. Br Med J. 2008;336(7659):1495–8.
80. Phillips BJ. Electrolyte replacement: a review. Internet J Intern Med. 2004;(5)1. doi:10.5580/1cf4

Chapter 13
Nutrition Support

Arlene A. Escuro and Mandy L. Corrigan

Key Points

- Nutrition support is of critical importance to both the ischemic and hemorrhagic stroke patient population due to dysphagia, altered mental status, and the possible need for intubation.
- Enteral nutrition (EN) is clearly established as the preferential route of nutrition support for this patient population, which should commence as early as feasible. Parenteral nutrition (PN) is indicated for the patient with a non-functioning and/or inability to access the gastrointestinal (GI) tract.
- The extent of neurological damage and recovery will affect nutrition requirements and the nutrition care plan.

Keywords Nutrition assessment • Enteral nutrition • Parenteral nutrition • Dysphagia • Stroke • Transitional feeding • Stroke rehabilitation

Abbreviations

ACTH	Adrenocorticotropin Releasing Hormone
ASPEN	American Society for Parentearl and Enteral Nutrition
BMI	Body Mass Index
EN	Enteral Nutrition
GI	Gastrointestinal

A.A. Escuro, M.S., R.D., L.D., C.N.S.C. (✉)
Nutrition Therapy, Cleveland Clinic, 9500 Euclid Avenue/M17, Cleveland, OH 44195, USA
e-mail: escuroa@ccf.org

M.L. Corrigan, M.P.H., R.D., L.D., C.N.S.C.
Nutrition Support Team, Cleveland Clinic, 9500 Euclid Avenue/TT2, Cleveland, OH 44195, USA
e-mail: mandycorrigan1@gmail.com

M.L. Corrigan et al. (eds.), *Handbook of Clinical Nutrition and Stroke*,
Nutrition and Health, DOI 10.1007/978-1-62703-380-0_13,
© Springer Science+Business Media New York 2013

ICP   Intracranial Pressure
IL-1RA   Interleukin-1 Preceptor Antagonist
IL-6   Interleukin-6
IVFE   Intravenous Fat Emulsion
LBM   Lean Body Mass
NDD   National Dysphagia Diet
PPN   Peripheral Parenteral Nutrition
PN   Parenteral Nutrition
TBI   Traumatic Brain Injury
TEE   Total Energy Expenditure

Metabolic Response Post Stroke

The intense catabolic response that occurs in patients who have sustained a traumatic brain injury (TBI) is well documented, but not well defined in the stroke
patient population. The earlier notion that stroke patients exhibit an initial hypermetabolic phase similar to TBI has been challenged over the past decade. Bardutzky
and colleagues evaluated 34 sedated, mechanically ventilated patients with ischemia and hemorrhagic stroke and found that total energy expenditure (TEE) as
determined by indirect calorimetry was low during the first 5 days after ICU admission [1]. In addition, the TEE did not differ between acute cerebral ischemia or
intracerebral hemorrhage. Brain injury resulting from stroke has metabolic and
physiologic consequences, and the presence of preexisting malnutrition and malnutrition that may develop after a stroke contributes to clinical outcomes [2–4]. The
obligatory mobilization of lean body mass (LBM) observed with brain injury is
estimated to be up to 25 g N per day, or triple the normal turnover rate, which would
cause a 70 kg man to lose 10% of LBM in a week [5]. Chalela and associates examined nitrogen balance in patients who had acute stroke (either ischemic or hemorrhagic) where enteral nutrition (EN) was initiated within 2 days of injury and
nitrogen balance was evaluated on day 5 [6]. The authors found that 44.4% of
patients were in negative nitrogen balance and concluded that patients were
underfed.

The injured brain stimulates the secretion of many hormones that affect metabolic function such as adrenocorticotrophin releasing hormone (ACTH), growth
hormone, prolactin, vasopressin, and cortisol as a natural response to stress. In addition, glucagon and catecholamines are released in excess. Although catecholamines
are released to help support blood pressure and cardiac output (and hence cerebral
perfusion), the surge of catecholamines after an acute brain injury leads to hyperglycemia and hyperinsulinemia, which impairs ketogenesis and promotes protein
catabolism. The resultant catabolic state can have significant detrimental effects on
systemic organ function [7].

After excluding patients with evidence of infection, Beamer and colleagues [8]
found higher levels of interleukin-6 (IL-6), a regulator of the acute phase response,

Table 13.1
Interpretation of BMI [9]

BMI	Interpretation
Below 18.5	Underweight
18.5–24.9	Normal
25–29.9	Overweight
30–34.9	Obesity (grade 1)
35–39.9	Obesity (grade 2)
Greater than 40	Obesity (grade 3)

and interleukin-1 receptor antagonist (IL-1RA), an anti-inflammatory mediator in the acute phase, in patients with acute stroke compared with healthy, community-living controls ($p<0.001$). Both IL-6 and IL-1RA were significantly correlated with the C-reactive protein, an acute phase protein, suggesting that there is an acute phase response to brain infarction. Exogenous substrates provided by EN or PN may reduce the need for the liberation of endogenous substrate stores, and thus reduce these catabolic effects.

Nutrition Assessment

Components

Components of a comprehensive nutrition assessment include evaluation of anthropometrics, biochemical markers, clinical examination, and the patient's recent diet history. Although the same four components of nutrition assessment are utilized regardless of the patient's injury or disease state, the focus of these components can be tailored to the unique nutritional needs of the stroke patient. Nutrition assessment identifies patients requiring nutrition intervention and the ideal timing of intervention.

Assessment of body weight and composition guides nutrition assessment, estimation of nutritional requirements (macronutrient needs), and development of a nutrition care plan. Body mass index (BMI, {weight (kg)/height (m)^2}) is often a starting point to a nutrition assessment. See Table 13.1 for interpretation of BMI [9]. Caution must be taken when interpreting BMI as it may be overinflated by altered weight from fluid resuscitation or fluid retention in the ICU setting. A recent, pre-morbid weight or edema free admission weight should be used for BMI calculations. Assessment of the patient's weight history pre-neurological injury will guide the nutrition clinician in assessment of the nutritional status.

Unfortunately, there is no universally accepted definition of malnutrition. Currently The American Society for Parenteral and Enteral Nutrition (A.S.P.E.N.) defines malnutrition as "an acute, sub acute, or chronic state of nutrition, in which a combination of varying degrees of overnutrition or undernutrition and inflammatory activity have led to a change in body composition and diminished function" [10].

Table 13.2

Predictive equation

Formula	Male	Female
Harris-Benedict equation	BMR = 66 + (13.7 × weight (kg)) + (5 × height (cm)) − (6.8 × age (years))	BMR = 655 + (9.6 × weight (kg)) + (1.8 × height (cm)) − (4.7 × age (years))

A new A.S.P.E.N. Taskforce is proposing a new method to diagnose malnutrition by taking into account the impact of the inflammatory response on nutritional status [11]. Once validated, this will be a tool to help universalize the diagnosis of malnutrition.

Obtaining a detailed nutrition history including intake and recent weight history is critical for nutrition assessment. A weight history that reveals involuntary weight loss of greater than 10% of usual body weight in 6 months or loss of 5% of usual body weight in 1 month indicates malnutrition. Cognitive function or intubation status may limit the patient from providing an accurate history and nutrition professionals may need to seek this information from family members or other caregivers. A nutrition focused physical exam will identify edema, muscle wasting, signs of nutrient deficiencies, and assist in assessment of nutritional status.

As equations to estimate nutritional requirements are fraught with inaccuracies (of either under- or overestimation of caloric needs), indirect calorimetry is the gold standard for determining caloric requirements. Unfortunately, indirect calorimetry is not routinely available for use in many institutions for a variety of reasons (largely due to cost and the need for skilled clinicians to preform and interpret the readings). No single predictive equation is available or has been validated with a large patient sample size in the stroke population. The presence of obesity may also further complicate calculation of nutritional requirements when indirect calorimetry is unavailable.

Finestone and colleagues used indirect calorimetry on day 7, 11, 14, 21, and 90 days post stroke to study energy demands over time after stroke [12]. Resting energy expenditure (REE) was shown to be approximately 10% higher than predicted by the Harris-Benedict equation, but energy needs did not differ by type of stroke, and changes in resting energy expenditures were not statistically significant over time [12]. These results confirm findings from a smaller study that measured REE 24–72 h following stroke and a repeated measurement of REE 10–14 days after [13]. The authors suggested that energy requirements were not elevated due to decreased physical activity and changes in muscle tone due to the neurological injury [13]. See Table 13.2 for predictive equations for nutrition assessment. The caloric content of medications such as propofol (1.1 cal/mL) or dextrose containing intravenous fluids should be taken into consideration for the nutrition feeding prescription to prevent overfeeding.

Protein needs should be individualized, but 1–1.5 g/kg is recommended [14]. Protein needs may be higher in rehabilitation patients in the presence of wounds. Mobility limitations may also predispose patients for skin breakdown and development of pressure ulcers. Routine skin assessment is required and provision of adequate protein is prudent.

Infection, mobility, activity levels, and weight status may alter caloric requirements leading to the need for frequent reassessment. When limitations in mobility or paralysis are present, caloric requirements will be lower due to decreased activity. Early medical treatments in the acute care setting with barbiturates or induced hypothermia as a method to decrease intracranial pressure also decreases caloric requirements [1, 15]. Indirect calorimetry is ideal for assessment of nutritional needs in these clinical scenarios.

Many professionals heavily rely on biochemical markers to quickly label nutritional status. Hepatic proteins such as albumin, prealbumin (transthyretin), and transferrin are commonly used as nutritional markers in clinical practice. Historically, the use of serum albumin was used to define malnutrition in hospitalized patients. Older studies, including the majority of those done in the stroke population, commonly placed a strong emphasis on equating low albumin levels to malnutrition without accounting for the role of the inflammatory cascade after injury. After neurological injury, metabolic demands are altered with elevation of peripheral plasma catecholamines, cortisol, glucagon, interleukin-6, interleukin-IRA, and acute phase proteins [12]. These alterations directly impact the way traditional biochemical markers of nutrition are assessed.

Now with the recent focus on the impact of inflammation on nutrition, clinicians understand that hepatic proteins are influenced by many non-nutritional factors and change rapidly in times of stress and in turn do not accurately reflect nutritional status. Mediators of inflammation have the largest effect on serum protein levels and contribute to an increase in net protein loss from catabolism [16]. Albumin, prealbumin, and transferrin are all negative acute phase proteins, thereby the liver decreases production of these components in the presence of inflammation regardless of pre-morbid nutritional status.

Albumin can be a good marker of nutritional status in the absence of inflammation and infection. Given the long half-life of albumin (20 days), it may only be ideal for long-term care or rehabilitation settings. Prealbumin (3 days) and transferrin (7 days) have much shorter half-lives compared to albumin and are more appropriately monitored in the acute care setting along with C-reactive protein levels for a decrease of inflammation. Following hepatic protein levels over time may be considered to be of more clinical significance by some clinicians than a single point in time measurement. Although commonly used in clinical practice, the use of prealbumin and C-reactive protein have not been validated.

Timing of Enteral Nutrition

Once it is determined that a stroke patient cannot be fed orally, EN should be initiated in the first 24–48 h, as it clearly becomes an important goal for the initial nutrition support plan. Early EN has been associated with beneficial effects such as attenuation of the hypercatabolic response, gut atrophy, muscle mass loss, and infection in brain injury patients [17]. Chiang and colleagues found EN initiated within 48 h post injury in patients with severe TBI is associated with greater survival rate, Glasgow Coma Score (GCS) recovery, and a better clinical outcome at 1 month post injury [18]. The provision of early nutrition forestalls the breakdown of protein and fat stores, blunts the innate inflammatory response, promotes immune competence, decreases intensive care unit (ICU) infections, limits the risk of bacterial translocation, and improves neurologic outcome at 3 months after injury [16, 19].

Enteral Nutrition

The major effect on the GI tract following stroke is impairment of oral, pharyngeal, and esophageal functions manifested as dysphagia. Swallowing requires multiple neurologic inputs to perform correctly and damage to these circuits may occur as a result of stroke in as many as 60% of patients [20]. The decision on how to feed a stroke patient should be made shortly after hospital admission and will be partially dictated by the patient's presenting condition and medical/surgical history [21]. See the enteral stroke feeding algorithm in Fig. 13.1 [21]. The selected route of nutrition support should commence as soon as the stroke patient is stabilized and adequately resuscitated. In addition, a patient who sustained a massive stroke may be vented initially and require specialized nutrition support. Appropriate candidates for EN have functional GI tracts and no contraindications to placement of a feeding tube, such as coagulopathy following tissue plasminogen activator (t-PA) administration or previous medical/surgical procedures such as gastrointestinal (GI) surgery that may alter normal anatomy [22].

Numerous challenges exist in providing adequate EN to critically ill stroke patients such as impaired gastric emptying due to vagus nerve damage, elevated levels of endogenous opioids and endorphins, or medications such as pentobarbital or narcotics, altered levels of consciousness, and overall neurologic function [7, 23, 24]. Patients who are in the ICU can have elevated intracranial pressure (ICP), which can delay gastric emptying. Thus, initial attempts to feed via a nasogastric tube may not be successful, and small bowel feeding should be considered. However, careful consideration of clinical status is warranted before endoscopically placing a feeding device in patients with ICP elevations [7, 25]. Monitoring the ICP is important during endoscopic procedures in critically ill stroke patients to minimize secondary insults to the brain (intracranial hypertension, seizures, and cerebral edema) [7]. As the ICP improves, patients often tolerate gastric feeding [21]. Tube feeding should be started as a continuous drip, full strength at 10–20 mL/h, and advanced to goal rate by 10–20 mL every 4–8 h. In the stable stroke patient who is tolerating gastric feedings, tube feeding regimens may be adjusted on an individual basis to a bolus or gravity controlled regimen to facilitate initiation of oral intake or to avoid food–drug interactions.

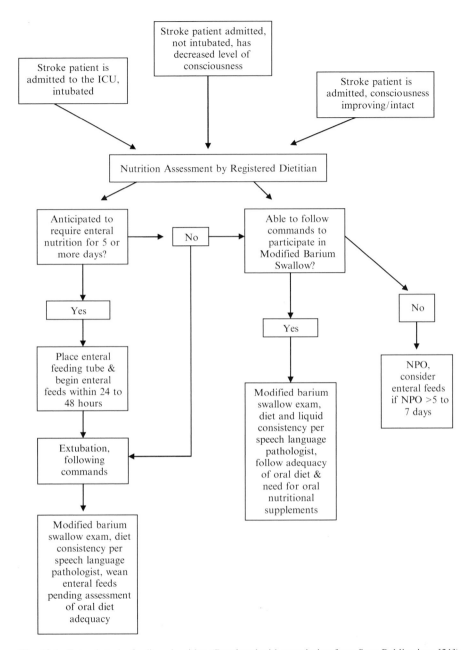

Fig. 13.1 Enteral stroke feeding algorithm (Reprinted with permission from Sage Publications [21])

Caution is also warranted in patients receiving EN and high doses of vasopressors due to case reports of ischemic bowel. EN should be withheld in patients who are hypotensive (mean arterial pressure <60 mmHg), particularly if clinicians are initiating use of catecholamine agents (norepinephrine, phenylephrine, epinephrine, dopamine) or escalating the dose of such agents to maintain hemodynamic stability. It appears that provision of EN with caution to patients on stable low doses of pressor agents is safer than initially thought. If a patient is on stable or declining doses of vasopressors, start trophic or trickle feeds of 10–20 mL/h of a polymeric, fiber-free solution and leave at that rate for 24 h then reassess. But any signs of intolerance (abdominal distention, increasing nasogastric tube output or gastric residual volumes, decreased passage of stool and flatus, hypoactive bowel sounds, rising lactate, increasing metabolic acidosis and/or base deficit), should be scrutinized as possible early signs of gut ischemia [26]. If the patient is tolerating slow rate EN and the clinical condition is improving, start to increase the feeding rate. A recent large scale, multicenter, observational study evaluated mechanically ventilated, vasopressor dependent patients who were classified as to whether they were fed within 48 h (early group) or after 48 h (after group). They used sophisticated statistical strategies (propensity scores) to adjust for potential confounding variables and showed that vasopressor dependent patients fed early (within 48 h) had a significant survival advantage compared to the delayed group (after 48 h) [27].

Nasally inserted small bowel feeding access devices are generally safe and easily inserted at bedside. Adequate anchoring of the tube is essential to prevent the tube from getting dislodged due to patient agitation, discomfort, or inadequate sedation. In these instances, use of a commercial retention system or nasal bridle has been associated with fewer displaced tubes [28–30]. Acosta-Escribano and associates evaluated the efficacy of small bowel feeding compared with gastric feeding in patients with severe TBI and found a decrease in the incidence of ventilator-associated pneumonia, low rate of GI complications, and tube malfunction [31]. Implementation of feeding protocols that specifically address the timing of establishing enteral access, tube placement confirmation, and route of feeding (EN or PN) could assist clinicians so patients are fed as quickly as possible [26].

Enteral Formula Selection

Enteral tube feeding formulas are generally well tolerated in the stroke patient population. Depending on calorie and protein needs, a 1 kcal/mL to a 2 kcal/mL, polymeric, standard intact protein formula is appropriate. Very limited data exists regarding any benefits or detriments of specialty products in the stroke patient population. The role of elemental and semi-elemental enteral tube feeding formulations is not well defined in this patient population. The use of fiber must be considered in light of the medical plan of care. Fiber is avoided in cases where pressors or paralytic agents are being used. Fiber-containing formulation is generally recommended for patients requiring long-term enteral feedings, especially during rehabilitation.

Most 2 kcal/mL formulas do not meet estimated protein requirements for this population. Therefore, patients will require use of a protein supplement to meet needs. Monitoring protein supplementation is difficult as albumin and prealbumin are both negative acute phase proteins and are more indicative of inflammation and not nutrition deprivation or recovery. Protein supplementation should be routinely reviewed and adjusted during the course of stroke recovery. A 2 kcal/mL formula may also be warranted during fluid restriction for control of the syndrome of inappropriate antidiuretic hormone (SIADH).

Complications of Enteral Nutrition

Diarrhea is the most commonly reported complication of enteral feeding. No universally accepted definition of diarrhea exists. However, a clinically useful definition is any abnormal volume or consistency of stool. Normal stool water content is 250–500 mL/day. Diarrhea has also been defined as >500 mL every 8 h or >3 stools per day for at least 2 consecutive days [32, 33]. Most standard EN formulas are lactose free, not excessively high in fat, and are not exceedingly hypertonic to cause diarrhea. Brain-injured patients often receive elixirs (containing sorbitol), electrolyte supplements, and other medications that are extremely hypertonic compared to the EN [7]. Patients with diarrhea should be evaluated and treated in a stepwise approach before using parenteral nutrition (PN). Once infection and medication-related factors have been eliminated as causes of diarrhea, changing to an enteral formula with added fiber or addition of soluble fiber to the medication regimen may lessen diarrhea. A semi-elemental EN product may improve absorption and minimize diarrhea. Antidiarrheal agents can be added once *Clostridium difficile* has been ruled out or is being treated. Constipation is common in the stroke patient receiving narcotics and should be given a standing bowel regimen when not experiencing diarrhea.

Gastric residuals have traditionally been used to assess tolerance to tube feeding and aspiration risk. Research has shown no correlation between the presence of high gastric residual volumes and gastric emptying, regurgitation, vomiting, and pneumonia [34]. An isolated incidence of a high gastric residual volume should not prompt enteral feeding to be held without other signs and symptoms of intolerance. Evidence suggests that a decision to stop tube feeding should be based on a trend in serial measurements and not on a single isolated high volume [35].

Implementation of a feeding protocol has been recommended by clinical practice guidelines as a key strategy to standardize the delivery of EN, maximize the benefits, and minimize the risks of EN in the critically ill patients [26]. Utilizing feeding protocols or algorithms not only improve the delivery of EN, but have also been shown to improve outcome. Results of a multicenter observational study showed that sites that used feeding protocol use more EN, started EN earlier, and used more motility agents in patients with high gastric residual volumes compared to sites that did not use a feeding protocol [36]. In addition, adequacy of EN was higher in sites with protocols compared to non-protocol sites. Components of feeding protocols may include orders for early initiation of EN, use of motility agents, gastric residual volumes, head of the bed elevation, and use of small bowel feeding tubes.

If delayed gastric emptying is suspected, appropriate interventions include elevating the head of bed by 30° to 45° to decrease reflux of gastric contents into the pharynx and esophagus and X-ray confirmation of feeding tube placement [26]. The use of small bowel feeding tubes (ideally the tip of the feeding tube located in the third portion of the duodenum or further distal) allows for increased feeding tolerance and to minimize pulmonary aspiration [37]. Small bowel access can be attained at the bedside, and a number of techniques that will be described on Chap. 14 (endoscopically, fluoroscopically, etc.). Continuous infusion of EN is better tolerated early in neurologic illness compared to bolus feedings. If nausea or vomiting occur as the rate of administration of the EN increases, the rate should be reduced to the last tolerated amount, with an attempt to increase the rate again after the symptoms abate. Promotility agents such as metoclopramide or erythromycin should also be considered to promote peristalsis and EN tolerance. Promotility agents are not without adverse effects, so these agents should be used for a short duration until the desired effect is obtained and maintained [7].

Abdominal distention and its associated symptoms of bloating and cramping, usually occurs as a result of ileus and obstruction. Critically ill stroke patients frequently require paralytic agents and narcotics which can contribute to poor GI motility and may prevent the patient from reaching their EN goal. Discontinuation of EN and initiation of PN may be necessary if the motility is poor or if the bowel is markedly dilated.

Parenteral Nutrition

The use of PN in the stroke population is rare, but when indicated is not without risk. The use of small bowel feeding tubes has alleviated many cases of inappropriate PN use. Common complications of PN used on a short-term basis include hyperglycemia, catheter related blood stream infection, and electrolyte imbalances.

Indications for Parenteral Nutrition

Delivery of enteral nutrients provides multiple benefits over delivery of nutrients via the parenteral route. Benefits of EN include decreased length of stay, lower risk of infection, decreased cost, and fewer hyperglycemia and infectious complications compared to PN, and also maintains integrity of the gut mucosa, preserves gut barrier function, and gut associated immune function [38–42].

Indications for PN require the patient to present with a nonfunctioning GI tract or unable to ingest or absorb adequate nutrients from EN (either orally or via a feeding tube). Indications for PN include diffuse peritonitis, intestinal obstruction, intractable vomiting or diarrhea, prolonged ileus, and GI ischemia [39], radiation enteritis, malabsorption from short bowel syndrome, high output GI fistulas, severe GI bleed, and pseudo-obstruction [38, 43]. These medical conditions necessitating use of PN are not routinely seen following stroke.

In the stroke population, the use of PN may be indicated with prolonged inability to access the GI tract depending on the patient's pre-morbid nutritional status. Every attempt to achieve enteral access should continue to be made after PN is initiated. The use of small bowel feeding tubes (ideally the tip of the feeding tube should be located in the third portion of the duodenum or beyond—see Chap. 14) can avoid the inappropriate use of PN for ileus or gastroparesis following stroke. Patients receiving PN therapy should exhibit presence of significant malnutrition. For the benefit of PN to be realized, PN should be used for at least 7 days [26]. Clinically, it may be challenging for clinicians to predict the length of use of PN therapy as each patient case and progress is unique.

The timing of PN initiation is important and is determined based on the patient's nutritional status. Published ICU nutrition guidelines from the Society for Critical Care Medicine (SCCM) and the American Society for Parenteral and Enteral Nutrition (A.S.P.E.N) in 2009 specifically address use and timing of PN in the critically ill population. In the presence of severe malnutrition (as identified from nutrition assessment), if EN is not possible, PN should be started early after adequate resuscitation to reduce complications compared to just providing standard therapy (intravenous fluids and no nutrition support) [41, 44]. Standard therapy (intravenous fluids and no nutrition support) in severely malnourished ICU patients leads to a higher risk of mortality and also a trend towards a higher rate of infection [44].

In the absence of malnutrition prior to ICU admission, where EN is not an option or indicated, standard therapy (intravenous fluids and no nutrition support) is superior to PN until after 7 days [26]. Standard therapy was associated with significantly less infectious morbidity, and a trend towards overall reduction in complications compared to use of PN [45]. When PN was provided in patients who were not malnourished, an increase in mortality and a trend towards increased rate of complications occurred [44].

Contraindications for Providing Parenteral Nutrition

The main contraindication to PN is a functional GI tract. Other contraindications include unstable cardiopulmonary parameters, aggressive therapy is no longer desired due to DNR status, or unstable fluid and electrolytes. Initiation of PN should be delayed until fluid and electrolyte disturbances are fully corrected as evidenced by normal serum values. Careful ongoing monitoring and correction of electrolyte abnormalities and glycemic control is prudent in patients receiving PN.

Vascular Access and Types of Parenteral Nutrition Solutions

There are a variety of vascular access devices through which PN may be infused. The choice for which vascular access device to use is dictated by the length of PN therapy. Peripheral catheters can be used on a short-term basis to provide peripheral PN (PPN); however, the patient's full nutritional requirements will not be met. PPN is generally only used for a maximum of 1–2 weeks due to the increased amount of fat provided. Fat contributes least to the osmolarity of a PPN solution leading to the higher amount of fat dosed in PPN. A PPN solution with a maximum of 900 mOsm can be infused through a peripheral catheter (see Chap. 19 for calculation of peripheral PN and osmolarity).

A peripheral catheter providing PPN may be useful while awaiting placement of central access or confirmation of the location of the tip of the catheter. Peripheral PN should not be used in patients with cardiac or renal dysfunction necessitating fluid restriction or in any patient requiring a low volume PN solution. Peripheral PN solutions deliver a large percentage of calories as isotonic fat emulsions and a smaller percentage of dextrose and protein calories, and are less hypertonic than central PN solutions (less than 900 mOsm).

Hospitalized patients commonly have temporary central venous catheters (either via the internal jugular or subclavian veins) or Peripherally Inserted Central Catheters (PICCs). When a vascular access device is used for PN, the tip of the central venous catheter should be placed with the tip located at the cavo-atrial junction to reduce the risk of catheter associated venous thrombosis [38, 46–48]. Other acceptable positions for the tip of the vascular access device include the mid to lower third of the superior vena cava. It is critical in the stroke patient especially to take any measure to avoid thrombosis as anticoagulation may be contraindicated in certain patients after a stroke [21]. A central PN solution has no limit on osmolarity as does peripheral PN and therefore can be customized to meet the patient's full nutritional requirements. For calculation of central PN solutions see Chap. 19.

Parenteral Nutrition Solutions

The three basic components of a PN solution include dextrose (as dextrose monohydrate providing 3.4 cal/g), protein (in the form of crystalline amino acids providing 4 cal/g), and intravenous fat emulsion ([IVFE] providing 10 cal/g). It is a general recommendation that IVFE be limited to provide no more than 1 g/kg of body weight of fat per day. PN solutions providing only dextrose and protein are called two-in-one PN solutions whereas three-in-one PN solutions contain dextrose, protein, and IVFE. The decision to incorporate IVFE into the PN solution is individualized based on the clinical judgment. SCCM and A.S.P.E.N. Guidelines suggest IVFE free PN solutions for ICU patients during the first week of therapy [26].

Additives

Electrolytes are added as salts for maintenance of serum electrolytes. Calcium, magnesium, potassium, sodium, and phosphorus may be added to PN solutions. Potassium and sodium salts come in the form of acetate or chloride and are manipulated based on that patients laboratory studies (serum bicarbonate and chloride levels). Standard intravenous multivitamin (MVI) and multiple trace element preparations are added to PN solutions daily. Some MVI solutions contain a small amount of vitamin K (150 µg), but the MVI should not be omitted from the PN solution when on anticoagulation therapy as the amount of vitamin K is consistent from day to day.

Iron is not routinely added to PN solutions and cannot be added to a PN solution containing IVFE due to the risk of destabilizing the solution [49]. The only form of iron compatible with fat free PN solutions is iron dextran and a test dose must be given outside the PN solution before it can be added due to the risk of anaphylaxis. Iron therapy via PN solutions is rarely used in the ICU setting and only with long-term PN patients outside the ICU setting. Iron should not be given in times of infection or sepsis [49].

Medications may be added to PN solutions; however, if the PN solution is stopped for any reason the patient does not receive the full dose of the medication. Commonly added medications include H2 blockers, octreotide, insulin, hydrocortisone, or heparin.

Parenteral Nutrition Administration

PN solutions are infused over 24 h in acute care settings. Calories are gradually increased over a few days to provide the patients full nutritional requirements while monitoring electrolytes and blood sugars. Cyclic PN solutions are typically only used in the home or long-term care setting.

Parenteral Nutrition Complications

Complications of PN include infectious (catheter sepsis or site infections), mechanical (catheter occlusions, breaks), and metabolic (hyperglycemia, electrolyte abnormalities, metabolic bone disease). Other complications include thrombosis and PN associated liver disease. Short-term PN complications seen in the acute care setting with short-term PN use are mainly hyperglycemia and electrolyte abnormalities, but also can include catheter sepsis and mechanical complications.

Hyperglycemia seen with initiation of PN solutions can be managed in many ways. Initiating PN with a gradual increase of the dextrose load is prudent along with frequent monitoring until blood sugars are stable on the goal calorie PN

Table 13.3
Parenteral nutrition monitoring for the hospital setting

Baseline (before PN initiation)	First 3 days (or until normal values on goal PN solution)	Weekly
CMP[a]	BMP[b]	CMP[a]
Magnesium and phosphorus	Magnesium and phosphorus	Magnesium and phosphorus
Complete blood count		Complete blood count
Glucose, serum	Every 6 h with continuous PN	On CMP

[a]Complete metabolic panel (sodium, potassium, chloride, bicarbonate, blood urea nitrogen, creatinine, glucose, total protein, albumin, AST, ALT, Alk phos, bilirubin)
[b]Basic metabolic panel (sodium, potassium, chloride, bicarbonate, blood urea nitrogen, creatinine, glucose)

solution. Insulin drips can be utilized in the ICU setting for severe hyperglycemia and insulin can be added to the PN solution to assist with glycemic control. Great debate continues on the ideal range to maintain glycemic control. Blood sugars may be elevated due to reasons other than PN solutions such as medications (steroids), past medical history (diabetes, pancreatitis), and in the presence of infection.

Refeeding syndrome or a shift of serum electrolytes from the serum to intracellular space may occur in malnourished patients when initiating a large number of calories through initial PN solutions. Hypomagnesemia, hypokalemia, and hypophosphatemia are frequently observed with excessive dextrose in initial PN solutions [50]. Gradual advancement of calories via PN solutions is prudent to avoid this metabolic complication.

Parenteral Nutrition Monitoring

See Table 13.3 for suggested monitoring of PN therapy in the hospital setting.

Dysnatremia

Disturbances of sodium balance, referred to as dysnatremia, are frequently observed in neurocritical patients. In the past, fluid restriction was a common practice in patients with elevated ICP to reduce ICP by decreasing total circulating volume. Today, however, most data suggest resuscitation to a normal intravascular volume, with the avoidance of hyponatremia and hypo-osmolarity [51]. Hyponatremia can occur due to the syndrome of inappropriate antidiuretic hormone (SIADH) or cerebral salt wasting syndrome (CSWS). The physiological response elicited by SIADH results in renal conservation of water and a dilutional hyponatremia that is treated with a water restriction. To facilitate a negative fluid balance, concentrated enteral or parenteral formulations should be provided.

The primary defect in CSWS is due to the kidney's inability to conserve salt due to intracranial disease, resulting to hyponatremia and volume depletion. CSWS is predominantly associated with subarachnoid hemorrhage (SAH), but has also been described in conjunction with traumatic brain injury, glioma, and tuberculous or carcinomatous meningitis [52]. Once the presence of CSWS is confirmed, treatment consists of volume and salt replacement which may be accomplished by intravenous (IV) normal saline, or rarely, hypertonic saline, and/or oral/enteral salt provision [53]. The initial finding of an abnormal sodium level should always prompt specific investigation into the underlying cause before management is initiated. The speed of the onset of the hyponatremia, as well as the presence of symptoms, is most important because patients with the most rapid onset are more likely to become symptomatic [54]. A differentiation must be made between hypervolemia with normal total body sodium (suggesting SIADH) and hypovolemia with disproportionately low total body sodium (suggesting CSWS). This differentiation is crucial because the managements of these two conditions are diametrically opposed, but will not be considered further here [53].

Hypernatremia and hyperosmolality due to diabetes insipidus (DI) may frequently develop in patients with severe cerebral disease or injury. DI is characterized by urinary output of more than 300 mL/h with a specific gravity of <1.005, along with a rising serum sodium [51]. These patients often require the aggressive use of desmopressin acetate (DDAVPP) via the intravenous (IV) or subcutaneous route.

Medication Considerations

Impaired absorption of phenytoin with patients on enteral feeding is probably the most commonly known drug–nutrient interaction. Phenytoin is an anticonvulsant often used for the prevention and treatment of posttraumatic seizures. Holding EN for 1 h before and after each dose of the acid suspension (adequately shaken to ensure even particle distribution) appears to be feasible and effective option for circumventing this interaction [7]. If EN is to be held for phenytoin delivery, adjust the EN infusion rate to avoid underfeeding and verify by checking actual EN delivered into the patient (see Chap. 19 for modifying EN schedule with oral/enteral phenytoin). To avoid routine EN interruptions, the IV route for phenytoin administration may be a better option.

Propofol, a short-acting anesthetic and sedative, is commonly used in neurocritical patients because it is easily titrated to desirable clinical effects, and its actions are rapidly terminated with drug discontinuation [55]. In vitro, propofol has been shown to be neuroprotective against oxygen and glucose deprivation brain injury [56]. The oil source is soybean, composed of long-chain triglycerides (LCTs) and omega-6 fatty acid. This 10% lipid vehicle provides 1.1 kcal/mL (0.1 g/mL) calories in the form of fat, primarily linoleic acid. Because propofol also contains egg lecithin, it should be used with caution in patients who have known allergy to soy or eggs. The extra calories provided should be considered when recommending nutrition support regimens. Institutions with sedation protocol in place should include a nutrition component, such as routine measurement of triglycerides and adjustment of nutrition support formulations to avoid overfeeding and ensure protein adequacy (see Chap. 19 for modifying EN regimen with propofol administration).

Metabolic suppression agents such as pentobarbital are used to induce a pharmacologic coma in an effort to decrease cerebral metabolism. Neurocritical patients receiving pentobarbital for refractory elevated ICP may have diminished energy requirement due to decreased cerebral and peripheral energy demands [57]. The use of these medications for the treatment of elevated ICP should be considered when estimating nutrition needs and plan of care. Pentobarbital-induced coma decreases the tone and amplitude of contractions of the GI tract; therefore, patients are more likely to not tolerate EN [58]. Routine use of bowel regimens with stool softeners and stimulants may delay or eliminate the development of a drug-induced ileus [7].

Nutrition in Stroke Rehabilitation

Enteral Nutrition

Swallowing difficulties that require placement of an enteral feeding tube to safely maintain adequate nutrition and hydration are common following a severe stroke. EN may represent a sole or supplemental source of nutrition support after stroke. Generally, EN as the sole source of nutrient intake is reserved for dysphagic patients for whom oral feeding is considered unsafe. However, failure to thrive non-dysphagic stroke patients may also be candidates for EN in the presence of prolonged and inadequate oral intake [59]. The use of feeding tubes in these stroke patients has been shown to reverse malnutrition [60]. A nasoenteric tube is often placed in patients who are expected to return to a full oral diet within 1 month. A permanent feeding access is indicated when a prolonged period of non-oral intake (>1 month) is anticipated (see Chap. 14).

There is a growing practice trend to refer more stroke patients who have high levels of medical severity and complexity to rehabilitation programs, a change that has shifted the management of many acute medical problems into the rehabilitation setting. This trend has brought to rehabilitation units more patients who need external support for nutrition, hydration, ventilation, and other physiological functions. One study showed that the presence of ≥1 medical tubes (enteral feeding tube, tracheostomy, or indwelling urethral catheter) is associated with more severe and disabling strokes, an increased number of medical complications, longer acute and rehabilitation hospitalizations, and greater resource use [61].

Ickenstein and colleagues investigated the predictors for removal of a feeding tube from stroke patients during rehabilitation and identified three negative predictors (bilateral stroke, aspiration during videofluoroscopic swallowing study, and age) [62]. A follow-up study by Ickenstein et al. reported that 11.6% of stroke patients admitted to a rehabilitation hospital required an enteral feeding tube secondary to dysphagia, and only 45% of the patients were able to resume oral diets and have their feeding tubes removed [63]. In the same study, the authors gave a conservative estimate that a large percentage of patients with a feeding tube placement in the acute period after stroke will return to oral feeding within 3 months of stroke onset [63]. In another study, 47% of stroke patients were able to return to three meals daily within 5.5 weeks from onset of stroke, and 20% of the patients were able to have their feeding tubes removed prior to discharge from inpatient rehabilitation [64]. Factors associated with returning to three meals daily included gender (i.e., female), longer inpatient rehabilitation length of stay, and higher admission Functional Independence Measurement (FIM) scores [64]. The removal of the feeding tube was associated with patients being more likely to be discharged to the home environment.

Specialized Diets for Dysphagia

Nutrition therapies for dysphagia have been standardized by the Academy of Nutrition and Dietetics through the National Dysphagia Diet Task Force. The National Dysphagia Diet (NDD) was instituted in April 2002 to standardize food consistencies and terminology throughout the health care continuum. Dietitians, speech-language pathologists, and food researchers from this task force developed the NDD. It includes three levels of solid foods (dysphagia pureed, dysphagia mechanically altered, dysphagia advanced) and four levels of fluids (thin, nectar-thick, honey-thick, spoon-thick) [65]. See Table 13.4 for an overview of the three levels of the NDD [21].

Liquids may need to be thickened to the appropriate consistency as recommended by the speech language pathologist. Some patients may be on a regular solid consistency but still require altered liquid consistencies. Commercially available gel and powder thickening agents can be added to liquids to achieve the recommended consistency (nectar-thick, honey-thick, or spoon-thick). See Chap. 19 for a list of commercial and household liquid thickening agents. Pre-thickened beverages are also available and provide less variation in consistency compared with gel or powder thickening agents. Of concern, is that the thicker the liquid is made, the less fluid is usually consumed by the patient. Dehydration can be a potentially overwhelming problem for patients with dysphagia. Many of these patients will require an additional source for hydration either by intravenous fluids or by a feeding tube.

The level 1 NDD (dysphagia pureed) is designed for patients who have moderate to severe dysphagia with poor oral phase abilities and reduced ability to protect their airway. The diet consists of pureed, homogenous, and cohesive foods that have "pudding-like" texture. Foods that require bolus formation, controlled manipulation, or mastication are excluded.

The level 2 NDD (dysphagia mechanically altered) is indicated for patients with mild to moderate oral and/or pharyngeal dysphagia. This level consists of foods that are moist, soft-textured, and easily formed into bolus. This diet is used in transition from the pureed texture to a more solid texture. All foods from NDD level 1 are appropriate at this level.

Table 13.4
The national dysphagia diet

Food type	Breads	Cereals/grains	Dairy/desserts	Fats	Fruits	Meat/meat substitutes	Soups	Vegetables	Other
Level 1 Pureed *Recommend*	Pureed breads (pancakes, muffins, bread, etc.)	Smooth cooked cereals (farina type), pureed noodles	Smooth pudding, custard, pureed desserts	Butter, strained gravy, mayo, cheese sauces	Pureed fruits, thickened juices (no pulp, seeds, chunks)	Pureed meat or eggs, hummus, legumes	Pureed, thickened soup broth	Pureed vegetables, mashed potatoes, tomato sauce	Sugar, salt, spices, ketchup, honey, smooth jelly
Level 1 Pureed *Avoid*	Non-pureed breads	Dry cereals, oatmeal, cooked cereal with lumps	Ice cream, gelatins, non-pureed baked goods, chewy candy	Fats with coarse, chunky additives	Whole fruit (frozen, fresh, canned, or dried)	Whole or ground meat, non-pureed eggs	Non-pureed soups or broth with chunks	Non-pureed vegetables, tomato sauce with seeds or chunks	Coarse pepper, jams with seeds, nuts, sticky foods
Level 2 Mechanically altered *Recommend*	Soft pancakes with syrup, slurried breads	Cooked cereal with texture (oatmeal), dumplings with gravy, noodles in sauce	Pudding, custard, cake with icing, canned fruit, soft chocolates	Butter, gravy, sour cream, mayo, cheese sauce	Soft canned or cooked fruit without skin, ripe bananas, gelatin with canned fruit	Moistened ground meats in gravy/sauce, pasta, scrambled eggs	Soup with veggies or meat (<½ in. in size)	Well-cooked vegetables, boiled or baked potatoes	Jams and preserves without seeds, salsa
Level 2 Mechanically altered *Avoid*	Dry breads	Dry, course cereals, cereals with flax, seeds, or nuts	Chewy candy, dry cakes/cookies, yogurt with nuts	Fats with coarse, chunky additives	Pineapple, fruit with skin or seeds, dried fruit	Dry meat, bacon, sausage, hot dogs	Large chunks of meat, rice, corn in soup	Broccoli, asparagus, celery, corn, peas, potato skins	Nuts, seeds, sticky foods, coconut

	Breads	Cereal/Rice/Pasta		Spreads	Fruit	Meats	Soups	Vegetables	Miscellaneous
Level 3 Advanced *Recommend*	Moist breads (butter, jam, syrup)	Moist cereal, rice, pasta	All others except those in avoid category	All others except those in avoid category	Canned or cooked fruit, peeled fresh fruit	Ground tender meats and tender fish	All others except those in avoid category	Tender vegetables, shredded lettuce, fried potatoes	Seasoning, sauces, jelly, jam, honey
Level 3 Advanced *Avoid*	Dry bread, toast, crackers	Dry cereals, shredded wheat bran	Dry baked goods, nuts, taffy, coconut	Course spreads with nuts	Dried fruit, fruit snacks, fruit with pulp/skin	Tough dry meat, fish with bones, chunky	Chowders, large pieces of vegetables	Raw, rubbery, stringy vegetables	Chunky peanut butter

Recommendations by type of food and consistency (Reprinted with permission from Sage Publications [21])

The level 3 NDD (dysphagia advanced) is a transition to a regular diet. This level consists of food of nearly regular textures except for very hard, crunchy, or sticky foods. The foods still need to be moist and should be in bite-size pieces. At this level, patients should be assessed for ability to tolerate mixed textures. This diet level is appropriate for patients with mild oropharyngeal dysphagia [65]. See Chap. 19 for dysphagia diet sample menus. Eating frequent, small meals may help increase food intake. After patients demonstrate the ability to tolerate these foods safely, the diet can be advanced to a regular diet without restrictions.

Weaning Enteral Nutrition

The goals of rehabilitation include enhancing function and returning to normal living, which includes oral eating. Weaning stroke patients from tube to oral feeding is a primary nutrition goal and can take place in the acute setting, during stroke rehabilitation, or at home. Transitional feeding requires an interdisciplinary approach involving the speech language pathologist, dietitian, nurse, and physician. Regularly scheduled evaluation of tube-fed patients by a speech language pathologist is necessary to identify positive changes in swallowing function that can permit transition from tube to oral feeding [21]. Feeding the stroke patient requires not only routine nutrition assessment by the dietitian, but also assistance from nursing for patients who cannot feed themselves, as well as assistance from occupational therapists for evaluation of assistive feeding devices. After clinical, diagnostic, and instrumental evaluations, the speech language pathologist will recommend the appropriate food and liquid consistencies for the initial oral diet. A modified barium swallow (MBS) study can help guide decisions about feeding regimens and estimate the stroke patient's risk of respiratory complications from oral feeding. It allows the speech-language pathologist to determine whether some type of compensatory swallowing strategy can circumvent a problem and actually experiment with that strategy during the examination to assess its benefit. In addition, an MBS study may also allow the patient to continue eating safely, even full nutrition and hydration cannot be maintained by mouth.

The weaning process, nutrition goals, and plan of action should be discussed thoroughly with the patient, family members, and the health care team. Continuous tube feedings are often transitioned to cyclic feedings at night and oral feedings during the day to potentially stimulate the hunger sensation. EN can infuse between 8 and 20 h and provide anywhere from 25 to 75% of the requirement during the time of transition. A calorie-dense EN formula may be needed to achieve this amount of calories in a shortened time frame. Bolus or intermittent feeds can be implemented to offer a more normal timing of meals and to accommodate other therapies. Oral nutrition supplements can be given between meals or as part of a meal to achieve caloric goals. Adequacy of oral intake dictates adjustment in tube feeding volume and consequent success of feeding tube removal [21]. Documenting the patient's intake during the transitional phase can be cumbersome, yet it is critical in deciding when to discontinue the tube feedings. The total time to wean from tube to oral feeding is patient dependent, and may not be a goal shared by all patients [66]. Crary and Groher described that the process of transitioning from tube to oral feeding can be challenging both cognitively and physically for some patients [67]. At a minimum, tube-fed patients with dysphagia who are candidates to return to oral feeding must be able to consume adequate oral nutrition and demonstrate a safe and efficient swallow on a consistent basis [67].

Buchholz proposed a 2-phase clinical algorithm, specific to patients with stroke or acquired brain injury, for transitioning tube-fed patients to oral feeding during acute rehabilitation [66]. The initial phase, termed the *preparatory phase*, focuses on medical and nutrition stability, swallowing assessment, and implementation of an intermittent tube feeding schedule. The *weaning phase* is a described as gradual progression in oral feeding with corresponding decreases in tube feeding. Once a patient is able to consume ≥75% of his or her nutrition requirements consistently for 3 days, all tube feedings are discontinued. Weight, hydration, and swallowing ability are closely monitored during these stages with a specific focus on respiratory complications.

A safe swallow function does not guarantee that the stroke patient, especially the elderly, will be able to ingest adequate oral nutrition. As with any change, the goal of transitional feeding is long-term success. If at any time in the progression toward oral intake a stroke patient is unable to maintain adequate consumption, other measures should be considered. In such cases, it is recommended that the patient's nutrition be maintained through partial oral feeding with supplemental tube feeding as required.

Summary

Malnutrition is a common finding following a stroke and nutrition support is common in patients with severe neurological injury. Whether the patient requires modified oral diets for dysphagia, enteral tube feedings, or PN, a registered dietitian is integral in managing the nutrition care of stroke patients. In addition to the dietitian, implementing the nutrition care plan relies on the interdisciplinary team of nurses, physicians, pharmacist, SLP, and occupational therapy as meeting nutritional goals relies on many non-nutritional factors.

References

1. Bardutzky J, Georgiadis D, Kollmar R, Schwarz S, Schwab S. Energy demand in patients with stroke who are sedated and receiving mechanical ventilation. J Neurosurg. 2004;100:266–71.
2. Davis JP, Wong AA, Schuter PJ, Nelson RJ. Impact of premorbid undernutrition on outcome of stroke patients. Stroke. 2004;35:1930–4.

3. Choi-Kwon S, Yang YH, Kim EK, Jeon MY, Kim JS. Nutritional status in acute stroke: under-nutrition versus overnutrition in different stroke subtypes. Acta Neurol Scand. 1998;98: 187–92.
4. Foley NC, Salter KL, Robertson J, Teasell RW, Woodbury MG. Which reported estimate of prevalence of malnutrition after stroke is valid? Stroke. 2009;40:e66–74.
5. Bratton S, Chestnut R, Ghajar J, Mc Connell Hammond F, Harris O, Hartl R, et al. Brain Trauma Foundation guidelines: nutrition. J Neurotrauma. 2007;24:S77–82.
6. Chalela J, Haymore J, Schillinger P, Kang D, Warach S. Acute stroke patients are being under-fed: a nitrogen balance study. Neurocrit Care. 2004;1:331–4.
7. Cook AM, Peppard A, Magnuson B. Nutrition considerations in traumatic brain injury. Nutr Clin Pract. 2008;23:608–20.
8. Beamer NB, Couli BM, Clark WM, Hazel JS, Silverstein MD. Interleukin-6 and interleukin-1 receptor antagonist in acute stroke. Ann Neurol. 1995;37:800–4.
9. Obesity education initiative task force. Clinical Guidelines on the identification, evaluation, and treatment of overweight and obesity in adults. National Institutes of Health. Available at: www.nhlbi.nih.gov/guidelines/obesity/prctgd_c.pdf. Accessed 12 Jan 2012.
10. A.S.P.E.N. Board of Directors and Clinical Practice Committee. Definition of terms, style and conventions used in A.S.P.E.N. board of directors—approved documents. 2010. www.nutritioncare.org.wcontent.aspx?id=4714. Accessed 12 Jan 2012.
11. Jensen GL, Mirtallo J, Compher C, Dhaliwal R, Forbes A, Grijalba RF, et al. Adult starvation and disease-related malnutrition: a proposal for etiology-based diagnosis in the clinical practice setting from the International Consensus Guideline Committee. JPEN J Parenter Enteral Nutr. 2010;34:156–9.
12. Finestone HM, Greene-Finestone LS, Foley NC, Woodbury MG. Measuring longitudinally the metabolic demands of stroke patients, resting energy expenditure is not elevated. Stroke. 2003;34:502–7.
13. Weekes E, Elias M. Resting energy expenditure and body composition following cerebro-vascular accident. Clin Nutr. 1992;11:18–22.
14. Brunner CS. Neurologic impairment. In: Matarese LE, Gottschlich MM, editors. Contemporary nutrition support practice: a clinical guide. 2nd ed. St. Louis, MO: Saunders; 2003. p. 384–95.
15. Bardutzky J, Georgiadis D, Kollmar R, Schwab S. Energy expenditure in ischemic stroke patients treated with moderate hypothermia. Intensive Care Med. 2004;30:151–4.
16. Fuhrman MP, Charney P, Mueller CM. Hepatic proteins and nutrition assessment. J Am Diet Assoc. 2004;104:1258–64.
17. Taylor SJ, Fettes SB, Jewkes C, Nelson RJ. Prospective, randomized, controlled trial to deter-mine the effect of early enhanced enteral nutrition on clinical outcome in mechanically venti-lated patients suffering from head injury. Crit Care Med. 1999;27:2525–31.
18. Chiang YH, Chao DP, Chu SF, Lin HW, Huang SY, Yeh YS, et al. Early enteral nutrition and clinical outcomes of severe traumatic brain injury patients in acute stage: a multi-center cohort study. J Neurotrauma. 2012;29:75–80.
19. Perel P, Yanagawa T, Bunn F, Roberts I, Wentz R, Pierro A. Nutritional support for head-injured patients. Cochrane Database Syst Rev. 2006;CD001530.
20. Mann G, Hankey GJ, Cameron D. Swallowing function after stroke: prognosis and prognostic factors at 6 months. Stroke. 1999;30:744–8.
21. Corrigan ML, Escuro AA, Celestin J, Kirby DF. Nutrition in the stroke patient. Nutr Clin Pract. 2011;26:242–51.
22. Brunner CS. Neurologic impairment. In: Gottschlich MM, DeLegge MH, Mattox T, Mueller C, Worthington P, editors. The A.S.P.E.N. nutrition support core curriculum: a case based approach—the adult patient. Silver Spring, MD: American Society for Parenteral and Enteral Nutrition; 2007. p. 424–39.
23. Magnuson B, Hatton J, Williams S, Loan T. Tolerance and efficacy of enteral nutrition for neurosurgical patients in pentobarbital coma. Nutr Clin Pract. 1999;14:131–4.
24. Zarbock SD, Steinke D, Hatton J, Magnuson B, Smith KM, Cook AM. Successful enteral nutritional support in the neurocritical care unit. Neurocrit Care. 2008;9:210–6.

25. de Aguilar-Nascimento JE, Kudsk KA. Clinical costs of feeding tube placement. JPEN J Parenter Enteral Nutr. 2007;31:269–73.
26. McClave SA, Martindale RG, Vanek VW, McCarthy M, Roberts R, Taylor B, et al. Guidelines for the provision and assessment of nutrition support therapy in the adult critically ill patient: Society of Critical Care Medicine (SCCM) and American Society for Parenteral Nutrition (A.S.P.E.N.). JPEN J Parenter Enteral Nutr. 2009;33:277–316.
27. Khalid I, Doshi P, DiGiovine B. Early enteral nutrition and outcomes of critically ill patients treated with vasopressors and mechanical ventilation. Am J Crit Care. 2010;19:261–8.
28. Popovich MJ, Lockrem JD, Zivot JB. Nasal bridle revisited: an improvement in the technique to prevent unintentional removal of small bore nasoenteric feeding tubes. Crit Care Med. 1996;24:429–31.
29. Seder CW, Janczyk R. The routine bridling of nasojejunal tubes is a safe and effective method of reducing dislodgement in the intensive care unit. Nutr Clin Pract. 2008;23:651–4.
30. Seder CW, Stockdale W, Hale L, Janczyk R. Nasal bridling decreases feeding tube dislodgement and may increase caloric intake for the surgical intensive care unit: a randomized controlled trial. Crit Care Med. 2010;38:797–801.
31. Acosta-Escribano J, Fernandez-Vivas M, Carmona TG, Caturla-Sach J, Garcia-Martinez M, Menendez-Meiner A, et al. Gastric versus transpyloric feeding in severe traumatic brain injury: a prospective, randomized trial. Intensive Care Med. 2010;36:1532–9.
32. Mobarhan S, DeMeo M. Diarrhea induced by enteral feeding. Nutr Rev. 1995;53:67–70.
33. Williams MS, Harper R, Magnuson B, Loan T, Kearney P. Diarrhea management in enterally fed patients. Nutr Clin Pract. 1998;13:225–9.
34. McClave SA, Lukan JK, Stefater JA, Lowen CC, Looney SW, Matheson PJ, et al. Poor validity of residual volumes as a marker for risk of aspiration in critically ill patients. Crit Care Med. 2005;33(2):324–30.
35. Parrish CR, McClave SA. Checking gastric residual volumes: a practice in search of science? Pract Gastroenterol. 2008;67:33–47.
36. Heyland DK, Cahill NE, Dhaliwal R, Sun X, Day AG, McClave SA. Impact of enteral feeding protocols on enteral nutrition delivery: results of a multicenter observational study. JPEN J Parenter Enteral Nutr. 2010;34:675–84.
37. Malone AM, Seres DS, Lord L. Complications of enteral nutrition. In: Gottschlich MM, DeLegge MH, Mattox T, Mueller C, Worthington P, editors. The A.S.P.E.N. nutrition support core curriculum: a case-based approach—the adult patient. Silver Spring, MD: American Society for Parenteral and Enteral Nutrition; 2007. p. 246–63.
38. A.S.P.E.N Board of Directors and Clinical Guidelines Task Force. Guidelines for the use of parenteral and enteral nutrition in adult and pediatric patients. JPEN J Parenter Enteral Nutr. 2002;26:1SA–37.
39. Mirtallo JM. Overview of parenteral nutrition. In: Gottschlich MM, DeLegge MH, Mattox T, Mueller C, Worthington P, editors. The A.S.P.E.N. nutrition support core curriculum: a case-based approach—the adult patient. Silver Spring, MD: American Society for Parenteral and Enteral Nutrition; 2007. p. 264–76.
40. Marik PE, Zaloga GP. Early enteral nutrition in acutely ill patients: a systematic review. Crit Care Med. 2001;29:2264–70.
41. McClave SA, Heyland DK. The physiologic response and associated clinical benefits from provision of early enteral nutrition. Nutr Clin Pract. 2009;24:305–15.
42. Jabbar A, Chang WK, Dryden GW, McClave SA. Gut immunology and the differential response to feeding and starvation. Nutr Clin Pract. 2003;18:461–82.
43. Skipper A. Parenteral nutrition. In: Matarese LE, Gottschlich MM, editors. Contemporary nutrition support practice: a clinical guide. 2nd ed. St. Louis, MO: Saunders; 2003. p. 227–62.
44. Heyland DK, MacDonald S, Keefe L, Drover JW. Total parenteral nutrition in the critically ill patient: a meta-analysis. JAMA. 1998;280:2013–9.
45. Braunschweig CL, Levy P, Sheean PM, Wang X. Enteral compared with parenteral nutrition: a meta-analysis. Am J Clin Nutr. 2001;74:534–42.

46. Mirtallo J, Canada T, Johnson D, Kumpf V, Petersen C, Sacks G, et al. Safe practices for parenteral nutrition. JPEN J Parenter Enteral Nutr. 2004;28(6):S39–70.
47. Steiger E. Dysfunction and thrombotic complications of vascular access devices. JPEN J Parenter Enteral Nutr. 2006;30:S70–2.
48. DeChicco R, Seidner DL, Brun C, Steiger E, Stafford J, Lopez R. Tip position of long-term central venous access devices used for parenteral nutrition. JPEN J Parenter Enteral Nutr. 2007;31(5):382–7.
49. Kumpf VJ. Update on parenteral iron therapy. Nutr Clin Pract. 2003;18:318–26.
50. Solomon SM, Kirby DF. The refeeding syndrome: a review. JPEN J Parenter Enteral Nutr. 1990;14(1):90–7.
51. Jimenez LL, Davis F. Traumatic brain injury and stroke. In: Cresci G, editor. Nutrition support for the critically ill patients: a guide to practice. 1st ed. Boca Raton, FL: CRC; 2005. p. 529–40.
52. Betjes MG. Hyponatremia in acute brain disease: the cerebral salt wasting syndrome. Eur J Intern Med. 2002;13:9–14.
53. Zafonte RD, Mann NR. Cerebral salt wasting syndrome in brain injury patients: a potential cause of hyponatremia. Arch Phys Med Rehabil. 1997;78:540–2.
54. Oh MS, Carroll HJ. Disorders of sodium metabolism: hypernatremia and hyponatremia. Crit Care Med. 1992;20:94–103.
55. de Leon-Knapp I. The effects of propofol on nutrition support. Support Line. 2009;31(6): 12–9.
56. Rossaint J, Rossaint R, Weis J, Fries M, Rex S, Coburn M. Propofol: neuroprotection in an in vitro model of traumatic brain injury. Crit Care. 2009;13:61–9.
57. Dempsey DT, Guenter PA, Mullen JL, Fairman R, Crosby LO, Spielman G, et al. Energy expenditure in acute trauma to the head with and without barbiturate therapy. Surg Gynecol Obstet. 1985;160:128–34.
58. Bochicchio GV, Bochicchio K, Nehman S, Casey C, Andrews P, Scalea TM. Tolerance and efficacy of enteral nutrition in traumatic brain-injured patients induced into barbiturate coma. JPEN J Parenter Enteral Nutr. 2006;30(6):503–6.
59. Foley N, Teasell R, Bhogal S, Speechley M. Nutritional interventions following stroke. 2010. www.ebrsr.com. Accessed 12 Jan 2012.
60. Finestone HM, Greene-Finestone LS, Wilson ES, Teasell RW. Malnutrition in stroke patients on the rehabilitation service and at follow-up: prevalence and indicators. Arch Phys Med Rehabil. 1995;76:310–6.
61. Roth EJ, Lovell L, Harvey RL, Bode RK, Heinemann AW. Stroke rehabilitation: indwelling urinary catheters, enteral feeding tubes, and tracheostomies are associated with resource use and functional outcomes. Stroke. 2002;33:1845–50.
62. Ickenstein GW, Kelly PJ, Furie KL, Ambrosi D, Rallis N, Goldstein R, et al. Predictors of feeding gastrostomy tube removal in stroke patients with dysphagia. J Stroke Cerebrovasc Dis. 2003;12:169–74.
63. Ickenstein GW, Stein J, Ambrosi D, Goldstein R, Horn M, Bogdahn U. Predictors of survival after severe dysphagic stroke. J Neurol. 2005;252:1510–6.
64. Krieger RP, Brady S, Stewart RJ, Terry A, Brady JJ. Predictors of returning to oral feedings after feeding tube placement for patients post stroke during inpatient rehabilitation. Top Stroke Rehabil. 2010;17(3):197–203.
65. National Dysphagia Diet Task Force. National dysphagia diet: standardization for optimal care. Chicago, IL: American Dietetic Association; 2002. p. 10–25.
66. Buchholz AC. Weaning patients with dysphagia from tube feeding to oral nutrition: a proposed algorithm. Can J Diet Pract Res. 1998;59:208–14.
67. Crary MA, Groher ME. Reinstituting oral feeding in tube-fed adult patients with dysphagia. Nutr Clin Pract. 2006;21:576–86.

Chapter 14
Enteral Access

Donald F. Kirby and Keely R. Parisian

Key Points

- Recognize the importance of enteral access for early nutrition in the appropriate stroke patient.
- Identify the clinical factors that are essential in deciding on how to feed a stroke patient.
- Discuss the short-term and long-term options for enteral access and understand the complications associated with each of them.

Introduction

This chapter will discuss the importance of early enteral feeding in the appropriate stroke patient and the factors that play a role in deciding how to feed a stroke patient. In addition, the chapter will discuss the options for enteral access which include the following: blind placement of nasoenteric and oroenteric feeding tubes, facilitated placement of nasoenteric feeding tubes, percutaneous gastrostomy and jejunostomy tubes, and surgical gastrostomy and jejunostomy tubes.

Keywords Enteral access • Enteral nutrition • Nasoenteric feeding tube • Jejunostomy tube

D.F. Kirby, M.D., F.A.C.P., F.A.C.N., F.A.C.G., A.G.A.F., C.N.S.C., C.P.N.S.
Center for Human Nutrition, Department of Gastroenterology, Cleveland Clinic,
9500 Euclid Avenue/A51, Cleveland, OH 44195, USA

K.R. Parisian, M.D. (✉)
Albany Gastroenterology Consultants, 1375 Washington Ave Suite 101,
Albany, NY 12206, USA

M.L. Corrigan et al. (eds.), *Handbook of Clinical Nutrition and Stroke*,
Nutrition and Health, DOI 10.1007/978-1-62703-380-0_14,
© Springer Science+Business Media New York 2013

Abbreviations

ASPEN	American Society for Parenteral and Enteral Nutrition
NDT	Nasoduodenal Tube
NGT	Nasogastric Tube
NIHSS	National Institute of Health Stroke Scale
NJT	Nasojejunal Tube
OGT	Oral Gastric Tube
PEG	Percutaneous Gastrostomy
PEG-J	Percutaneous Placed Gastrojejunostomy Tube

Background

As discussed in Chap. 11, malnutrition is common both before and after stroke. Nutritional intervention, including enteral feeding, is an essential part of the interdisciplinary approach to the care and treatment of stroke patients. Studies have shown the importance of providing nutrients to the intestinal absorptive surface to stimulate gut immune function and to prevent deterioration of intestinal integrity [1, 2]. This loss of intestinal integrity may lead to bacterial translocation and the potential for spread of bacteria from the gut. Therefore, enteral nutrition should be used as early as possible in the acute phase of stroke (during the first 24–48 h) and continued during the rehabilitation phase of stroke until the patient can be safely transitioned to an oral diet.

Mental status and the presence or absence of dysphagia are the predominant factors that dictate the decision on how to feed a stroke patient; however, the patient's presenting condition, past medical and surgical history, presence of a functional gastrointestinal tract (ileus does not preclude enteral feeding), and anticipated length of time that the patient will require enteral nutrition are also important (Table 14.1). For example, approaches to feeding a patient who is comatose from a massive stroke and is in an intensive care unit (ICU) will differ from a patient with mild dysarthria following a stroke.

Table 14.1

Factors that dictate how to feed a stroke patient

Patient factors
Mental status[a]
Dysphagia[a]
Presenting condition
Past medical and surgical history
Presence of a functional gastrointestinal tract
Anticipated length of time that enteral nutrition is required
Predicted prognosis
Patient and family expectations

[a]Key factors that dictate how to feed a stroke patient

Enteral Stroke Feeding Algorithm

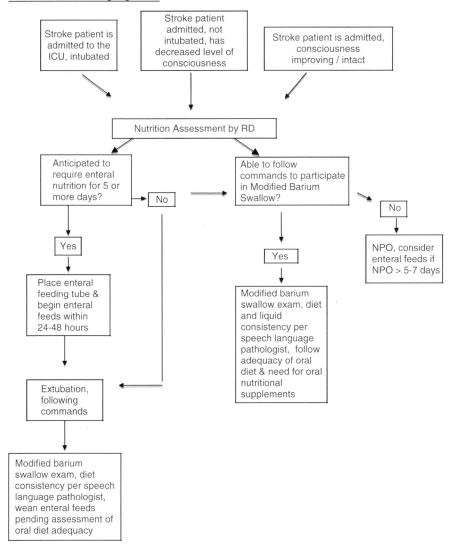

Fig. 14.1 Enteral stroke feeding algorithm. Reprinted from Ref. [3] with permission from American Society of Parenteral and Enteral Nutrition

    This chapter will discuss the following mechanisms for enteral access: blind placement of nasoenteric or oroenteric feeding tubes, facilitated placement of naso-enteric feeding tubes, percutaneous gastrostomy and jejunostomy tubes, and surgical gastrostomy and jejunostomy tubes. Corrigan et al. designed an algorithm for enteral feeding in stroke patients upon admission to the hospital to assist with risk stratification (Fig. 14.1) [3].

Table 14.2
Enteral access options

Enteral access	Placement technique	Anticipated length of time for enteral support
Nasoenteric tube (NGT, NDT, NJT, OGT)	Blind or facilitated via the Cortrak® enteral access system[a], Gabriel™ feeding tube[b], fluoroscopy, endoscopy	<3 weeks
Percutaneous gastrostomy and gastrojejunostomy	Endoscopy or radiologically placed	>4 weeks
Surgical gastrostomy and jejunostomy	Surgically	>4 weeks

[a]CORPAK MedSystems, Inc., Buffalo Grove, IL
[b]Syncro Medical Innovations, Inc., Macon, GA

Nasoenteric and Oroenteric Access

A nutritional assessment by a registered dietitian or physician is the initial step in determining enteral access type. Requirements for nasoenteric feeding include appropriate access, a functional gut, no other medical contraindications (i.e., intestinal obstruction), and an estimated length of use of less than 3 weeks of enteral nutritional support [4, 5]. Enteric feedings include nutrition delivered by way of a nasogastric tube (NGT), orogastric tube (OGT), nasoduodenal tube (NDT), or nasojejunal tube (NJT) (Table 14.2 and Fig. 14.2). OGTs may be used in the setting of facial trauma that precludes passage of an NGT, but may be a problem in patients who are more alert and have an intact gag reflex.

The placement of a NGT is the initial preferred method to provide nutrition in stroke patients, unless a particular ICU follows a specific enteral feeding protocol in critically ill patients. Nasoenteric tubes are commonly made of polyurethane or silicone, both of which remain soft and flexible over time. NDTs or NJTs are typically smaller than NGTs (#8 to #10 French), which leads to less patient discomfort, but are associated with a higher risk of tube clogging. Common enteral tube complications include local nasal irritation, epistaxis, sinusitis if used long-term, tube dislodgement, tube clogging, and feeding intolerance (Table 14.3) [6, 7].

Delayed gastric emptying has been shown in some patients following stroke and acute brain injury who have elevated intracranial pressure that can lead to high gastric residuals and intolerance of nasogastric feeding [8]. In this setting, it is appropriate to consider NDT (placement is ideal within the third portion of the duodenum or beyond) or NJT feedings. In addition, concomitant use of promotility agents and enteral feeds may be beneficial in providing nutrition to stroke patients with gastroparesis. Metoclopramide is currently the only FDA-approved promotility agent; however, its use is limited by the potential for central nervous system side effects and resultant black box warning. Further caution should be exercised in prescribing metoclopramide to patients with epilepsy and in patients taking medications that

Examples of Enteral Access

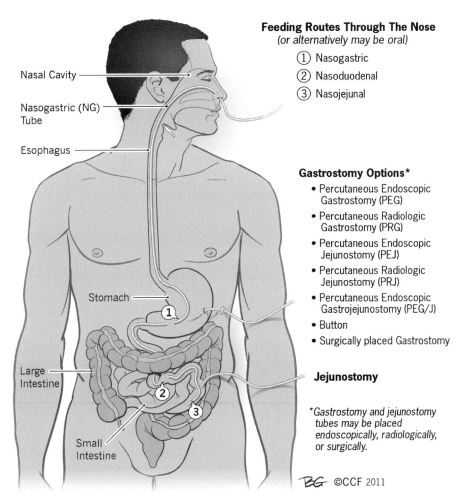

Feeding Routes Through The Nose
(or alternatively may be oral)

① Nasogastric
② Nasoduodenal
③ Nasojejunal

Nasal Cavity

Nasogastric (NG) Tube

Esophagus

Gastrostomy Options*

- Percutaneous Endoscopic Gastrostomy (PEG)
- Percutaneous Radiologic Gastrostomy (PRG)
- Percutaneous Endoscopic Jejunostomy (PEJ)
- Percutaneous Radiologic Jejunostomy (PRJ)
- Percutaneous Endoscopic Gastrojejunostomy (PEG/J)
- Button
- Surgically placed Gastrostomy

Stomach

Jejunostomy

Large Intestine

*Gastrostomy and jejunostomy tubes may be placed endoscopically, radiologically, or surgically.

Small Intestine

BG ©CCF 2011

Fig. 14.2 Examples of enteral access. Reprinted with permission, Cleveland Clinic Center for Medical Art & Photography © 2011–2012. All rights reserved

can increase the risk for extrapyramidal side effects. A case series showed improvement in gastric motility (based upon a radionuclide gastric emptying study) following administration of metoclopramide therapy in patients with traumatic brain injury [9]. Although not FDA-approved for gastroparesis, erythromycin has been used off-label very effectively as a promotility agent. A retrospective study of patients with and without traumatic brain injury admitted to a trauma or neurosurgical ICU with gastric feeding intolerance showed efficacy rates for metoclopramide 10 mg, metoclopramide 20 mg, and 10 mg metoclopramide–250 mg erythromycin

Table 14.3
Complications associated with enteral access

Enteral access	Complications
Naso-oroenteric tubes (NGT, NDT, NJT, OGT)	Local oral or nasal irritation, epistaxis, sinusitis, tube dislodgement, tube malposition, tube clogging, tube kinking, feeding intolerance
Percutaneous gastrostomy (PEG) and gastrojejunostomy (PEG-J)	*Minor complications*: stoma leakage, wound infection, bleeding, tube dislodgement, pain, gastroesophageal reflux, tube blockage
	Major complications: gastrocolocutaneous fistula, necrotizing fasciitis, tumor implantation at the stoma site, cardiac failure with hypoxia, gastric hemorrhage, peritonitis, cellulitis, hematoma, internal bleeding, catheter dislodgement into the peritoneal cavity, buried bumper syndrome, pressure necrosis from internal or external bumpers, aspiration pneumonia
Surgical gastrostomy and jejunostomy	Same as above (percutaneous gastrostomy and gastro-jejunostomy)

of 55 %, 62 %, and 79 %, respectively [9]. Patients with gastric residual volume >200 mL or emesis were given intravenous metoclopramide 10 mg every 6 h followed by a dose escalation to 20 mg every 6 h if gastric residual volume did not improve. Combination therapy with metoclopramide and intravenous erythromycin 250 mg every 6 h was instituted if increased gastric residual was observed after dose escalation of metoclopramide alone. The authors reported metoclopramide failure more frequently in patients with traumatic brain injury, and therefore they recommended combination therapy with erythromycin as first-line therapy for patients with gastric feeding intolerance [10].

Nasoenteric tubes may be placed blindly or facilitated by means of the Cortrak® enteral access system (CORPAK MedSystems, Inc., Buffalo Grove, IL), Gabriel™ feeding tube (Syncro Medical Innovations, Inc., Macon, GA), fluoroscopy, or endoscopy. Although tubes may be passed at the bedside, poor positioning of the tube often requires either fluoroscopic or endoscopic guidance. Success rates vary widely as a result of operator skill, tube type or available equipment, patient mental status and cooperation, and patient anatomy. Ugo et al. placed #8 or #10 French small-bore, weighted feeding tubes past the pylorus of 103 patients at bedside in an ICU [11]. Patients were placed in the left lateral decubitus position with auscultation to track the tube into the small intestine. Postpyloric placement was achieved in 83 % of patients; however, only 43 % of the tubes were in the preferred positions of the third portion of the duodenum or beyond.

A technique using computer technology to facilitate efficient placement of nasoenteric tubes was developed in 2008 in an attempt to reduce clinical risk, financial costs, and need for X-ray exposure to confirm tube placement. A retrospective study of data from the first 14 months of the Cortrak® system use in the United Kingdom showed successful NGT placement in 100 % of cases and successful post-pyloric tube placement in 70 % (20/29) of cases [12]. In addition, the authors showed a reduction in clinical risks and cost avoidance related to X-ray exposure and initiation of parenteral nutrition. In another study, Rivera et al. compared the overall agreement between feeding tube tip location as determined by an electromagnetic tube placement device vs. an abdominal radiograph [13]. There were a significantly greater number of tubes found by radiograph to be distal (18.6 %) vs. proximal (15.3 %) to the suspected location by an electromagnetic tube placement device ($p<0.0001$). The authors concluded that there was strong agreement between radiograph and an electromagnetic tube placement device when tubes were believed to be in the second part of the duodenum or beyond, and that a radiograph is necessary only when the feeding tube tip is suspected to be in the proximal duodenum. Currently, the American Society for Parenteral and Enteral Nutrition (ASPEN) states that a radiograph that visualizes the entire course of the tube is the gold standard for confirming correct placement of a blindly inserted enteral access device; however, there are no recommendations for confirming placement of electromagnetic sensing devices such as the Cortrak® feeding system [14]. A more recent study by Hemington-Gorse et al. evaluated the use of the Cortrak® system in burn ICU patients who had encountered problems with blind tube placement previsouly [15]. They showed that 37/44 (84 %) of tubes were post-pyloric and 7/44 (16 %) were NG. Additionally, the location of 38/44 (86 %) of cases were correctly determined by the Cortrak® system when compared to an X-ray position. Of the 6/44 (14 %) that were thought to be NG on the Cortrak® system monitor, all were in fact post-pyloric on X-ray. The study concluded that the Cortrak® system is safe and effective in burn ICU patients.

The Gabriel™ feeding tube (Syncro Medical Innovations, Inc, Macon, GA) is another device that was designed to facilitate placement of nasoenteric feeding tubes with use of a small magnet in the distal tip. After a tube is inserted through the nares into the esophagus, an external magnet is used to draw the tube tip beyond the pyloric sphincter and further into the duodenum or jejunum. In a case series of critically ill patients who required placement of an enteral feeding tube, 293/329 cases (89 %) were placed beyond the pyloric sphincter when confirmed by abdominal X-ray [16]. It is important to note that absolute exclusion criteria included the presence of an implanted automatic defibrillator or a Greenfield inferior vena cava filter placed in the preceding 2 weeks. Additionally, the Gabriel™ tube should be removed before performing a magnetic resonance image (MRI) examination. The study demonstrated that the Gabriel™ tube is a reliable and safe bedside technique for placing enteral feeding tubes in patients without an implanted automatic defibrillator or Greenfield inferior vena cava filter.

As a result of inconsistent performance with blind placement and few data on facilitated placement, fluoroscopy is as a useful technique to assist in placement of nasoenteric tubes. Procedures may be performed in the radiology department or at bedside in the ICU with a portable C-arm fluoroscopy device. The average time for fluoroscopically guided tube placement has been reported as 30–40 min [Standard Deviation (SD)±14 min] [17, 18]. The rates of success and complications were evaluated in a study of 882 fluoroscopically guided feeding tube placements [19]. Twenty-nine percent of patients included had neurologic impairment. An 8-French, weighted feeding tube was advanced under fluoroscopic guidance (with the patient in the right decubitus position) through the pylorus and into the proximal jejunum with use of air insufflation. Initial tube placement was successful (the tip was distal to the third portion of the duodenum) in 87 %, partially successful (the tip was beyond the pylorus but proximal to the fourth portion of the duodenum) in 5 %, and unsuccessful (the tip was proximal to the pylorus) in 7.4 %. The tube was dislodged from its jejunal position in 77 % of cases due to an uncooperative and unrestrained patient, coughing, or vomiting. A well-positioned tube became clogged in 23 % of cases. Rare complications included aspiration pneumonia in 27 patients, arrhythmias leading to cardiac arrest in 3 patients, and tube malposition in the tracheobronchial tree in one patient. The authors concluded that fluoroscopically guided nasoenteric tube passage is safe, easily performed, and highly successful [18]. A study by Thurley et al. supports this data and showed successful placement of a tube in the distal duodenum or jejunum in 92 % of patients, placement in the proximal duodenum or distal stomach in 3 %, and failure to insert a tube in 5 % [20]. The authors concluded that radiological placement of post-pyloric feeding tubes is quite safe and has a success rate comparable with endoscopically placed tubes.

Without bedside fluoroscopy, it becomes difficult to transport critically ill, ventilated patients to a fluoroscopy unit. Endoscopic placement of nasoenteric tubes is another technique to provide enteral nutrition to patients. There have been numerous modifications to the original "drag and pull" endoscopic method including the following: a push technique with a stiffened tube, use of a distal suture tie, and placement using an ultrathin transnasal endoscopic technique compared with fluoroscopic placement. All of these techniques have shown similar outcomes in nasoenteric feeding tube placement. Patrick et al. evaluated 54 consecutive critically ill patients referred for endoscopic NJT placement [21]. The NJT with guidewire was advanced, under direct visualization, through the pylorus and to the appropriate position in the small bowel. An X-ray was obtained after each case to confirm placement on day 1 and then also on day 3, day 7, and then weekly thereafter until the tube was removed or needed to be replaced. Placement was successful in 51/54 (94 %) of tubes, which was defined as radiologically verified placement of the tube in the distal duodenum or proximal jejunum. The average length of time to complete the procedure was 12 min. The longevity of the tube ranged from 1 to 42 days, with an average of 9 days. Negative outcomes following endoscopic NJT placement included adapter cracking in 6/54 (11 %), clogging in 5/54 (9 %), kinking in 3/54 (6 %), inadvertent removal by patient or staff in 11/54 (21 %), aspiration in 1/54 (2 %), and epistaxis in 1/54 (2 %). The authors concluded that endoscopic placement of nasoenteric tubes in critically ill patients offered several advantages including the following: ability to directly visualize the placement of the tube reducing the complications associated with blind placement, reduction in the need for repeat radiographs to confirm correct placement, ease of performing the procedure in the ICU at bedside, high success rate, and low procedure time.

Mahadeva and coworkers later evaluated the utility of transnasal endoscopic placement of nasoenteric tubes in 22 non-critically ill patients [22]. Patients with persistent gastrocutaneous fistula, gastroparesis, gastric outlet obstruction, duodenal stenosis, acute pancreatitis, and gastroesophageal reflux after surgery were referred for endoscopic placement of a nasoenteric tube. Postpyloric placement was achieved in 19/22 (86 %) of patients. Of those, 37 % were placed in the jejunum, 47 % in the distal duodenum, and 16 % in the second part of the duodenum. Nasoenteric tubes remained in place for a median of 24 days (Range 2–94 days). Complications included tube dislodgement in 3/22 (14 %) and tube clogging in 5/22 (23 %). The authors concluded that transnasal endoscopy has a role in the placement of nasoenteric tubes in non-critically ill patients requiring post-pyloric feeding but there may be limitations in patients with altered duodenal anatomy.

A bridle may be anchored to the nasal septum to diminish the likelihood of enteric tube dislodgement in a confused or uncooperative patient; which, in turn, may reduce restraint use, patient discomfort, and overall health care costs including radiography, procedural, and tube expenses. The bridle was first described in 1980 by Armstrong et al [23]. There have been several variations in this technique that have followed. Popovich and colleagues illustrated an umbilical tape bridle procedure in 26 critically ill patients who received enteral nutrition and either had removed or were at risk for removing their nasoenteric feeding tubes [24]. There were no episodes of bleeding, infection, sinusitis, or nasal septal trauma caused by the umbilical tape bridle. The authors reported that the umbilical tape bridle was a safe and effective method to prevent accidental removal of nasoenteric feeding tubes. In another study, Seder et al. randomized 80 patients to have their nasoenteric tubes secured with either a magnetically placed nasal bridle or an adhesive device [25]. Bridled tubes were less likely to be unintentionally removed than unbridled tubes (18 % vs. 63 %, $p<0.0001$). Bridled patients received a significantly greater percentage of goal calories than unbridled patients (median, 78 % vs. 62 %, $p=0.016$). Complications associated with the bridle included mild epistaxis and superficial nasal ulceration. The authors concluded that bridling in critically ill patients is a low-morbidity practice that reduced the rate of accidental tube dislodgement and may improve caloric intake [25].

Endoscopic Gastrostomy and Gastrojejunostomy

In stroke patients who may require long-term enteral access (>4 weeks) and in stroke patients with recurrent nasoenteric tube complications as described above, a percutaneously placed gastrostomy tube (PEG) or percutaneously placed gastrojejunostomy tube (PEG-J) may be inserted. In a 28 day randomized controlled trial, Park et al. compared PEG and NGT feeding in patients with persisting neurological dysphagia [26]. The proportion of prescribed feed received by the PEG group and the NGT group was 93 % and 55 %, respectively ($p<0.001$). Patients in the PEG group also gained significantly more weight after 7 days of feeding compared to the NGT group (1.4 kg vs. 0.6 kg, $p<0.05$). The authors concluded that PEG feeding was a safe and effective method for providing long-term enteral nutrition to patients with neurological dysphagia and offered important advantages over NGT feeding. In a similar study design, Norton et al. compared PEG and NGT feeding in patients after acute dysphagic stroke [27]. They showed that mortality was lower in the PEG group compared to the NGT group (12 % vs. 57 %, $p<0.05$). Patients in the NGT group received a significantly smaller proportion of prescribed feed compared to the PEG group (78 % vs. 100 %, $p<0.001$). The mean albumin concentration in the PEG group increased from 27.1 to 30.1 g/l at 6 weeks whereas the mean albumin concentration in the NGT group decreased from 31.2 to 22.3 g/l at 6 weeks ($p<0.003$). The study indicated that early gastrostomy tube feeding is superior to NGT feeding and should be the nutritional treatment of choice for patients with acute dysphagic stroke. These studies show that some patients benefit from early PEG placement (within 2–4 weeks), and PEG is acceptable for long-term nutrition (more than 4 weeks).

Despite low published mortality rates in patients post-PEG placement, numerous studies have documented associated complications. Complications have been divided into minor and major categories [28]. Minor complications, referred to as local and non-life-threatening, are composed of such categories as stoma leakage, wound infection, bleeding, tube dislodgement, pain, gastroesophageal reflux and tube blockage. Major complications are those that are systemic and life-threatening, and include gastrocolocutaneous fistula, necrotizing fasciitis, tumor implantation in the stoma site, cardiac failure with hypoxia, gastric hemorrhage, peritonitis, cellulitis, hematoma, internal bleeding, catheter dislodgement into the peritoneal cavity and aspiration pneumonia. Koc et al. studied 31 patients who underwent PEG tube placement in the neurosurgical ICU [29]. Indications for PEG included absent gag reflex in 10 patients and low Glasgow Coma Scale (GCS, 9-12) score in 21 patients. Complications after PEG placement were as follows: accidental removal of the PEG in 2 patients, buried bumper syndrome in 1 patient, death in 2 patients due to underlying diseases. Procedure-related mortality, 30-day mortality, and overall mortality were 0 %, 6 %, and 45 %, respectively. The authors concluded that PEG was a safe and well-tolerated method for neurosurgical ICU patients with depressed neurologic state or severe lower cranial nerve palsies.

Alshekhlee et al. evaluated the relationship between the NIH Stroke Scale (NIHSS) score and the need for PEG tube placement in hospitalized patients with acute ischemic stroke [30]. A PEG tube was placed in 33/187 patients (17.6 %). Patients with a PEG tube placed were slightly older (73 vs. 66 years), had severe stroke (median NIHSS score, 19 vs. 4), and a longer hospital stay (median 12 vs. 4 days). Patients with aspiration pneumonia and NIHSS score ≥12 has the highest likelihood [Relative Risk (RR)=4.67; $p<0.0001$] of requiring a PEG tube. In the absence of pneumonia, NIHSS score ≥16 yielded a moderate likelihood of requiring a PEG (RR=1.80; $p<0.0001$). The findings suggested that the presence of aspiration pneumonia and high NIHSS score were the best predictors for requiring PEG tube insertion in patients with ischemic stroke; this may prompt early decision making, lead to shorter hospitalization, and possible cost savings.

Well-selected stroke patients may benefit from a PEG-J, as a reasonable alternative to a PEG. In a critical appraisal, prospectively collected data of 268 patients with a PEG and 38 patients with a PEG-J were collected over a 7 year period [31].

Indications for a PEG-J include documented history of reflux esophagitis or previous aspiration, the presence of gastroparesis, pancreatitis, diminished gag, swallow, or cough reflexes in obtunded patients, or post-lung transplant. Overall mortality was 53 % in patients with a PEG and 50 % in patients with a PEG-J. Major procedure-related complications (abscesses, aspiration, and tube dysfunction) and minor procedure-related complications (including bleeding, peristomal infection, and wound problems) occurred in 8.4 % of cases and 24 % of cases, respectively in the first 28 days. In prolonged follow-up, complications were most commonly the result of tube dysfunction (clogging and fracture occurred after a median of 347 days). Aspiration occurred in 10 PEG-treated patients and 2 PEG-J patients. Complaints of nausea and vomiting were similar in PEG and PEG-J; however, there was a significantly higher rate of dumping symptoms (nausea, shaking, diaphoresis, and diarrhea shortly after initiation of enteral feeds) seen in PEG-Js as compared to PEGs. The authors concluded that a PEG-J offers tube durability, acceptable tube dysfunction rate, and an impressive reduction in aspiration. Therefore, PEG-J was an option for enteral access reserved for well-selected patients at risk for aspiration, but may be associated with a higher number of overall complications.

Surgical Gastrostomy and Jejunostomy

A surgically placed gastrostomy tube or jejunostomy may be inserted if endoscopic or fluoroscopic attempts have been unsuccessful. It may also be convenient to place a jejunostomy feeding tube during an operative procedure so that enteral nutrition can be started soon after surgery. There are multiple surgical techniques performed, which are dictated by individual surgeon experience and specific institution. In a study of patients in the surgical ICU undergoing laparotomy, Moore et al. compared patients randomized to either total enteral nutrition via jejunostomy within 12 h of surgery or total parenteral nutrition after post-operative day 5 [32]. The total enteral nutrition group showed improved nitrogen balance ($p < 0.001$) and had significantly less septic outcomes ($p < 0.025$). The authors concluded that early enteral nutrition via jejunostomy tube provided additional clinical benefit compared to early parenteral nutrition in high-risk surgical patients.

Conclusion

Enteral feeding in stroke patients requires a functional gastrointestinal tract and appropriate access. This chapter has discussed the numerous modalities by which enteral nutrition may be delivered and the complications associated with each modality. The decision for enteral access in stroke depends ultimately on the patient's mental status and the presence or absence of dysphagia; however, the patient's past medical and surgical history, clinical presentation, length of anticipated feeding time, and previous complications associated with enteral access devices must also be considered. It is essential that the patient and/or family and the physician together assess the risks and benefits of enteral access options in all stroke patients.

References

1. Alverdy J, Chi HS, Sheldon GF. The effect of parenteral nutrition on gastrointestinal immunity: the importance of enteral stimulation. Ann Surg. 1985;202:681–4.
2. Deitch EA, Winterton J, Li M, et al. The gut as a portal of entry for bacteria. Role of protein malnutrition. Ann Surg. 1987;205:681–92.
3. Corrigan ML, Escuro AA, Celestin J, Kirby DF. Nutrition in the stroke patient. Nutr Clin Pract. 2011;26:242–52.
4. Kirby DF. Decisions for enteral access in the intensive care unit. Nutrition. 2001;17:776–9.
5. Kirby DF, Opilla M. Enteral access and infusion equipment. In: Merritt R, DeLegge MH, Holcombe B, Mueller C, Ochoa J, Ringwald Smith K, Schwenk II WF, editors. The ASPEN nutrition support practice manual. 2nd ed. Silver Spring: American Society for Parenteral and Enteral Nutrition; 2005. p. 54–62.
6. Kirby DF, DeLegge MH. Enteral nutrition in the neurologic patient. In: Enteral and tube feeding. Third Edition. Rombeau JL, Rolandelli RH, eds. Philadelphia: WB Saunders - 1997;286–299.
7. Kirby DF, DeLegge MH, Fleming CR. American Gastroenterological Association technical review on tube feeding for enteral nutrition. Gastroenterology. 1995;108:1282–301.
8. Crome P, Rizeg M, George S, et al. Drug absorption may be delayed after stroke: results of the paracetamol absorption test. Age Ageing. 2001;30:391–3.
9. Jackson MD, Davidoff G. Gastroparesis following traumatic brain injury and response to metoclopramide therapy. Arch Phys Med Rehabil. 1989;70:553–5.
10. Dickerson RN, Mitchell JN, Morgan LM, et al. Disparate response to metoclopramide therapy for gastric feeding intolerance in trauma patients with and without traumatic brain injury. JPEN J Parenter Enteral Nutr. 2009;33:646–55.
11. Ugo PJ, Mohler PA, Wilson GL. Bedside postpyloric placement of weighted feeding tubes. Nutr Clin Pract. 1992;7:284–7.
12. Windle EM, Beddow D, Hall E, et al. Implementation of an electromagnetic imaging system to facilitate nasogastric and post-pyloric feeding tube placement in patients with and without critical illness. J Hum Nutr Diet. 2010;23:61–8.
13. Rivera R, Campana J, Hamilton C, et al. Small bowel feeding tube placement using an electromagnetic tube placement device: accuracy of tip location. JPEN J Parenter Enteral Nutr. 2011;35:636–42.
14. Bankhead R, Boullata J, Brantley S, et al. Enteral nutrition practice recommendations. JPEN J Parenter Enteral Nutr. 2009;33:122–67.
15. Hemington-Gorse SJ, Sheppard NN, Martin R, et al. The use of the Cortrak Enteral Access System™ for post-pyloric (PP) feeding tube placement in a burns intensive care unit. Burns. 2011;37:277–80.
16. Gabriel SA, Ackermann RJ. Placement of nasoenteral feeding tubes using external magnetic guidance. JPEN J Parenter Enteral Nutr. 2004;28:119–22.
17. Zaloga GP. Bedside method for placing small bowel feeding tubes in critically ill patients—a prospective study. Chest. 1991;100:1643–6.
18. Ott DJ, Mattox HE, Gelfand DW, et al. Enteral feeding tubes: placement by using fluoroscopy and endoscopy. Am J Roentgenol. 1991;157:769–71.

19. Gutierrez ED, Balfe DM. Fluoroscopically guided nasoenteric feeding tube placement: results of a 1-year study. Radiology. 1991;178:759–62.
20. Thurley PD, Hopper MA, Jobling JC, et al. Fluoroscopic insertion of post-pyloric feeding tubes: success rates and complications. Clin Radiol. 2008;63:543–8.
21. Patrick PG, Marulendra S, Kirby DF, DeLegge MH. Endoscopic nasogastric-jejunal feeding tube placement in critically ill patients. Gastrointest Endosc. 1997;45:72–6.
22. Mahadeva S, Malik A, Hilmi E, et al. Transnasal endoscopic placement of nasoenteric feeding tubes: outcomes and limitations in non-critically ill patients. Nutr Clin Pract. 2008;23: 176–81.
23. Armstrong C, Luther W, Sykes T. A technique for preventing extubation of feeding tubes: "The bridle" (abstract). JPEN J Parenter Enteral Nutr. 1980;3:603.
24. Popovich MJ, Lockrem JD, Zivot JB. Nasal bridle revisited: an improvement in the technique to prevent unintentional removal of small-bore nasoenteric feeding tubes. Crit Care Med. 1996;24:429–31.
25. Seder CW, Stockdale W, Hale L, et al. Nasal bridling decreases feeding tube dislodgment and may increase caloric intake in the surgical intensive care unit: a randomized, controlled trial. Crit Care Med. 2010;38:797–801.
26. Park RH, Allison MC, Lang J, et al. Randomised comparison of percutaneous endoscopic gastrostomy and nasogastric tube feeding in patients with persisting neurological dysphagia. BMJ. 1992;304:1406–9.
27. Norton B, Homer-Ward M, Donnelly MT, et al. A randomised prospective comparison of percutaneous endoscopic gastrostomy and nasogastric tube feeding after acute dysphagic stroke. BMJ. 1996;312:13–6.
28. Galaski A, Peng WW, Ellis M, et al. Gastrostomy tube placement by radiolgical versus endoscopic methods in an acute care setting: a retrospective review of frequency, indications, complications and outcomes. Can J Gastroenterol. 2009;23:109–14.
29. Koc D, Gercek A, Gencosmanoglu R, et al. Percutaneous endoscopic gastrostomy in the neurosurgical intensive care unit: complications and outcome. JPEN J Parenter Enteral Nutr. 2007;31:517–20.
30. Alshekhlee A, Ranawat N, Syed TU, et al. National Institutes of Health Stroke Scale assists in predicting the need for percutaneous endoscopic gastrotomy tube placement in acute ischemic stroke. J Stroke Cerebrovasc Dis. 2010;19:347–52.
31. Mathus-Vliegen LMH, Koning H. Percutaneous endoscopic gastrostomy and gastrojejunostomy: a critical reappraisal of patient selection, tube function and the feasibility of nutritional support during extended follow-up. Gastrointest Endosc. 1999;50:746–54.
32. Moore EE, Moore FA. Immediate enteral nutrition following multisystem trauma: a decade perspective. J Am Coll Nutr. 1991;10:633–48.

Chapter 15
Dysphagia in Stroke

Brian J. Hedman and Amy Calhoun Rosneck

Key Points

- The development of oropharyngeal dysphagia following stroke can lead to serious pulmonary complications.
- The Bedside Swallow Evaluation and Modified Barium Swallow are examples of assessments of oropharyngeal swallowing function that are completed by a Speech-Language Pathologist.
- Therapeutic interventions and diet modifications are utilized to decrease aspiration risk in patients who have had a stroke.

Keywords Dysphagia • Stroke • Speech-language pathologist • Aspiration • Aspiration pneumonia • Swallowing • Swallowing evaluation • Swallowing therapy

Abbreviations

BSE	Bedside swallow evaluation
FEES	Fiberoptic endoscopic evaluation of swallowing
FFWP	Frazier free water protocol
GI	Gastrointestinal
LIP	Licensed independent practitioner
MEBDT	Modified evans blue dye test
NDD	National dysphagia diet
RT	Respiratory therapist
SLP	Speech-language pathologist

B.J. Hedman, M.A., C.C.C.-S.L.P. (✉) • A.C. Rosneck, M.A., C.C.C.-S.L.P.
Head and Neck Institute, The Cleveland Clinic, 9500 Euclid Avenue, A71,
Cleveland, OH 44195, USA
e-mail: hedmanb@ccf.org; rosneca@ccf.org

M.L. Corrigan et al. (eds.), *Handbook of Clinical Nutrition and Stroke*,
Nutrition and Health, DOI 10.1007/978-1-62703-380-0_15,
© Springer Science+Business Media New York 2013

Incidence of Dysphagia Following Stroke

Swallowing, or deglutition, is the neuromuscular act involving sensory and motor components controlling the movement of food from the oral cavity through the pharynx and esophagus to the stomach. Dysphagia is difficulty in the act of swallowing due to weakness, impaired coordination or obstruction. The incidence of dysphagia following stroke is reported to be between 19 and 81 % [1, 2]. The lower range reflects unilateral hemispheric strokes and the higher range is reflective of bilateral brainstem strokes. In general the larger the area of infarct, the more impaired the swallowing [3]. Dysphagia is more prevalent when the stroke involves the brainstem. According to Flowers and colleagues, the incidence of dysphagia in the midbrain is 6 %, 43 % in the pons, 40 % in the medial medulla, and 57 % in the lateral medulla [4].

Aspiration and Aspiration Pneumonia

"Laryngeal penetration" is the entrance of food, liquid, or secretions into the laryngeal vestibule which remains above the level of the vocal folds. The term "aspiration" is used to describe food, liquid, or secretions which fall below the vocal folds and enter into the trachea (*see* Figs. 15.1 and 15.2).

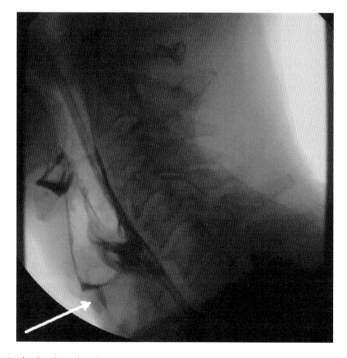

Fig. 15.1 Aspiration into the airway

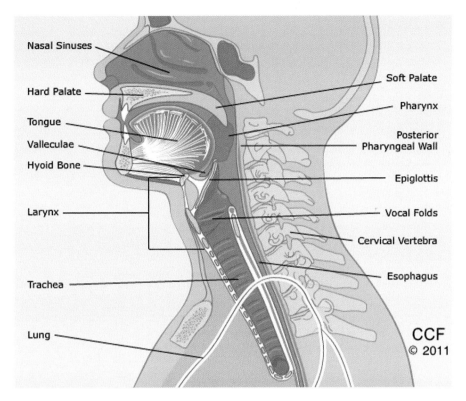

Fig. 15.2 Anatomy of the swallowing mechanism. (Reprinted with permission, Cleveland Clinic Center for Medical Art & Photograpy © 2011–2012. All Rights Reserved)

Pulmonary conditions related to aspiration include acute respiratory distress syndrome (ARDS), lipid pneumonia, aspiration pneumonia, and chronic pneumonitis [3].

Aspiration pneumonia is a pulmonary infection which results from the entrance of food, liquid, oral secretions, or stomach contents into the bronchi of the lungs [3]. Data from Cameron and colleagues' study reported that the right lower lobe is most frequently involved following aspiration, followed by the left lower lobe and least likely in the left upper lobe [5].

The most common cause of oropharyngeal neurogenic dysphagia is cerebrovascular disease [3]. A systematic database review of articles addressing the frequency of dysphagia or pneumonia completed by Martino et al. confirms there is a high incidence of dysphagia following stroke which is also associated with an increased risk for pneumonia in adults [6]. The presence of dysphagia following a stroke increased a patient's hospital length of stay, and those patients with dysphagia were more likely to develop pneumonia as a complication of their stroke [7]. Katzan et al. found that pneumonia occurred in 5.6 % of patients hospitalized with acute stroke resulting in a per patient increased hospital cost of $15,000 [8]. Therefore it is important to assess a patient's risk for aspiration following a stroke.

The Phases of Swallowing

The three primary phases of swallowing are oral, pharyngeal, and esophageal (*see* Figs. 15.3–15.5).

1. *Oral Phase*: A voluntary activity involving cranial nerves V (trigeminal), VII (facial) and XII (hypoglossal). The preparatory portion of this phase includes mastication and manipulation of food, liquid, and saliva in the mouth and formation of a bolus with the tongue. Then, as lip (labial) tension increases, the tongue presses up against the hard palate propelling the bolus posteriorly with greatest positive lingual pressure in the anteriomedian area of the tongue, resulting in clearance of the oral cavity [9, 10].
2. *Pharyngeal Phase*: Once the swallow is initiated, an involuntary rapid sequence of events occurs involving cranial nerves V, IX (glossopharyngeal), X (vagus), XI (spinal accessory), and XII. The soft palate elevates and retracts to close off the nasopharynx to avoid nasal regurgitation. The pharyngeal constrictor muscles contract sequentially to assist bolus transfer inferiorly. The anterior-superior movement of the hyoid bone and larynx assists in relaxation of the cricopharyngeus muscle for bolus passage into the esophagus. The retraction and downward tilting of the epiglottis over the arytenoid cartilages and the tight closure of the aryepiglottic folds results in closure of the laryngeal vestibule. The true and false vocal folds adduct during the swallow causing cessation of respiration and an increase in subglottic pressure.
3. *Esophageal Phase*: Involuntary bolus passage occurs through the upper esophageal sphincter and into the esophagus. Peristaltic motion and gravity propels the bolus distally, through the lower esophageal sphincter, and into the stomach.

Swallowing Mechanisms

Oral Phase

This phase begins when the food or liquid is prepared for swallowing.

Solid particles are moved around in the mouth, chewed, mixed with saliva, and formed into a bolus.

During the oral phase, food or fluids are voluntarily manipulated backward toward the pharynx by the muscles of the tongue against the palate.

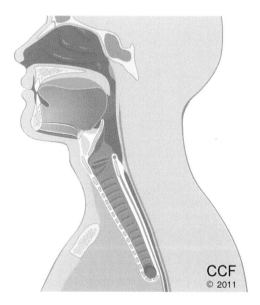

Fig. 15.3 Oral phase of the swallow. (Reprinted with permission, Cleveland Clinic Center for Medical Art & Photograpy © 2011–2012. All Rights Reserved)

Swallowing Mechanisms

Pharyngeal Phase

This phase begins at the time the food reaches the back of the mouth and the swallow reflex is triggered. It is at this point the act of swallowing becomes automatic and can not be stopped.

During this second phase, the trachea closes, the esophagus opens, and food passes into the pharynx as the larynx closes to prevent food from entering the lungs.

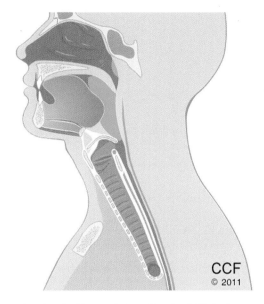

Fig. 15.4 Pharyngeal phase of the swallow. (Reprinted with permission, Cleveland Clinic Center for Medical Art & Photograpy © 2011–2012. All Rights Reserved)

Swallowing Mechanisms

Esophageal Phase

This phase begins when food or liquid enters the esophagus where peristaltic activity moves the food from the pharynx to the stomach.

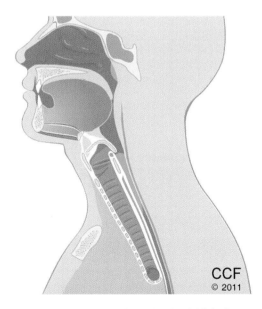

Fig. 15.5 Esophageal phase of the swallow. (Reprinted with permission, Cleveland Clinic Center for Medical Art & Photograpy © 2011–2012. All Rights Reserved)

Neuronal Control of Swallowing

The process of transferring food safely from the oropharynx into the esophagus requires activation of 55 muscles via 6 cranial nerves [11]. The oral and pharyngeal phases of swallowing were once believed to occur sequentially, but evidence now suggests that these phases are interdependent and occur simultaneously [3]. The initiation of the swallow was once classified as a reflex. It is now generally agreed that swallowing is a sequenced response (a central pattern generator), coordinated by a collection of brainstem motor nuclei in the nucleus tractus solitarius, a descending tract of nerve fibers that is situated near the dorsal surface of the medulla, and in the nucleus ambiguus, located in the lateral portion of the rostral medulla [12]. Sensory input from the trigeminal, facial, and glossopharyngeal nerves and motor information from the muscle spindles in the tongue via the hypoglossal nerve is carried to the swallowing center in the medulla.

Swallowing is then regulated by the cerebral cortex [13]. It is likely that the cortex has a significant modulatory role in the control of the brainstem swallowing center and may have an initiating responsibility in the development of a voluntary swallow [9]. According to Shaker, there are three types of swallowing: subconscious, (occurs about once every minute); reflexive (an airway protective mechanism); and nutritional or volitional (which occurs when eating). A swallowing network in the cerebral cortex which includes the insula, cingulate gyrus, prefrontal gyrus, somatosensory cortex, and precuneus regions are all activated when a volitional swallow is produced [14].

Dysphagia Assessments

Nursing Swallow Screen

Many hospitals are utilizing a Nursing Swallow Screen as the initial bedside tool to evaluate a stroke patient's ability to swallow upon hospital admission. At Cleveland Clinic, the bedside nurse assesses the level of alertness and the patient's ability to follow commands. If they are determined to have an adequate level of consciousness, the nurse then presents sips of water, eventually progressing to a trial of three ounces of water. If the patient demonstrates difficulty at any level, the evaluation is stopped and the physician is notified. When appropriate, the physician then places a consult to Speech-Language Pathology for a formal Bedside (Clinical) Swallowing Evaluation.

Observations by other caregivers (Physicians, Dietitians, Physical Therapist, etc.) that might warrant a consult for a formal swallow assessment would include the following:

- Sialorrhea–excessive oral secretions.
- Coughing/choking when eating or drinking.

- Pocketing of food in the mouth.
- Complaints of food sticking in throat.
- Globus sensation–sensation of lump in the throat.
- Excessive oropharyngeal secretions.
- Xerostomia–lack of saliva.
- Wet vocal quality.
- Frequent pneumonia.
- Complaints of trouble swallowing.
- Odynophagia–painful swallowing.
- Presence of a tracheostomy tube.

Clinical Evaluations of Swallowing

Bedside Swallow Evaluation

Upon receiving the orders for a bedside swallow evaluation (BSE), the speech-language pathologist (SLP) completes a thorough chart review noting any preexisting history of dysphagia or diagnosis in which dysphagia might be included in the sequelae. Some of these include prior stroke, neuromuscular diseases, esophageal and other GI disorders, head and neck cancer and radiation, autoimmune disorders and cervical spine disease. It is also beneficial to review the patient's current medications to see if they might have a negative impact the patient's ability to swallow. These may include medications with anticholinergic or antimuscarinic effects, medications that cause xerostomia, antipsychotic/neuroleptic medications, medications that depress the CNS and drugs that may cause esophageal injury [15]. The SLP would then see the patient at the bedside and assess basic cognitive skills including orientation and current level of alertness and awareness. If the patient is able to follow simple commands, an oral motor examination would be completed. Assessment would include inspection of the oral cavity for quantity and quality of oral secretions, lip pursing and retraction, tongue strength and range of motion, velar movement and vocal quality. It is also important to determine if the patient is able to cough on command and if the cough appears strong and productive. Although a gag reflex may be tested, its absence does not predict aspiration in acute stroke [16].

The SLP would then initiate oral trials including ice chips, water from the spoon, straw, and/or cup, a pureed food, and a solid, chewable food item. However, if the patient was experiencing significant difficulty at any time, the swallow evaluation would be discontinued for the safety of the patient. Adequacy of mastication, oral manipulation of the presented consistencies, promptness of the pharyngeal swallow and laryngeal elevation via palpation, coughing/choking, excessive throat clearing, and changes in vocal quality are assessed.

Modified Evans Blue Dye Test

"Evans blue" is a blue-green dye extensively used to study cellular membrane permeability [17]. To study the incidence of aspiration in patients with endotracheal and tracheostomy tubes, Cameron and colleagues placed 4 drops of a 1 % solution of Evans blue dye on the tongues of patients every 4 h and monitored tracheal secretions for blue color which would indicate evidence of aspiration [18].

This procedure was modified and called "The Modified Evans Blue Dye Test (MEBDT)," and is used to assess for aspiration in tracheostomed patients by mixing the dye with liquids and foods [19]. It is an inexpensive and relatively simple procedure that can be completed at the bedside, but whose reliability has been questioned. Winklmaier and colleagues in 2007 studied tracheostomized patients following treatment of head and neck squamous cell carcinoma (HNSCC) and determined the sensitivity of the MEBDT in predicting aspiration was 95.24 % and the specificity was 100 % [20]. They concluded that the MEBDT in the HNSSC population offers a quick and reliable method of identifying aspiration risk and is more sensitive than in tracheostomied neurological patients where studies have ranged in MEBDT sensitivity from 0 to 79.3 % and specificity from 0 to 82 % [19, 21, 22]. Donzelli and colleagues indicated a 50 % false-negative error rate for the detection of aspiration when done simultaneously during a video nasal endoscopy examinations [23].

If the patient has undergone a tracheostomy due to respiratory and ventilator needs, a MEBDT can be completed at the bedside by a speech pathologist and respiratory therapist (RT). During this procedure at Cleveland Clinic, the RT will deflate the cuff of the tracheostomy tube and suction the patient prior to feeding. A few drops of green food coloring are added to food and liquids and the patient is given multiple sips of green water and green colored apple sauce or vanilla pudding. The patient is monitored for any overt signs of aspiration. After the trials have been given, the RT thoroughly suctions the patient. The SLP, RT, and nurse monitor for any green colored food, liquid or secretions over the next several hours. If colored material matching what was consumed is observed from or around the tracheostomy tube at the neck, it represents a test that is positive for food or liquid aspiration.

When blue dye is used by speech pathologists in swallowing studies, this usually refers to FD&C Blue No.1 (blue food coloring) which is a Food and Drug Administration (FDA) approved water-soluble dye used in foods, drugs and cosmetics. This has a different chemical composition than Methylene blue [24]. Following the death of two patients with sepsis whose enteral tube feeding was colored blue to identify pulmonary aspiration, Maloney in 2002 raised concerns in light of the apparent toxic effects of FD&C Blue #1 on mitochondria and advises to avoid its use in patients with active conditions that increase gut permeability. These include cardiac bypass, major vascular surgery, renal failure, severe burns, cystic fibrosis and nonsteroidal inflammatory drug use [25].

After completion of a clinical swallow evaluation, the SLP must determine whether the patient is ready to begin an oral diet with or without diet modification or compensatory techniques to maximize safety of oral intake. If the SLP subjectively determines the patient's ability to protect the airway is questionable, then further assessment via instrumental means will likely be recommended. An enteral feeding tube, if not already placed, may also be recommended for initiation of enteral nutrition.

The decision on when to repeat a BSE in the acute stage of a stroke will depend on the patient's overall progress and current medical condition. The Speech Pathologist together with the medical team will determine the appropriate time to repeat the evaluation.

The Nursing Swallow Screening and BSE are not sensitive tests to rule out silent aspiration or aspiration not resulting in obvious overt signs such as coughing, throat clearing or increased vocal wetness. Stroke patients have an increased risk of silent aspiration due to decreased laryngeal and pharyngeal sensation [26]. An order is required by a licensed independent practitioner (LIP) for the SLP to perform a videofluoroscopic swallow study (VFSS) or an endoscopic swallow study.

Instrumental Evaluations of Swallowing

Fiberoptic Endoscopic Evaluation of Swallowing

A fiberoptic endoscopic evaluation of swallowing (FEES) is an instrumental examination that can be completed at the patient's bedside. Procedures and protocols for completing the FEES were developed and documented by Langmore [27]. Procedures can also be found in the American Speech-Language-Hearing Association's (ASHA) "Guidelines for Speech-Language Pathologists Performing in the Performance and Interpretation of Endoscopic Evaluation of Swallowing: Guidelines" [28].

The FEES is done by an SLP with one other person assisting with feeding the patient. A flexible endoscope is placed through the patient's nares and into the oropharynx. Due to complaints of discomfort, some patients may require a small amount of topical anesthetic (2 % viscous lidocaine gel) along the floor of the nose, but it is best not to use a spray anesthetic in order to minimize the effects of the anesthesia on the swallow. The SLP is able to visualize velum elevation, the base of tongue, the laryngopharyngeal structures and the proximal trachea. How the patient is managing their own secretions is also noted. Any concern of structural abnormalities would require a referral for a formal examination by an otolaryngologist.

Food and liquids with reflective properties such as milk and peaches are then fed to the patient. Food coloring is also utilized by some speech pathologists to enhance the visualization of bolus trials during a FEES [29]. Though Leder and colleagues concluded that the reliability of FEES to detect aspiration is high whether food coloring is used or not and therefore dismissed the need to use food coloring [30]. The scope then remains in place as the patient swallows. In real time, with real foods, the

SLP is able to assess delay of the swallow onset, degree of spillage into the pharynx, pharyngeal contraction and aspiration before the swallow is triggered. After the swallow is complete, residual food/liquid in the valleculae and pyriform sinuses, along the pharyngeal walls, and along the epiglottis and in the proximal larynx is noted. The scope can then briefly be passed into the larynx for a better view of any material that had fallen deep into the larynx and coated the vocal folds or aspirated into the proximal trachea. During the swallow, the base of tongue retracts to the posterior pharyngeal wall causing a brief "white out" period at which time the swallow is not visualized.

An advantage of FEES is that it is completed at the patient's bedside in a more natural eating environment. An entire meal could be evaluated if desired, as long as the patient tolerates the scope in their nose. It also allows for frequent repetition (serial FEES) if needed to monitor effectiveness of compensatory strategies over a number of days or weeks without exposing the patient to radiation. FEES cannot be used to assess esophageal function [23]. Unfortunately, not all healthcare centers have the resources, equipment, and personnel available to conduct FEES.

Videofluoroscopic Swallow Study

A VFSS, also known as a Modified Barium Swallow study (MBS) or "Cookie Swallow" has been considered the "gold standard" of swallowing assessments [31]. It is a dynamic assessment of the oral and pharyngeal phases of swallowing and is completed by a SLP. It allows the SLP to view bolus transit from the oral cavity through the pharynx and into the cervical esophagus during swallowing. This study should not be confused with another similarly named radiographic study, the Barium Swallow, which is completed by a GI radiologist. This study, also known as an Esophagram or Upper GI series is used to assess abnormalities in the esophagus, stomach and small intestine.

Procedures and protocols for completing the VFSS have been documented by Logemann [32] and the American Speech-Language-Hearing Association's (ASHA) "Guidelines for Speech-Language Pathologists Performing Videofluoroscopic Swallowing Studies" [34]. The speech pathologist and referring LIP must decide if the patient is appropriate for transfer to the radiology department. The patient must not only be alert and cooperative enough to assess the oropharyngeal swallow function and aspiration risk, but ideally they would be able to attempt postural and compensatory swallowing strategies to see which will be most useful later on during a real eating situation. During the VFSS, swallowing is assessed with the patient in the most optimal position for swallowing. In the acute phase of a stroke, when a patient may have mobility and trunk control difficulty, they will likely be seated as upright as possible in either the Hausted® or VESS chair (VESS Chairs Inc., Milwaukee, WI, USA), which are specially designed for this procedure. The patient may also be assessed in a reclined, supine or standing position as well. Patients are typically assessed in the lateral view but the

Table 15.1

The 8-point penetration-aspiration scale

1. Material does not enter the airway
2. Material enters the airway, remains above the vocal folds, and is ejected from the airway
3. Material enters the airway, remains above the vocal folds, and is not ejected from the airway
4. Material enters the airway, contacts the vocal folds, and is ejected from the airway
5. Material enters the airway, contacts the vocal folds, and is not ejected from the airway
6. Material enters the airway, passes below the vocal folds, and is ejected into the larynx or out of the airway
7. Material enters the airway, passes below the vocal folds, and is not ejected from the trachea despite effort
8. Material enters the airway, passes below the vocal folds, and no effort is made to eject

Reprinted with permission from Ref. [34]

anterior-posterior projection may also be studied [33]. The radiologist or radiology technician operates the fluoroscopy equipment while the SLP gives verbal instructions to the patient. Varibar® is a contrast agent manufactured by E-Z-EM Inc. specifically designed for use in the VFSS to correlate with consistencies consumed by the patient during meal time. It is a 40 % weight/volume concentration radiopaque material produced in different viscosities; thin liquid, nectar, thin honey, honey, pudding. Barium contrast can also be mixed with food items to assess the patient's mastication and swallowing ability with solid consistencies.

The patient is given the different consistencies of barium in varying quantities and at varying rates of intake to assess the oral and pharyngeal phases of swallowing. Compensatory strategies (discussed later in this chapter) are attempted to determine their effectiveness on swallowing safety. A VFSS assesses the patient's risk of aspiration as well as quantifies the degree of aspiration, before, during and after the swallow.

In 1996, Rosenbek and colleagues developed the 8-Point Penetration-Aspiration Scale to quantify the laryngeal penetration and aspiration events observed during VFSS (*see* Table 15.1) [34]. The Penetration-Aspiration Scale is a widely utilized measure which is helpful to standardize subjective ratings among clinicians.

The modified barium swallow should be repeated as clinically indicated depending on the patient's status and severity of the previous modified barium swallow. The SLP working with the patient will make the recommendation as to when to repeat the modified barium swallow. This may be once the patient exhibits neurological improvement, better tolerance of their secretions or once the patient is successfully utilizing swallow controls or techniques.

Diet Modifications

Based on the results of clinical or instrumental evaluations, the SLP may suggest diet modifications.

Liquids

Thin liquids are often the most difficult consistency for a person to swallow safely, especially in patients with neurogenic swallowing disorders as a result of a stroke which can compromise muscular power and control [35, 36]. The liquid consistencies from least to greatest difficulty to swallow are as follows:

- Pudding thick liquids–liquids tha' are as thick as pudding. This texture would generally need to be eaten with a spoon.
- Honey thick liquids–liquids that are the consistency of honey. These would drip slowly from a spoon.
- Nectar thick liquids–liquids that are the consistency of nectar. Some liquids are naturally a nectar thick consistency such as fruit nectar juices (peach nectar, mango nectar, etc.), tomato juice, and some oral supplements such as Boost Plus® or Ensure Plus®.
- Thin liquids—all liquids which are thin in their natural state such as water, juice, coffee, etc.

Thickeners

Commercial thickeners are readily available to be added to liquids to make them nectar or honey thickness. The thickeners are either as starch based, such as ThickenUp® or Thick-it®, or gum based products, such as SimplyThick®. Care providers should carefully follow the specific manufacturers mixing instructions for the individual thickening agent to ensure the proper consistency.

Frazier Free Water Protocol

Developed in 1984 by Panther at The Frazier Rehab Institute in Louisville, Kentucky, the Frazier free water protocol (FFWP) allows patients water without thickener for their comfort, quality of life, and to help with hydration needs [37]. It was reported that patients who required thickened liquids did not feel their thirst was adequately quenched and also felt that patients who are allowed some thin liquids are more likely to follow the recommendation for thickened liquids and remain adequately hydrated [38]. No other thin liquids (coffee, tea, milk, etc.) are allowed during the FFWP. Water is considered nearly pH neutral and close to the pH of body fluids (pH 7.2), and does not pose the same risk as liquids that are very low, or very high in pH [39]. Langmore concludes that since the bacteria in water is not pathogenic to the lungs and can be easily absorbed into the bloodstream that the only ways water can cause pneumonia is by drowning resulting in asphyxiation or the washing of bacteria laden oropharyngeal secretions into the lungs [40].

The protocol includes the following:

- Allowing the patient sips of water throughout the day except with meals.
- All liquids taken with meals should be thickened to the appropriate consistency.
- Thirty minutes after the meal, the patient may resume sips of water.
- Aggressive oral hygiene is necessary to prevent colonization of oral bacteria and contamination of the secretions [37].

In 2011, Frey and Ramsberger in a retrospective cohort study found that a group of stroke patients in an acute neurorehabilitation hospital who were known aspirators of thin liquid and on a thickened liquid diet did not have an increased incidence of aspiration pneumonia when placed on a water protocol. The incidence of aspiration pneumonia was actually higher in the group that were not given water and continued only with thickened liquids [39].

A study by Karagiannis et al. reported that acute patient's with degenerative neurologic dysfunction who are immobile or have low mobility are at higher risk to develop lung complications if given access to water [41]. They concluded that these patients should be encouraged to continue to adhere to the suggested thickened liquids. Subacute patients with relatively good mobility should be allowed a choice as long as they are well informed of the possible risk of developing bronchopulmonary pneumonia and its sequelae [41].

Diet Textures

In 2002, the Academy of Nutrition and Dietetics (formerly the American Dietetic Association) endorsed utilizing National Dysphagia Diet (NDD) levels [42]. Many facilities have adopted the National Dysphagia Diet.

- Regular diet—generally there are no restrictions to what the patient can eat. However, the physician may choose to limit sodium, added sugar, or fat as the patient requires.
- Level 3 NDD/advanced—foods are nearly a regular texture. However, hard, crunchy, or sticky foods would not be included.
- Level 2 NDD/mechanically altered—foods that are easy to masticate and have a soft, moist texture. Usually excludes tougher or chewy meats, fresh fruits, and fresh vegetables.
- Level 1 NDD/pureed diet: all foods are smooth and cohesive and have a pudding-like consistency which requires minimal mastication. Some facilities utilize food molds to shape the pureed foods to look like the original product to improve the presentation of this diet level.

Compensatory Swallow Strategies

During the bedside and/or instrumental swallowing evaluations, the SLP will attempt some compensatory swallowing strategies to determine their effectiveness in preventing or reducing aspiration. The SLP determines why the patient is aspirating and the timing of aspiration; before, during, or after the swallow; to identify which strategy is most effective. Recommended compensatory strategies then may be combined with dietary modifications.

Common examples of compensatory strategies may include the following:

Head Postures

- Chin Tuck: The chin is lowered to their chest prior to swallowing. It assists in controlling the rate of bolus transfer into the pharynx.
- Head Turn toward the Affected Side: The patient turns their head toward the side of their body affected by the stroke. This will close off the weaker side and reduce residuals.
- Head Tilt and Back: Used to increase oral control, manipulation of the bolus to the stronger side, and to assist with oral transfer.

Maneuvers

- Effortful Swallow: Utilized to improve base of tongue retraction and reduce vallecular residue.
- Mendelsohn Maneuver: The patient attempt to hold the larynx at its highest point during the swallow to assist with the opening of the upper esophageal sphincter for improved bolus clearance into the esophagus.
- Supraglottic Swallow Sequence: To improve vocal fold closure before and during the swallow; the instructions include having the patient hold his breath, swallow, cough, and then re-swallow.

Therapeutic Intervention

During the acute phase of the stroke, therapy may be limited due to the patient's severity of illness. However, once the patient is transferred to a rehabilitation or skilled facility, the patient may be more appropriate to participate and benefit from dysphagia therapy.

Common examples of dysphagia therapy include the following:

- Oral Motor Exercises: Exercises targeted to improve strength and agility of the oral structures and to improve oropharyngeal muscle function. These are generally completed without presentation of food or liquid.
- Shaker Exercise: Goal is to strengthen the suprahyoid muscles used for opening of the upper esophageal sphincter by lying flat on the back and raising the head without lifting the shoulders, multiple times.
- Neuromuscular Electrical Stimulation (NMES) or VitalStim®: Involves the placement of electrodes on the throat with electrical stimulation provided to the muscles involved in swallowing. NMES is provided while simultaneously working with the patient on swallowing exercises. VitalStim® is a Food and Drug Administrative (FDA) approved device [43].

It is important to note that there is limited research data on many of the therapeutic interventions of swallowing, though further investigation is ongoing. However, the usefulness of therapeutic maneuvers during an instrumental exam may be more beneficial as their effect on swallowing can be immediately determined.

Conclusion

The primary goal of the SLP assessing a stroke patient's swallowing ability is to determine the least restrictive diet while minimizing their risk of aspiration. A swallowing evaluation is not a "pass/fail" test. Careful attention must be paid not only to a patient's limitations, but also to their capabilities in order to allow for initiation of at least quality of life oral nutrition. Although at times, NPO (nothing by mouth) status needs to be recommended, it is not satisfying to the clinician, patient, or their family to not allow some oral intake if possible.

Although the diagnosis and treatment of dysphagia following a stroke is primarily the SLP's responsibility, the entire stroke care team is essential in managing dysphagia. The physician is needed to coordinate the medical care; nursing professionals for the daily management and effective use of swallowing strategies; occupational therapists for adaptive equipment; physical therapist for positioning assistance; nutrition therapist for ensuring adequate nutritional intake; as well as various other bedside caregivers. Everyone must work together toward managing dysphagia and having a positive outcome for the patient.

References

1. Barer DH. The natural history and functional consequences of dysphagia after hemispheric stroke. J Neurol Neurosurg Psychiatry. 1989;52:236–41.
2. Sharma JC, Fletcher S, Vassallo M, Ross I. What influences outcome of stroke-pyrexia or dysphagia? Int J Clin Pract. 2001;55:17–20.

3. Teasell R, Foley N, Fisher J, Finestone H. The incidence, management, and complications in patients with medullary strokes admitted to a rehabilitation unit. Dysphagia. 2002;17: 115–20.
4. Flowers HL, Skoretz SA, Streiner DL, Silver FL, Martino R. MRI-based neuroanatomical predictors of dysphagia after acute ischemic stroke: a systemic review and meta-analysis. Cerebrovasc Dis. 2011;32(1):1–10.
5. Cameron JL, Mitchell WH, Zuidema GD. Aspiration pneumonia: clinical outcome following documented aspiration. Arch Surg. 1973;206:49–52.
6. Martino R, Foley N, Bhogal S, Diamant N, Speechley M, Teasell R. Dysphagia after stroke: incidence, diagnosis, and pulmonary complications. Stroke. 2005;36:2756–63.
7. Murray T, Carrau RL. Clinical management of swallowing disorders. 2nd ed. San Diego: Plural Publishing, Inc.; 2006.
8. Katzan IL, Dawson NV, Thomas CL, Votruba ME, Cebul RD. The cost of pneumonia after acute stroke. Neurology. 2007;68:1938–43.
9. Shaker R, Cook JS, Dodds WJ, Hogan WJ. Pressure-flow dynamics of the oral phase of swallowing. Dysphagia. 1988;3:79–84.
10. Ono T, Hori K, Takashi N. Pattern of tongue pressure on hard palate during swallowing. Dysphagia. 2004;19:259–64.
11. Hambdy S. Review: role of cerebral cortex in the control of swallowing. GI Motility online. [Internet] 2006 May 16 [cited 2012 Feb 4]: [about p. 15]. Available from: http://www.nature.com/gimo/contents/pt1/full/gimo8.html.
12. Jean A. Brain stem control of swallowing: neuronal network and cellular mechanisms. Psychol Rev. 2001;81:929–69.
13. Ramsey DJ, Smithard DG. Assessment and management of dysphagia. Hosp Med. 2004;65(5): 274–9.
14. Shaker R. Management of dysphagia in stroke patients. J Gastroenterol Hepatol. 2011;7(5): 308–32.
15. DMR Health Standard 07-1 [Internet]. Guidelines for identification and management of dysphagia and swallowing risks. Attachment a. [cited 2012 Jul 08]. Available from http://www.ct.gov/dds/lib/dds/health/attacha_med_dsyphagia_swallowing_risks.pdf.
16. Davies AE, Stone SP, Kidd D, MacMahon J. Pharyngeal sensation and gag reflex in healthy subjects. Lancet. 1995;345(8948):487–8.
17. Hamer PW, McGeachie JM, Davies MJ, Grounds MD. Evans blue dye as an in vivo marker of myofibre damage: optimizing parameters for detecting initial myofibre membrane permeability. J Anat. 2002;200:69–79.
18. Cameron JL, Reynolds J, Zuidema GD. Aspiration in patients with tracheostomies. Surg Gynecol Obstet. 1973;136:68–70.
19. Thompson-Henry S, Braddock B. The modified Evans blue dye procedure fails to detect aspiration in the tracheostomized patient: five case reports. Dysphagia. 1995;10:172–4.
20. Winklmaier U, Wust K, Plinkert PK, Wallner F. The accuracy of the modified Evans blue dye test in detecting aspiration in head and neck cancer patients. Eur Arch Otrhinolaryngol. 2007;264:1059–64.
21. Belafsky PC, Blumenfeld L, LePage A, Nahrstedt K. The accuracy of the modified Evans blue dye test in predicting aspiration. Laryngoscope. 2003;113(11):1969–72.
22. O'Neil-Pirozzi TM, Lisiecki DJ, Jack Momose K, Connors JJ, Milliner MP. Simultaneous modified barium swallow and blue dye tests: a determination of the accuracy of blue dye test aspiration findings. Dysphagia. 2003;18(1):32–8. Winter.
23. Donzelli J, Brady S, Wesling M, Craney M. Simultaneous modified Evans blue dye procedure and video nasal endoscopic evaluation of the swallow. Laryngoscope. 2001;111(10):1746–50.
24. Swigert N. Blue dye in the evaluation of dysphagia: is it safe? The ASHA Leader [serial on the internet]. 2003 Mar 8 [cited 2012 Jul 8] Available from: http://www.asha.org/Publications/leader/2003/030318/030318c.htm.
25. Maloney JP, Ryan TA. Detection of aspiration in enterally fed patients: a requiem for bedside monitors of aspiration. J Parenter Enteral Nutr. 2002;26(6):34–42.

26. Aviv JE, Murray T. FEEST: flexible endoscopic evaluation of swallowing with sensory testing. San Diego: Plural Publishing, Inc.; 2005.
27. Langmore S. Endoscopic evaluation and treatment of swallowing disorders. New York: Thieme Medical Publishers Inc.; 2001.
28. American Speech-Language-Hearing Association [Internet]. The role of the speech-language pathologist in the performance and interpretation of endoscopic evaluation of swallowing: Technical Report [Technical Report]; 2004 [cited 2012 Feb 27]. Available from www.asha.org/policy.
29. Matthews CT, Coyle J. Reducing pneumonia risk factors in patients with dysphagia who have a tracheotomy: what role can SLPs play? The ASHA Leader [serial on the internet]. 2010 May 18 [cited 2012 Jul 7] Available from: http://www.asha.org/Publications/leader/2010/100518/Reducing-Pneumonia-Risk-Factors.htm.
30. Leder SB, Acton LM, Lisitano HL, Murray JT. Fiberoptic endoscopic evaluation of swallowing (FEES) with and without blue-dyed food. Dysphagia. 2005;20(2):157–62. Spring.
31. Palmer JB, Kuhlemeier KV, Tippett DC, Lynch C. A protocol for the videofluorographic swallowing study. Dysphagia. 1993;8(3):209–14.
32. Logemann JA. Evaluation and treatment of swallowing disorders. San Diego: College-Hill Press; 1983.
33. American Speech-Language-Hearing Association [Internet]. Knowledge and skills needed by speech-language pathologists performing videofluoroscopic swallowing studies [knowledge and skill]; 2004 [cited 2012 Feb 4]. Available from www.asha.org/policy.
34. Rosenbek JC, Robbins JA, Roecker EB, Coyle JL, Wood JL. A penetration-aspiration scale. Dysphagia. 1996;11:93–8.
35. Strowd L, Kyzima J, Pillsbury D, Valley T, Rubin B. Dysphagia dietary guidelines and the rheology of nutritional feeds and barium test feeds. Chest [serial online]. 2008 June [cited 6 Jan 2012];133(6):1397–401. Available from Chest Online.
36. O'Leary M, Hanson B, Smith C. Viscosity and non-Newtonian features of thickened fluids used for dysphagia therapy. J Food Sci. 2010;75(6):E330–8.
37. Panther K. Frazier Water Protocol [Internet] 2010 [cited 2012 Feb 28]. Available from: http://www.jhsmh.org/Health-Services-Rehab-Services-Frazier-Rehab/Specialties/Frazier-Water-Protocol.aspx.
38. Garon B, Engle M, Ormiston C. A randomized control study to determine the effects of unlimited oral intake of water in patients with identified aspiration. Neurorehabil Neural Repair. 1997;11(3):139–48.
39. Frey KL, Ramsberger G. Comparison of outcomes before and after implementation of a water protocol for patients with cerebrovascular accident and dysphagia. J Neurosci Nurs. 2011; 43(3):165–71.
40. Langmore S. Why I like the free water protocol. ASHA Perspectives on Swallowing and Swallowing Disorders©. 2011;20:116–20.
41. Karagiannis MJ, Chivers L, Karagiannis TC. Effects of oral intake of water in patients with oropharyngeal dysphagia. BMC Geriatr. 2011;11:9.
42. National Dysphagia Diet Task Force. National dysphagia diet: standardization for optimal care. Chicago: American Diabetic Association; 2002.
43. VitalStim® Therapy [Internet] 2011 [cited 2012 Feb 28]. Available from: http//vitalstim.com.

Chapter 16
Stroke Nursing Care

Stacey Claus and Malissa Mulkey

Key Points

- Patient education is fundamental to primary and secondary stroke prevention.
- Nurses most often are the liaison between pre-hospital and hospital care.
- Protocols and checklists are an effective way to guide the team to meet time targets when caring for a stroke patient.
- Nurses must be knowledgeable about current stroke guidelines.
- Nursing care focuses on monitoring for progression of stroke, prevention of secondary injury and hospital acquired conditions, patient education and discharge planning.
- The process of moving the patient from the hospital to the next level of care or home is an extremely important time for patients and their caregivers.
- Specialized, comprehensive nursing care provided in designated stroke units is vital to improving and maintaining positive stroke outcomes.
- As the knowledge base for stroke continues to grow, nurses will not only contribute to the growing body of evidence but also continue the transition of evidence to practice.

Keywords Nursing care • Stroke • Transition • Rehabilitation • Acute care • Emergency

S. Claus, M.S.N., C.N.R.N., G.C.N.S.-B.C. (✉)
Nursing Education and Professional Practice Development, Cleveland Clinic,
9500 Euclid Avenue, Cleveland, OH 44195, USA
e-mail: clauss@ccf.org

M. Mulkey, M.S.N., R.N., C.C.N.S., C.C.R.N.
Neuroscience Clinical Nurse Specialist, Department of Advanced Clinical Practice,
Duke University Hospital, DUMC 3677/Durham, NC 27710,
DS/ Red Zone/ 4th floor/ Rm 4112

M.L. Corrigan et al. (eds.), *Handbook of Clinical Nutrition and Stroke*,
Nutrition and Health, DOI 10.1007/978-1-62703-380-0_16,
© Springer Science+Business Media New York 2013

Abbreviations

APN	Advance Practice Nurse
CLABSI	Central Line Associated Blood Stream Infection
CSF	Cerebral Spinal Fluid
EMS	Emergency Medical Services
ICP	Increased Intracranial Pressure
NIHSS	National Institute of Health Stroke Scale
NINDS	National Institute for Neurological Disorders and Stroke
SLP	Speech Language Pathology
tPA	Tissue Plasminogen Activator
UTI	Urinary Tract Infection
VAP	Ventilator Associated Pneumonia
VTE	Venous Thromboembolism Prophylaxis

Introduction

Stroke knowledge has grown exponentially in the past 40 years. More has been learned about stroke prevention and care in this time than ever before. A landmark paper from the 1970s was the first to identify hypertension as primary risk factor for all types of stroke and ignited new research with regard to stroke cause and management [1]. This new way of thinking gave rise to the development of the first comprehensive stroke unit and moved the focus of stoke care from palliative to preventive [1].

The rapidly changing, ever growing body of evidence for stroke care has brought about an environment of public awareness of stroke, standardization of stroke order sets, policy and protocol development as well as disease specific accreditation for stroke. Nurses across the stroke care continuum are in the position to impact stroke care through a variety of roles: educator, change agent, researcher, content expert, committee member, innovator, collaborator, and others.

With stroke the fourth leading cause of death and the leading cause for disability in the USA and the second leading cause of death worldwide, health care providers play a major role in prevention, management, and rehabilitation of stroke [2–4]. Stroke patients require specialized care and the role of the nurse is vital in achieving high quality outcomes. Nursing care of the stroke patient begins prior to admission to the hospital and continues across the acute care continuum into rehabilitation and recovery.

Nursing's Role in Primary Stroke Prevention

Stroke is considered a preventable disease given the number of modifiable risk factors associated with stroke. Modifiable risk factors are those that when identified and treated can significantly reduce an individual's risk of stroke. Modifiable risk factors include the following: hypertension, smoking, hypercholesterolemia, post menopausal hormone therapy, obesity, physical inactivity, diabetes, cardiac conditions, oral contraceptives, diet and nutrition [5–7]. Other potentially modifiable risk factors include drug use, sleep disordered breathing, hypercoagulable states, inflammation, and infection [6]. Non-modifiable risk factors are not the focus of stroke prevention education. The non-modifiable risk factors include the following: gender, age, race, and genetics [5–7].

Education is fundamental to primary stroke prevention and modification of stroke risk factors. Despite increased knowledge of stroke risk factors, these most readily treated, affordably managed conditions continue to be neglected. Although risk factors are well defined, knowledge is poor among the general public as well as among stroke survivors [1, 7]. As a result, over 70 % of strokes could have been prevented with improved modifiable risk factor management [5].

Risk factor management varies widely despite the volume of evidence based research suggesting several beneficial therapies designed to greatly decrease the risk for stroke. It is thought that this gap in transitioning evidence into practice stems from a lack of knowledge about proven therapies and inconsistencies in the approach to care and prevention by healthcare providers and their patients [8].

Education is most effective when patient's education needs are considered and perceptions of the education provided are understood. Equally important is the recognition of potential barriers to risk modifying behavior. Sullivan and Katajamaki [9] determined there was a significant positive association between susceptibility beliefs and severity beliefs, meaning the individual's perceived seriousness of stroke led a higher perceived susceptibility to stroke. There was also a significant positive association between intention and severity, meaning that the more severe an individual perceives stroke the greater the intention to change behavior. They determined that using a social cognitive framework in stroke prevention education provided positive effects on stroke beliefs. Beliefs regarding stroke provide a metric of the degree to which the individual may find the material relevant and internalize stroke education [9].

Nurses must be aware of and investigate differences in health beliefs, motivation and culture in order to impact risk modification. It is important to recognize that disparities exist across race, age, gender, socioeconomic status and impact an individuals' access to healthcare services, healthcare information and research [10].

Nursing's Role in Pre-hospital Care

The nurses' role in pre-hospital care varies. Though pre-hospital stroke care is typically provided by Emergency Medical Services (EMS), nurses may find themselves in the role of first responder with or without the presence of EMS. The nurse is most often the liaison between pre-hospital and hospital care and may provide stroke education to first responders [11].

Depending upon stroke severity, assessment of circulation, airway and breathing with the initiation of cardiopulmonary resuscitation may be necessary. Goals of supplemental oxygen in stroke are to keep the oxygen saturation greater than 92 % [11]. Rapid identification of stroke symptoms via the Cincinnati Prehospital Stroke Scale or the Los Angeles Prehospital Stroke Screen leads to the quick activation of EMS and early stroke intervention [11]. It is important to obtain a description of the event by witnesses, determine whether medications are present and locate telephone numbers of those who may be able to provide necessary health information or consent for treatment. The most beneficial information that can be obtained from the first responder and witnesses is the time the individual was last known to be without symptoms or "well" [11–13].

Nursing Care of the Stroke Patient in the Emergency Department

Once the individual is assessed by EMS and transported to the closest primary stroke center, hospital care begins. Nursing care begins with a handoff communication from the EMS personnel, including all pertinent information obtained in the field. Considering the time sensitive nature of stroke, typically multiple hospital based interventions occur simultaneously. Nurses certified to perform the National Institute of Health Stroke Scale (NIHSS) rapidly obtain the stroke score. The NIHSS score allows team members to clearly communicate using the same language so identified changes in stroke severity or patient decline can be shared. The NIHSS score is also a guide to determining further treatment decisions [11].

Protocols and checklists are an effective way to guide the team in the care of a stroke patient especially activation of a stroke team alert or neurology consult within the designated 10 min time frame. The emergency room nurse initiates cardiac monitoring, obtains a 12 lead ECG, and obtains vital signs including temperature and oxygen saturation. Vital signs with temperature assessment are completed at a minimum of every 30 min or more frequently depending upon the patient presentation [11]. Lab specimens are drawn and intravenous access is obtained in preparation for a CT scan of the brain to assess for possible intracerebral or subarachnoid hemorrhage. Measurement of actual body weight and rapid management of blood pressure must be obtained in preparation for the possibility of tissue plasminogen activator (tPA) administration in the presence of ischemic stroke [11]. The nurse is in a position to help gather key components of the medical and surgical history that are needed for the determination of other potential causes of symptoms like hypoglycemia and Todd's Paralysis that can mimic stroke as well as other factors that may impact the decision to administer tPA [11]. Information obtained in this process must be shared with team members for safe patient care.

Nurses familiar with the recommendations of the National Institute for Neurological Disorders and Stroke (NINDS) facilitate the assessment and movement of the stoke patient through the emergency room process. The rapid fire interventions of the emergency room are all completed under strict time constraints based on the NINDS study time targets of door to CT in 25 min and CT read within 45 min. Upon completion of the CT scan, if not medically contraindicated and the

CT scan is negative for hemorrhage, tPA administration is initiated within 60 min of arrival to the emergency department if the patient has arrived within 3–4.5 h of symptom onset [11–13]. The goal is to move the patient through the emergency department process to an inpatient hospital bed within 3 h [11–13].

In addition to understanding the time targets for stroke, emergency nurses must be knowledgeable about current stroke guidelines for the following: volume replacement; vital sign monitoring with temperature; tPA administration; post infusion monitoring; assessment for dysphagia; medications used to treat stroke and the effects of hypoxemia, hyperthermia and blood glucose levels.

The importance of communication cannot be understated during the high stress time of stroke and is necessary to perfect along the continuum of care. Communication occurs at multiple levels: EMS to healthcare providers; healthcare providers to healthcare providers; healthcare providers to patients and those involved in the decision making process. Clear communication during handoff reports is vital for patient safety. Communication with the patient and decision maker is most effective when provided in a timely manner and delivered in a calm, reassuring way using easily understood non-medical terminology. Communications are followed by open ended questions to evaluate understanding.

Nursing Care of the Acute Stroke Patient

The transition of care from the emergency department to the hospital begins with a thorough but concise nurse to nurse handoff communication. Transfer to a designated stroke unit when possible is preferred. Designated stroke units are associated with better patient outcomes with fewer complications like venous thromboembolism (VTE) and pressure ulcers [14, 15].

The most recent set of vital signs including temperature, blood pressure trends, cardiac rhythm, and NIHSS are included so the receiving nurse understands the baseline assessment and can identify and communicate changes. Completed lab results, all medications given and completed tests are helpful to communicate in the event that the patient is quickly transferred to the inpatient setting while time sensitive targets are still in process.

Stroke admission order sets are used to ensure complete and comprehensive care once the patient is admitted to the hospital. Basic stroke order sets typically include orders for diagnostic testing, cardiac monitoring, frequency of vital sign and neurological assessment, blood pressure and temperature parameters, blood glucose monitoring, dysphasia screen, VTE prophylaxis, and multidisciplinary consults [11].

Above and beyond the stroke order sets, nursing care is guided by stroke policies and protocols and the care is focused on the following: monitoring for cardiac events and progression of stroke; prevention of secondary brain injury; prevention of hospital acquired conditions; multidisciplinary collaboration; patient education and discharge planning.

Monitoring for cardiac events and stroke progression leading to patient deterioration is accomplished by the ongoing nursing assessment that includes a comprehensive neurological examination, continued telemetry monitoring and vital signs with temperature monitoring. Stroke patients are at risk of developing cardiac arrhythmias, heart attack or cardiac arrest which can further compromise the patient's ability to maintain adequate blood flow and cerebral perfusion [11–13]. The nurse frequently assesses the cardiac rhythm for changes from baseline and quickly notifies the team with deviation from baseline.

Stroke patients are at great risk of changing quickly. Though the patient may be stable upon admission, evidence suggests that approximately 1/3 of stroke patients will decline within the first 24 h [11]. These patients require frequent assessments and monitoring for a minimum of 24 h, especially those receiving tPA who are at risk for bleeding. Care is best provided in a location equipped to handle this high acuity patient [11]. Additional post tPA safety measures must be implemented to ensure bleeding risk is minimized and trauma or fall related injuries are avoided.

The rapidly changing stroke patient is at risk for increased intracranial pressure (ICP) related to hemorrhagic transformation of an ischemic stroke, hydrocephalus, cerebral edema, seizures and vasospasm, a complication seen in hemorrhagic stroke [11–13]. Nurses must be diligent in performing the comprehensive neurological examination in order to detect the subtle changes associated increased intracranial pressure (ICP), vasospasm and brain herniation [11–13]. The comprehensive neurological exam includes the assessment of the patients' level of consciousness, mood and behavior, cranial nerves, movement and strength, and NIHSS score. A complete NIHSS is scored on admission to the hospital or when deterioration occurs, followed by an abbreviated version of the NIHSS routinely performed with more frequent assessments [11–13]. Diligence in assessing the stroke patient frequently and thoroughly allows the nurse to alert the team when more aggressive interventions might be needed like intubation, surgical intervention, endovascular intervention or ICP monitoring [11–13].

Critical care management is necessary for the patient suffering from hemorrhagic conversion, cerebral edema with or without vasospasm. While in the ICU, an ICP monitor, placement of an external ventricular device with or without brain tissue oxygenation monitoring may be warranted to measure ICP and manage cerebral spinal fluid (CSF) volumes. Nurses monitor the ICP, oxygenation levels and collaborate with the healthcare team to manage ICP exceeding 20 mmHg. If an external ventricular drain is present, nurses assess the CSF drainage for amount, color and clarity, ensure appropriate level of the drainage device and assess for signs of over and under drainage via the hourly neurological assessment. Hypothermia therapy may be indicated to further manage cerebral edema and prevent damage to the brain tissue. Nurses knowledgeable in handling these devices assess for and help prevent intracranial infection. Nursing policies and protocols help guide the nurse in the assessment and management of the patient with these advanced monitoring devices and management therapies.

Aside from recognition of increased ICP, nursing management includes head of bed elevation to approximately 30°, neutral head and neck positioning to allow venous drainage and airway assessment for patency [11, 13]. Increased cognitive and environmental stimulation of the patient during this time can impact the patient negatively. Education to the patient or visitors includes methods of minimizing increases in intracranial pressure. Visitors eager to interact with their loved ones may require polite reminders from nurses that a calm, supportive, healing environment allowing for rest periods is necessary.

Prevention of secondary brain injury is supported by the ongoing assessment and management of vital signs, temperature and blood glucose by the nurse. Vital sign and temperature parameters provided in stroke order sets and protocols determine the point at which the nurse will administer prescribed medications or provide interventions. Assessment and monitoring of blood pressure with heart rate trends alert the nurse to physiological compensation measures or possible complications indicating an intracranial process like increased ICP due to hemorrhagic transformation or brain edema [11–13]. Recognizing the effects of pain, discomfort, noise, stimulation, infection, and bowel and bladder dysfunction can have on blood pressure and heart rate; nurses need to evaluate all possible causes of vital sign changes [11–13]. Nurses must be familiar with the most current guidelines for blood pressure management in stroke patients, treat when recognized and alert the team when the parameters cannot be maintained.

Increased temperature in the stroke patient increases the patients' metabolic demand and is associated with worse outcomes in stroke by hastening the damage to neurons [11–13]. A slight elevation in temperature, as little as 1°, is enough to impact the patients' outcome. The longer the temperature is elevated, the risk of secondary brain injury increases leading to increased morbidity and mortality [11–13]. Early recognition of elevated temperature leads to early intervention and investigation of cause. Determination of the fever causing source is helpful in decreasing the length of time the patient will experience temperature elevation [11–13]. The nurse must be knowledgeable about the importance of maintaining normothermia. Normothermia protocols guide the nurse in the use of antipyretics or combination therapy of antipyretics plus temperature control cooling systems [11–13].

Nurses play a vital role in protecting the patient from hospital acquired conditions like infection or VTE through the provision of comprehensive nursing care. Routine nursing interventions cannot be minimized. It is the important work of the nurse that will minimize a patient's risk of developing complications while hospitalized. The role of prevention and early identification impact patient outcomes, decreases length of stay and decreases costs incurred by hospitals. Indredavik et al. [14] found that stroke patients experienced at least one or more medical complication in the first week of hospitalization and was most often associated with stroke severity. Common complications in this study included pain, fever, urinary tract infection and stroke progression which provided more evidence in support of designated stroke units where complications like VTE and pressure ulcers are nearly nonexistent [14].

Nurses assess for the presence of fever and intervene quickly. Sources of fever in the stroke patient vary, however common reasons include pneumonia, infections related to presence of lines and drains, and urinary tract infection (UTI). While patients may present to the hospital with pneumonia, nurses assist in the prevention of hospital acquired pneumonia by screening for dysphagia prior to oral intake, identifying aspiration risks, implementation of early mobilization protocols, aggressive pulmonary and oral care in both intubated and non-intubated patients, patient positioning, and treatment of nausea or vomiting [11]. Initial dysphagia screen by the nurse occurs prior to any oral medications, food or liquids. Patients are kept NPO until the swallow screen is completed using an evidence based tool (See Fig. 16.1). Oral medications, food or liquids are not provided in the pre-hospital or emergency department until the same measures are taken to protect the patient from aspiration [11–13]. Patients at risk for aspiration are maintained at the NPO status, hydration is initiated, and a speech language pathology (SLP) consultation order is requested and obtained. Since stroke patients may experience a variety of changes that put them at risk for dysphagia, it is important for nurses to assess for signs of malnutrition and dehydration in order to promote early nutrition and hydration intervention for healing [11–13]. The registered dietitian is consulted to assess nutritional status and needs. The SLP completes a formalized swallow evaluation and provides recommendations to the healthcare team about safe oral feeding consistencies and interventions [11–13].

The presence of lines and drains also increases the risk for secondary infections such as ventilator associated pneumonia (VAP) and central line associated blood stream infections (CLABSI). To reduce the risk of VAP, continuous subglottic suction tubes assist with removal of secretions above the endotracheal tube. Meticulous oral care utilizing not only sponges with antiseptic, such as chlorhexidine, but also toothbrushes to remove bacteria harboring plaque is extremely important in the intubated and non-intubated patient.

CLABSI prevention is a primary role for the nurse. As a member of the healthcare team, nurses are encouraged to interrupt the placement of a central line if sterile technique is not maintained. The greatest impact the nurse can make in CLABSI prevention is the daily assessment of continued need for as well as proper care and maintenance of the line. Maintenance requires meticulous scrubbing of the access port prior to each use, diligent pulsatile flushing and facilitation of removal of lines that are clotted or are no longer necessary.

The use of an indwelling urinary catheter may be needed in acute stroke care, particularly when fluid balance by strict intake and output are being monitored. UTI is another potential source of fever and infection that can be minimized by meticulous care and daily assessment of the need for indwelling urinary catheter. Other treatment options like intermittent or external catheterization carry less risk [11]. Urinary incontinence is the most common urinary complaint; however an indwelling urinary catheter is not placed as a measure to control incontinence, but may be placed to keep pressure ulcers clean and dry or provide comfort to patients at end of life. Nursing protocols designed to guide bladder management assist nurses in the decision making process.

Poor outcomes in stroke are associated with hyperglycemia. Stroke order sets and hospital protocols typically guide the nurse in the management of hyperglycemia, a common finding in stroke patients. Current evidence supports frequent blood

Pre-screening checklist:

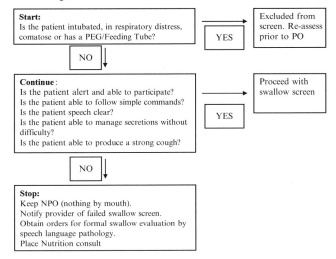

Swallow Screen:

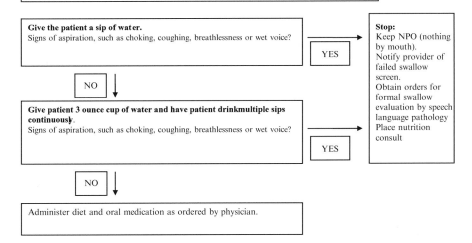

Fig. 16.1 Cleveland Clinic nursing swallow screen for patients at risk for dysphagia protocol

glucose monitoring every 1–2 h in patients with a blood glucose level above 140 who have also received tPA due to the risk associated with hemorrhage [11]. Most stroke patients are monitored every 6 h for the first 24–48 h [11]. Nurses must be knowledgeable in the effects of hyperglycemia in stroke including stroke expansion and hemorrhagic transformation, leading to prolonged hospitalization, morbidity and mortality [11–13].

Nursing interventions related to early mobilization of stroke patients minimize a number of potential complications. Hemodynamic stability in the acute stroke patient determines how quickly mobilization can happen and often bed rest is ordered until stability is achieved. Nurses must be knowledgeable about the effects of bed rest and are in a position to advocate for advancement of activity orders and seek orders for physical therapy as well as occupational therapy.

Prolonged immobilization leads to disuse atrophy of muscles and other physiologic changes that decrease the patient's ability to tolerate physical activity. Muscle atrophy begins within hours of immobilization, leading to a 4–5 % loss of muscle strength for each week of bed rest. Functional decline is often associated with other complications that can be severe and long-lasting [16].

Delirium is a common and serious condition that affects as high as 30–40 % of stroke patients and is associated with higher mortality rates [17, 18]. Delirium is defined as an acute disorder of attention and global cognitive function characterized by acute onset and fluctuating symptoms that occurs in the face of underlying organic etiology, such as medical illness or drug use or withdrawal [19–21]. Delirium can present as hypoactive, hyperactive, or a mixed delirium. Early recognition of delirium and screening by nurses is necessary to minimize its detrimental effects.

Aphasia, described as the change in ability to communicate through speech, writing or reading, affects up to 40 % of stroke patients and nurses are in a position to screen for this difficult and challenging cognitive change [22]. Communication disturbances, once recognized, can be evaluated by the SLP and interventions implemented. Stroke nurses, knowledgeable about communication therapies, reinforce and provide ongoing communication support [22].

Additional general nursing care considerations include the implementation of the following: fall minimization interventions; VTE prophylaxis; skin care and prevention protocols; range of motion activities; bladder and bowel management care plans; and supportive measures for mobility and sensory changes. Patient education about signs and symptoms of recurrent stroke, activation of EMS, medications, risk factor modification, and follow-up appointments are important before discharge. Nurses also advocate for consultation to palliative medicine, hospice, bioethics, as well as provide support at the end of life.

Nursing's Role in the Transition from Acute Care

Transitioning the patient from acute care setting is not a simple task for nurses working in the role of care manager. The process of moving the patient from the hospital to the next level of care or back to the home environment is an extremely important time for patients and their caregivers. The transition from acute care to home has been recognized as the most common and also the most stressful transitions for patients and caregivers to make. Patients express feelings of fear, lack of support, and poor or incomplete communication among providers [23]. Additionally, patients and caregivers express differences in the format and timing of education or information, ultimately impacting how prepared they are for next steps [24]. If patients are not successfully transitioned or well supported, the consequences are significant and can include readmission to the hospital setting, recurrent stroke, reduced quality of life for patients and their caregivers and even fatality [23].

Upon discharge, patients and their caregivers must be armed with a firm understanding of the ongoing plan of care, available services and access to medical providers for ongoing management or concerns [23]. All aspects of the patients potential care needs, not only physical, must be considered in the discharge planning process. Nursing collaboration and consultation with social work is beneficial to ensuring the needed supports are in place.

Great opportunities exist for advance practice nurses (APN) to research and define best practices in the management of post acute and effective stroke follow-up care. APNs must define their role as the primary contact for stroke care coordination and management. Additional areas of study would need to include interventions to improve patients understanding of stroke, sustainability of lifestyle and risk management modification, as well as the development of effective educational tools.

Nursing's Role in Stroke Rehabilitation

Stroke rehabilitation essentially begins once the patient stabilizes in the acute care setting. Like acute stroke care, stroke rehabilitation is best provided in a multidisciplinary, designated stroke rehabilitation unit with the primary focus of the patient reaching their highest level of functional independence. This care is provided in an acute care inpatient rehabilitation setting, skilled nursing facility, within the home or as an outpatient. Specialized rehabilitation nurses across the continuum of rehab care, along with the rehabilitation team using functional assessment tools, develop goal oriented plans of care designed to prevent complications, improve and maximize function, achieve maximal independence, and minimize risk factors to provide the patient with the highest quality of life possible [5, 25].

Rehabilitation nurses continue to focus not only on the pathophysiological process of stroke and education associated with the patient's understanding of disease process, prevention of recurrent event, and medication adherence, but also on the psychosocial aspects of disease adaptation [25]. Consideration for the overall impact of stroke on the individual and caregivers is essential to the success of rehabilitation especially when both personal and financial resources are evaluated [26]. Additional goals of nursing care are identification of available resources, clearly defined contacts in the event ongoing assistance is needed and caregiver stress and burden assessment [5, 25, 26].

Table 16.1 Stroke measures [27]

Measure	Definition	Stroke type
Venous thromboembolism prophylaxis (VTE)	• VTE prophylaxis by end of hospital day 2 • Documentation of contraindication	Ischemic Hemorrhagic
Anti-thrombotic therapy	• Anti-thrombotic therapy prescribed at discharge	Ischemic
Anticoagulation	• Diagnosis of atrial fibrillation or atrial flutter • Anticoagulant prescribed at discharge	Ischemic
Thrombolytic therapy	• Hospital arrival within 2 h of symptom onset (last known well) • Initiation of IV tPA within 3 h of symptom onset (last known well)	Ischemic
Anti-thrombotic therapy	• Administered an anti-thrombotic by the end of hospital day 2	Ischemic
Statin therapy	• Statin ordered at discharge if: – LDL ≥100 mg/dL or – On statin prior to admission	Ischemic
Stroke education	• Education provided on all of the following: – Activation of emergency medical system – Need for follow-up after discharge – Medications prescribed at discharge – Risk factors for stroke – Warning signs and symptoms of stroke	Ischemic Hemorrhagic
Assessed for rehabilitation	• Assessed for rehabilitation services prior to discharge	Ischemic Hemorrhagic

General rehabilitation nursing care incorporates a variety of evidence based treatment interventions to improve or maintain function and patients are readily encouraged to be as independent as possible. Nurses are active in the process of assessing and evaluating interventions related to stroke disease management, mood, sensory and cognitive changes as well as education and management of other chronic disease processes. Nursing care also includes ongoing assessment and evaluation of swallowing and communication, diet and nutritional intake, bowel and bladder function, skin care, mobility, pain, and spasticity. Stroke rehabilitation builds the foundation for continued recovery and disease adaptation allowing successful transition to this highest level of independence [5, 25, 26].

Nursing's Role in Stroke Center Certification

The need for disease specific primary stroke center accreditation was first acknowledged in June, 2000 and became a reality in 2004 when the Joint Commission, American Heart Association and American Stroke Association developed certification criteria largely based on the recommendations of the Brain Attack Coalition white paper [11]. Currently, eight evidence based performance measures exist (See Table 16.1) [27]. For example, application of intermittent pneumatic compression stockings (IPCs) by the end of hospital day 2 are ordered by the medical provider but carried out and maintained by nurses. Many of the certification criteria are impacted by the nursing care provided.

Since the days of Florence Nightingale, nurses have been the drivers of quality improvement for hospitalized patients. With regard to disease specific accreditation, nurses continue to maintain this passion for providing and driving high quality care, implementing quality improvement initiatives, and evaluation of outcomes [11]. Nursing plays a vital role in obtaining and maintaining primary stroke center certification. While many of the measures are physician driven, knowledgeable nurses, through collaboration and consultation with the multidisciplinary team, ensure highest quality care is delivered and patients' needs are met using best practices [11]. This can only happen when core hospital staff is trained and knowledgeable about primary stroke certification criteria and best practices.

The future of stroke care is evolving based on advancements in technology and the knowledge to develop an all encompassing coordinated program equipped to care for these high acuity patients. This is being realized through the development of criteria for comprehensive stroke center accreditation. Advanced accreditation requires high volume advanced care, research, dedicated care units, and peer review process [28].

Conclusion

Specialized, comprehensive nursing care, preferably provided in designated stroke units is vital to improving and maintaining positive stroke outcomes. The widely varied role of the nurse supports the patient across the continuum of care and even begins prior to hospital admission. Nurses are not only involved in the important work of direct patient care but also actively involved in improving all aspects of patient quality through policy and protocol development, quality improvement projects, research, education, and multidisciplinary collaboration. As the knowledge base for stroke continues to grow, nurses will not only contribute to the growing body of evidence, but will continue the transition of evidence to practice.

References

1. Hachinski V, Donnan GA, Gorelick PB, Hacke W, Cramer SC, Kaste M, et al. Stroke: working toward a prioritized world agenda. Stroke. 2010;41(6):1084–99.
2. Cerebrovascular Disease or Stroke [Internet]. Center for Disease Control and Prevention (CDC); 2012 [updated 2012 May 16; cited 2012 Jul 11]. Available from: http://www.cdc.gov/nchs/fastats/stroke.htm
3. Top 10 Causes of Death [Internet]. World Health Organization. [updated 2012; cited 2012 Jul 11]. Available from: http://www.who.int/mediacentre/factsheets/fs310/en/index.html
4. Knight AJ, Wiese N. Therapeutic music and nursing in poststroke rehabilitation. Rehabil Nurs. 2011;36(5):200–4; 215.

5. Barker EM, editor. Neuroscience nursing: a spectrum of care. St. Louis, MO: Mosby; 2008. p. 403–7; 522, 523; 558.
6. Goldstein LB, Bushnell CD, Adams RJ, Appel LJ, Braun LT, Chaturvedi S, et al. Council on Epidemiology and Prevention. Council for High Blood Pressure Research, Council on Peripheral Vascular Disease, and Interdisciplinary Council on Quality of Care and Outcomes Research. Guidelines for the primary prevention of stroke: a guideline for healthcare professionals from the American Heart Association/American Stroke Association. Stroke. 2011; 42(2):517–84.
7. Maasland L, Koudstaal PJ, Habbema JD, Dippel DW. Knowledge and understanding of disease process, risk factors and treatment modalities in patients with a recent TIA or minor ischemic stroke. Cerebrovasc Dis. 2007;23(5–6):435–40.
8. Ovbiagele B. Pessin award lecture 2008: lessons from the Stroke PROTECT program. J Neurol Sci. 2008;275(1–2):1–6.
9. Sullivan KA, Katajamaki A. Stroke education: promising effects on the health beliefs of those at risk. Top Stroke Rehabil. 2009;16(5):377–87.
10. Cruz-Flores S, Rabinstein A, Biller J, Elkind MS, Griffith P, Gorelick PB, et al. Racial-ethnic disparities in stroke care: the American experience: a statement for healthcare professionals from the American Heart Association/American Stroke Association. Stroke. 2011;42(7): 2091–116.
11. Summers D, Leonard A, Wentworth D, Saver JL, Simpson J, Spilker JA, et al. Comprehensive overview of nursing and interdisciplinary care of the acute ischemic stroke patient: a scientific statement from the American Heart Association. Stroke. 2009;40(8):2911–44.
12. Adams HP, del Zoppo G, Alberts MJ, Bhatt DL, Brass L, Furlan A, et al. Guidelines for the early management of adults with ischemic stroke. Stroke. 2007;38:1655–711.
13. Bederson JB, Connolly Jr ES, Batjer HH, Dacey RG, Dion JE, Diringer MN, et al. Guidelines for the management of aneurysmal subarachnoid hemorrhage: a statement for healthcare professionals from a special writing group of the Stroke Council, American Heart Association. Stroke. 2009;40(3):994–1025.
14. Indredavik B, Rohweder G, Naalsund E, Lydersen S. Medical complications in a comprehensive stroke unit and an early supported discharge service. Stroke. 2008;39(2):414–20.
15. Hanger C, Fletcher V, Fink J, Sidwell A, Roche A. Improving care to stroke patients: adding an acute stroke unit helps. N Z Med J. 2007;120(1250):U2450.
16. Korupolu R, Gifford J, Needham D. Early mobilization of critically ill patients: reducing neuromuscular complications after intensive care. Contemp Crit Care. 2009;6(9):1–12.
17. Shi Q, Presutti R, Selchen D, Saposnik G. Delirium in acute stroke: a systematic review and meta-analysis. Stroke. 2012;43:645–9.
18. Mitasova A, Kostalova M, Bednarik J, Michalcakova R, Kasparek T, Balabanova P, et al. Poststroke delirium incidence and outcomes: validation of the confusion assessment method for the intensive care unit (CAM-ICU). Crit Care Med. 2012;40(2):484–90.
19. Pisani MA, Araujo KL, Van Ness PH, Zhang Y, Ely EW, Inouye SK. A research algorithm to improve detection of delirium in the intensive care unit. Crit Care. 2006;10(4):R121.
20. McNicoll L, Pisani MA, Ely EW, Gifford D, Inouye SK. Detection of delirium in the intensive care unit: comparison of confusion assessment method for the intensive care unit with confusion assessment method ratings. J Am Geriatr Soc. 2005;53(3):495–500.
21. Otter H, Martin J, Bäsell K, von Heymann C, Hein OV, Böllert P, et al. Validity and reliability of the DDS for severity of delirium in the ICU. Neurocrit Care. 2005;2(2):150–8.
22. Poslawsky IE, Schuurmans MJ, Lindman E, Hafsteinsdottir TB. A systematic review of nursing rehabilitation of stroke patients with aphasia. J Clin Nurs. 2010;19:17–32.
23. Fitzpatrick M, Dawber S. Best practice in management of stroke: effective transfer of care from hospital to community. Br J Neurosci Nurs. 2008;4(12):582–7.
24. Hoffmann T, McKenna K, Herd C, Wearing S. Written education materials for stroke patients and their carers: perspectives and practices of health professionals. Top Stroke Rehabil. 2007; 14(1):88–97.

25. Hickey JV, editor. The clinical practice of neurological and neurosurgical nursing. Philadelphia, PA: Wolters Kluwer Health/Lippincott Williams & Wilkins; 2009. p. 213–6, 609.
26. Miller EL, Murray L, Richards L, Zorowitz RD, Bakas T, Clark P, et al. Comprehensive overview of nursing and interdisciplinary rehabilitation care of the stroke patient: a scientific statement from the American Heart Association. Stroke. 2010;41(10):2402–48.
27. Specifications Manual for National Hospital Inpatient Quality Measures. 2012. http://www. jointcommission.org/stroke/. Accessed Jun 2012.
28. Leifer D, Bravata DM, Connors JJ, Hinchey JA, Jauch EC, Johnston SC, et al. Metrics for measuring quality of care in comprehensive stroke centers: detailed follow up to brain attack coalition comprehensive stroke center recommendations: a statement for healthcare professionals from the American Heart Association/American Stroke Association. Stroke. 2011; 42:849–77.

Chapter 17
Stroke Rehabilitation

J. Patrick McGowan

Key Points

- While stroke can initially limit patient's functional abilities, rehabilitation can help improve function and strength.
- Proper selection of patients for rehabilitation programs can maximize benefits of rehabilitation.
- Nutrition is an integral therapy to assist patients in maximizing their rehabilitation potential.

Keywords Stroke • Rehabilitation • Function

Abbreviations

ADLs	Activities of Daily Living
DVT	Deep Venous Thrombosis
FIM	Functional Independence Measures
LMWH	Low Molecular Weight Heparin
OT	Occupational Therapy
PT	Physical Therapy
ROM	Range of Motion
SCD	Sequential Compression Devices
SNF	Skilled Nursing Facility

J.P. McGowan, M.D. (✉)
Consultative and Rehabilitation Unit, Physical Medicine and Rehabilitation,
Virginia Commonwealth University, 1223 E Marshall St., Richmond, VA 23298, USA
e-mail: jmcgowan@mcuh-vcu.edu

M.L. Corrigan et al. (eds.), *Handbook of Clinical Nutrition and Stroke*,
Nutrition and Health, DOI 10.1007/978-1-62703-380-0_17,
© Springer Science+Business Media New York 2013

ST   Speech Therapy
UFH   Unfractionated Heparin
UTI   Urinary Tract Infections

Introduction

Stroke is a sudden disruption to the brain's blood supply. In the USA, there are approximately 780,000 new strokes annually [1]. About one-fifth, or 160,000 per year are fatal. The fourth leading cause of death in the USA is from stroke [2], and is the second leading cause of death worldwide [3]. While strokes are more common with increasing age, strokes can occur at any age. Nearly 25 % of people who experience and survive their first stroke will have another in 5 years [1].

The previous chapters have reviewed the etiology and risk factors for stroke and therefore will not be discussed further in this chapter. Once a patient has survived a stroke, rehabilitation to optimize function and quality of life become paramount. The goal of rehabilitation is to improve patient's function enough to allow return to home, typically with support. The family or caregivers will be involved in training just prior to discharge. Patients will typically need to continue additional therapies with home health or outpatient therapies following an inpatient rehabilitation stay.

Anatomic Considerations

The majority of strokes occur in the anterior circulation of the brain, involving the carotid arteries to the anterior and middle cerebral arteries. Much of the current intervention is geared towards strokes in the anterior circulation. Symptoms suggestive of anterior stroke are unilateral vision loss and aphasia. Posterior circulation comes from the basilar artery, which is formed from bilateral vertebral arteries. These supply the cerebellum and brainstem, and symptoms include balance/coordination problems, cranial nerve involvement including cranial nerve involvement opposite from arm/leg involvement. Strokes involving the left hemisphere cause right weakness, with aphasia if the dominant hemisphere is involved. However, these patients have intact visuospatial functions and can learn by observing others, and typically do not need supervision. Strokes involving the right hemisphere have left sided weakness, along with neglect and impaired visuospatial function. These patients are typically verbally fluent and downplay their deficits. They will often need supervision 24 hours per day, and should not drive or have access to dangerous equipment such as power tools, guns, etc. They may need neuropyschological assessment to see if they have had sufficient recovery to allow driving or other non-supervised activities.

Rehabilitation

Once a patient has stabilized on the acute care service, they should be evaluated for rehabilitation to determine if patient will require an inpatient rehabilitation stay or other therapies prior to returning home. The rehabilitation physician will assess the patient on acute care to determine the best level of rehabilitation. Patients should begin therapies on the acute care setting as soon as they can. Physical Therapy (PT) will work on bed mobility, transfers including sit to stand and bed to wheelchair, ambulation, strength and endurance as applicable. Occupational Therapy (OT) will work on Activities of Daily Living (ADLs). ADLs include feeding, grooming, bathing, dressing, and toileting. Speech therapy (ST) works on communication, swallowing, and cognition.

Inpatient Rehabilitation may be an option for patients who require at least two of the three therapies (PT, OT, ST), can participate in 3 hours of intensive therapies daily, and plan to return to the community. Inpatient rehabilitation facilities require close medical supervision by a physiatrist or physician with specialty training and experience, 24 hours nursing care in rehabilitation [4]. The typical length of stay for inpatient rehabilitation patients is 2–3 weeks. The rehabilitation team works as an interdisciplinary team, with physician, nurse, dietitian, PT, OT, ST, and psychologist all working to improve patient's function (Fig. 17.1).

The rehabilitation physician plays an important role in monitoring and adjusting medications and treating medical conditions to ensure the patient can participate in 3 hours of therapy each day. The physician will attend weekly conferences and provide leadership for the team. The team will use the patient's improvement in function to guide length of stay. Patients are assessed daily by the physician and periodic reexaminations monitor the patient's overall recovery after a stroke. Poor prognosis for recovery and outcomes include severe memory problems, prior stroke, inability to understand commands, medical or surgical instability, advanced age, urinary and/or bowel incontinence, and visual spatial deficits [5].

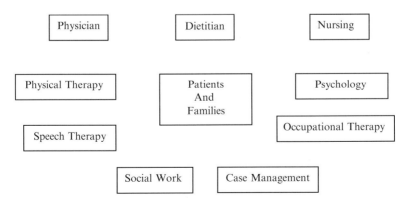

Fig. 17.1 The stroke rehabilitation team

Other sites for rehabilitation follow stroke include a skilled nursing facility (SNF), home therapy, or outpatient rehabilitation therapy. SNFs can provide up to an hour and a half of PT, OT and/or ST for patients unable to return home or unable to tolerate more intensive rehabilitation setting (i.e., 3 hours of therapy required for an inpatient rehabilitation program). For patients able to return home (often with assistance), home health therapies or outpatient therapies can help improve function. Home health is reserved for homebound patients whereas outpatient therapy is for patients that are not homebound and have transportation to and from the therapy site. Both of these types of programs are typically 2–3 times a week and with 30 min therapy sessions.

Regaining Function

Jorgenson and colleagues studied 1,000 patients with stroke and the majority of neurological and functional recovery occurred within the first 6 months [6]. They used the Barthel index as an outcome measure, and found functional recovery was "completed" within 12.5 weeks in 95 % of patients [6]. Eighty percent of patients reached their maximum functional recovery in 6 weeks [6]. A study by Hendricks and colleagues indicated the initial grade of motor paresis is a key prognosticator of motor recovery [7]. The Barthel Index is a measure of activity of daily living skills, including feeding, transfers, personal hygiene, toileting, bathing, ambulation, stair climbing, dressing, bladder and bowel control [8]. The Barthel has been largely replaced by the Functional Independence Measures (FIM). The FIM is composed of 18 items addressing the functional areas of self care, transfers, ambulation, sphincter control, communication and social cognition [8].

Stroke Complications

Spasticity

The increased tone in muscles following a stroke can prevent or seriously reduce patient's mobility and ADLs. Some patients will respond to stretching exercises, and modalities including heat and ice. However, medications are often needed to help reduce spasticity (Table 17.1). Lioresal is a gamma amino butyric acid agonist which works at the spinal cord level to reduce spasticity. Dosing is divided fashion up to four times a day, typically to 120 mg/day. Common side effects include sedation and confusion. Lioresal can be given via intrathecal pump for patients unable to tolerate oral Lioresal yet showing good response to spasticity. Dantrolene works at the muscle at the sarcoplasmic reticulum. As it works peripherally, it can cause weakness on the uninvolved side. Liver function should be monitored through

Table 17.1
Medications for spasticity in stroke
rehabilitation

Lioresal (Baclofen)
Dantrium (Dantrolene)
Tizanidine (Zanaflex)
Diazepam (Valium)
OnabotulinumtoxinA injection (Botox)

hepatic panels as this medication has been associated with liver toxicity. Tizanidine is also another treatment option. Diazepam has also been used, but central side effects can limit its utility in this patient population. Intramuscular injection of botulinum toxin is effective for localized spasticity. However, it is not FDA approved for this indication. Botulinum toxin works at the neuromuscular junction inhibiting release of acetylcholine from the presynaptic membrane. Botulinum toxin injection has a low side effect profile, has dose dependant response, and can be easy to administer [9]. Stimulation at the motor point with needle during injection can help localize the involved muscle.

Aphasia

Communication dysfunction is common after stroke, typically involving the dominant hemisphere. The types of aphasia are typically divided into fluent versus non fluent. Non-fluent include Global and Broca's aphasia. Global aphasia causes difficulty in reception as well as expression while Brocas's causes non-fluent or expressive aphasia, but good comprehension. Fluent aphasias include Wernicke's, involving the left posterior superior temporal region. Patients are often described with "word salad" with expression of words, but difficulty with reception/comprehension.

Dysphagia

Dysphagia is common following a stroke. An initial bedside swallow evaluation may help determine if patients could begin swallowing with therapy provided by the ST. Often a Modified Barium Swallow (MBS) is needed to determine which patients can safely swallow, if liquids need to be thickened, and if solids need to be modified. ST will work with patients to improve the swallow function. The physician will consult with the dietitian to ensure good nutrition and hydration for patients. Alternative measures for feeding, such as nasogastric or percutaneous endoscopic gastrostomy tubes, may be needed in cases of severe dysphagia with risk of aspiration. Enteral tube feedings will often be given nocturnally with concentrated formulas. Delivery of enteral tube feedings at night allows patients to participate in therapies during the day without limiting their mobility with enteral feeding pumps and poles. After tolerance is established to enteral feedings and discharge is approaching, the dietitian and physician may consider switching to bolus feeds during the day to help caregiver administration at home.

Pain

Pain can be a common symptom after stroke. Shoulder pain on the hemiplegic side can be seen in 20 % of patients 1 month after stroke [10]. Due to weakened muscles at the shoulder, the scapula changes orientation so the Glenoid fossa is pointing inferiorly, and gravity pulls the upper extremity downwards, leading to inferior subluxation. Proper positioning and range of motion (ROM) can help reduce pain. Slings can be useful during ambulation, but care needs to be used to prevent immobility at the shoulder. Caution and care should be used during transfers and other positioning of patients. Simple analgesics including non steroidal anti inflammatory drugs can help with alleviating pain [10]. Taping by an experienced therapist may also help. Therapists use tape to help support weakened muscles, particularly in the shoulder by running tape in different planes from the supraclavicular area into the upper arm.

Complex Regional Pain Syndrome has been reported in 12–25 % of stroke patients [11]. Besides pain in the hand and shoulder, patients often have hyperesthesias, vasomotor changes, distal edema, skin and muscle atrophy. The best imaging for the diagnosis of Complex Regional Pain Syndrome is done with bone scans [12]. The most effective treatment is sympathetic blockade at the stellate ganglion. However, some studies have shown that oral corticosteroids can be effective [12]. Thalamic pain can occur in patients with thalamic strokes. Amytriptyline, Gabapentin or other medicines can help with thalamic pain.

Medical Complications

Deep Venous Thrombosis

Deep venous thrombosis (DVT) occurs in approximately 11 % of patients on a Rehabilitation Unit [13]. Venous Duplex study is the test of choice to diagnosis DVT. There is controversy regarding use of Low Molecular weight Heparin (LMWH) versus Unfractionated Heparin (UFH). LMWH was found to have better efficacy preventing DVT in patients with ischemic stroke [14, 15]. A recent study showed enoxaparin 40 mg daily subcutaneously was superior to UFH 5,000 U subcutaneously every 12 h preventing DVT. Both agents had a similar rate of intracranial bleeding, but enoxaparin had a slightly higher risk of major extracranial bleeding [16].

Mechanical devices have been studied in patients with hemorrhagic strokes. Elastic stockings or sequential compression devices (SCD) were evaluated in one study of 151 patients admitted with intracerebral hemorrhage to an acute hospital SCD along with elastic stockings reduced the risk of DVT by 71 % compared to stockings alone [17]. However, SCDs may have a limited role on a stroke rehabilitation unit where patients are spending a significant amount of time out of bed.

The American College of Chest Physician Guidelines recommend against use of aspirin alone as a thromboprophylaxic agent for any patient group [18], but recommend mechanical methods of thromboprophylactic be used primarily for patients at high bleeding risk or possibly as an adjunct to anticoagulation [18]. For acutely ill medical patients admitted to hospital with congestive heart failure or respiratory disease, or who are confined to bed and have one or more additional risk factors, including active cancer, prior venous thromboembolic disease, sepsis, acute neurological disease or inflammatory bowel disease, recommend thromboprophylaxis with LMWH, LDUH or fondaparinux [18]. For medical patients with risk factors for venous thromboembolic disease, and for whom therapy is a contraindication to anticoagulant thromboprophylaxis, recommend the optimal use of mechanical thromboprophylaxis with graded compression stockings or intermittent pneumatic compression devices [18].

Stroke Syndromes

The vertebrobasilar system supplies the pons and medulla, and symptoms can be bilateral as lesions can cross the midline. Lateral medullary syndrome or Wallenberg syndrome causes contralateral pain and temperature decrease in the body, ipsilateral on the face, ipsilateral Horner's syndrome, ipsilateral ataxia, vertigo, nystagmus and nausea, along with hoarseness and dysphagia [19]. Locked in syndrome is a rare syndrome caused by lesions to the basilar artery to bilateral pons, causing tetraplegia, bilateral facial weakness, dysarthria and lateral gaze weakness. However, the patient can blink and has upward gaze intact [19].

Seizures

Patients with both ischemic and hemorrhagic strokes can have seizures. A study by Bladin et al. found seizures occurred in 10.6 % of hemorrhagic strokes and 8.6 % of ischemic stroke in the acute hospital stay [20]. Cortical location of bleeding was the major risk factor for seizures. Recurrent seizures occurred in 2.5 % of total patient population [20]. Patients are monitored by nursing and therapists for potential seizure activity, and an EEG may be needed to diagnosis seizure. Seizures are treated with standard antiseizure medications.

Urinary Function

Urinary tract infections (UTI) are common after stroke [21]. UTI are often seen with female sex, higher NIHSS score and advanced age [21]. UTI and pneumonia have independent association with worse scores on the Barthel index and have higher mortality rates seen 3 months after stroke [21]. Patients can have incontinence due to uninhibated bladder, but also due to decreased mobility, communication or cognition [22]. Patients with UTI may show increased lethargy, decreased ability to work with therapies. A simple urine culture with sensitivities can guide proper treatment based on the causative bacteria.

Depression

Depression is commonly seen after stroke. One study showed incidence of 25–30 % in the first 3 months after stroke, 16–19 % 1–2 years after stroke, and 29 % at 3 years after stroke [23]. One study of patients with stroke who had untreated depression had lower mobility scores compared to patients not depressed [24]. Tricyclic antidepressants were the primary treatment before selective serotonin reuptake inhibitors (SSRIs), but both have been shown to be helpful in post stroke depression [25]. SSRIs have fewer side effects [25]. The physician will commonly consult the clinical psychologist to help with depression and medication adjustment during rehabilitation stay. Following discharge from an inpatient rehabilitation program, patients can follow up with a psychologist and a primary care physician if depression continues.

Carotid Endarterectomy

Carotid Endarterectomy is a surgical procedure where fatty deposits are removed from the carotid arteries, the main source of blood for the brain [1]. This surgery is highly beneficial who have either already had a stroke or had stroke symptoms and have a severe stenosis of 70–99 % [1]. Surgery can reduce the estimated 2 year stroke risk by over 80 %, from greater than 1 in 4 to less than 1 in 10 [1]. If patients have had transient or mild stroke symptoms due to moderate carotid stenosis (50–69 %), surgery reduces the 5-year risk of stroke or death by 6.5 % [1]. The failure rate for the medical group is 22.2 % and is 15.7 % in the surgical group for ipsilateral stroke or death [1]. The Asymptomatic Carotid Atherosclerosis Study (ACAS) showed patients with carotid stenosis of 60–99 % but symptom free and have a reduction in 5 year stroke risk by about one half, from about 1 in 10 to less than 1 in 20 [1].

Conclusion

Stroke rehabilitation focuses on a team approach to assisting patients regain function and return back to the community. Collaboration between the stroke rehabilitation physician, PT, OT, ST, nutrition, and psychology is key. Dysphagia is common in these patients and relies on the registered dietitian, ST, and OT to help the patient achieve nutritional autonomy.

References

1. National Institute of Neurological Disorders and Stroke. Brain basics: preventing stroke. www.ninds.nih.gov
2. Kirby et al. Stroke: hope through research. 2004. http://www.cdc.gov/nchs/fastats/lcod.htm, http://www.cdc.gov/nchs/data/nvsr/nvsr60/nvsr60_04.pdf
3. Kirby et al. Stroke: Challenges, progress and Promise. 2009. http://www.who.int/mediacentre/factsheets/fs310/en/index
4. Medical Inpatient Rehabilitation Criteria Task Force. John L Melvin, chairman. Standards for assessing medical appropriateness criteria for admitting patients to Rehabilitation hospitals and units. Chicago, IL: American Academy of Physical Medicine and Rehabilitation. Sept 2006. Available from: http://www.aapmr.org/hpl/legislation/mirc.htm
5. Jougblood L. Prediction of function after stroke: a critical review. Stroke. 1986;17:765–76.
6. Jorgenson HS, Nakayama H, Raaschou HO, Viv-Larsen J, Stoier M, Olsen TS. Outcome and time course of recovery in stroke. Part II: time course of recovery. The Copenhagen Stroke Study. Arch Phys Med Rehabil. 1995;76:406–12.
7. Hendricks HT, van Limbeek J, Geurts AC, Zwarts MJ. Motor recovery after stroke: a systemic review of the literature. Arch Phys Med Rehabil. 2002;83:1629–37.
8. Mahoney F, Barthel DW. Functional evaluation: the Barthel Index. Md State Med J. 1965;14:61–5.
9. Harvey R, Roth EJ, Yu D. Rehabilitation of stroke syndromes. In: Braddom RL, editor. Physical medicine and rehabilitation. 3rd ed. Philadelphia, PA: Elsevier; 2007. p. 1175–212.
10. Ratnasabaphthy Y, Broud J, Baskett J, Pledger M, Marshall J, Bonita R. Shoulder pain in people with stroke: a population based study. Clin Rehabil. 2003;17:304–11.
11. Lo SF, Chen SY, Lin HC, Jim YF, Meng NH, Kao MJ. Arthrographic and clinical findings in patients with hemiplegic shoulder pain. Arch Phys Med Rehabil. 2003;84:1786–91.
12. Turner-Stokes L, Jackson D. Shoulder pain after stroke: a review of the evidence base to inform the development of an integrated care pathway. Clin Rehabil. 2002;116:276–98.
13. Oczkowski WJ, Ginsberg JS, Shin A, Panju A. Venous thromboembolism in patients undergoing rehabilitation for stroke. Arch Phys Med Rehabil. 1992;73:712–6.
14. Andre C, de Freitas GR, Fukujima MM. Prevention of deep venous thrombosis and pulmonary embolism following stroke: a systemic review of published articles. Eur J Neurol. 2007;14: 21–32.
15. Kamphusien PW, Agnelli G. What is the optimal pharmacological prophylaxis for the prevention of deep-vein thrombosis and pulmonary embolism in patients with acute ischemic stroke? Thromb Res. 2007;119:265–74.
16. Sherman DG, Albers GW, Bladin C, Fieschi C, Gabbai AA, Kase CS, et al. The efficacy and safety of enoxaparin versus unfractionated heparin for the prevention of venous thromboembolism after acute ischaemic stroke (PREVAIL Study): an open-label randomized comparison. Lancet. 2007;369:1347–55.

17. Lacut K, Bressollette L, Le Gal G, Etienne E, De Tinteniac A, Renault A, et al. Prevention of venous thrombosis in patients with acute intracerebral hemorrhage. Neurology. 2005;65: 865–9.
18. Geerts W, Bergqvist D, Pineo GF, Heit JA, Samama CM, Lassen MR, et al. Prevention of venous thromboembolism. American college of chest physician evidence-based clinical practice guidelines (8th Ed). Chest. 2008;133(6 Suppl):381S–433.
19. Blumenfeld H. Neuroanatomy through clinical cases. Sunderland, MA: Sinauer; 2002.
20. Bladin CF, Alexandrov AV, Bellance A, Bornstein N, Chambers B, Coté R, et al. Seizures after stroke: a prospective multicenter study. Arch Neurol. 2000;57:1617–22.
21. Aslanyan S, Weir CJ, Diener HC, Kaste M, Lees KR. Pneumonia and urinary tract infection after acute ischaemic stroke: a tertiary analysis of the GAIN International trial. Eur J Neurol. 2004;11:49–53.
22. Marinkovic S, Badlani G. Voiding and sexual dysfunction after cerebrovascular accidents. J Urol. 2001;165:359–70.
23. Astrom M, Adolfsson R, Asplund K. Major depression in stroke patients. A 3-year longitudinal study. Stroke. 1993;24:976–82.
24. Gainotti G, Antonucci G, Marra C, Paolucci S. Relation between depression after stroke, antidepressant therapy, and functional recovery. J Neurol Neurosurg Psychiatry. 2001;71:258–61.
25. Turner-Stokes L, Hassan N. Depression after stroke: a review of the evidence base to inform the development of an integrated care pathway. Part 2. Treatment alternatives. Clin Rehabil. 2002;16:248–60.

Chapter 18
Ethical Issues in Stroke Patients

Martin L. Smith

Key Points

- Clinical ethics provides important resources for patients, surrogates, and health care professionals facing difficult decisions and dilemmas after a patient has experienced a stroke.
- Because of the significance of the ethical principle of respect for patient autonomy, wishes and preferences, assessment of a stroke patient's decision-making capacity is an important first step for identifying goals of care and clinical management of the patient.
- Decisions to forgo life-sustaining treatment, including artificial nutrition and hydration, should be based on patient wishes and preferences as well as burden-to-benefit analyses.

Keywords Artificial nutrition and hydration • Best interest • Clinical ethics • Decision-making capacity • End-of-life care • Ethics consultation • Forgoing treatment • Informed consent • Patient autonomy • Substituted judgment

Abbreviations

ACE	Aid to capacity evaluation
AMA	American Medical Association
ACP	American College of Physicians
ANA	American Nurses Association
AND	Allow natural death

M.L. Smith, S.T.D. (✉)
Department of Bioethics, Cleveland Clinic, 9500 Euclid Ave, JJ60, Cleveland, OH 44195, USA
e-mail: smithm24@ccf.org

M.L. Corrigan et al. (eds.), *Handbook of Clinical Nutrition and Stroke*,
Nutrition and Health, DOI 10.1007/978-1-62703-380-0_18,
© Springer Science+Business Media New York 2013

ANH	Artificial nutrition and hydration
ASBH	American Society for Bioethics and Humanities
CPR	Cardiopulmonary resuscitation
DMC	Decision-making capacity
DNAR	Do not attempt resuscitation
DNR	Do not resuscitate
ECS	Ethics Consultation Service
ICU	Intensive care unit
MMSE	Mini mental state examination
MOLST	Medical orders for life-sustaining treatment
PEG	Percutaneous endoscopic gastrostomy
POLST	Physician orders for life-sustaining treatment
TLT	Time-limited trial
TPN	Total parenteral nutrition

Introduction and Background

Clinical ethics has been a developing field of practice since the late 1960s. During the past 50 years, core ethical principles and methods for "thinking ethically" have been identified and applied to critical care as well as to routine health situations, both at the bedside and in ambulatory care settings. Ethics resources to assist health care professionals, patients and their families have also emerged during this time (e.g., ethics committees and ethics consultation services; ethics-related policies and procedures; books and journals; clinical ethics conferences, workshops, and academic courses). The evolving history of clinical ethics has paralleled technological, scientific and medical advancements that have improved the quality and extended the quantity of life for many people—while generating a significant number of ethical issues, concerns, and questions.

Among the technical-medical advancements that have created ethical concerns and questions are the multiple ways to "artificially" or "medically" provide nutrition and hydration to patients who can consume very little food or who are unable to eat and drink by mouth, often after brain injuries such as stroke, head trauma, or anoxic injury. Artificial nutrition and hydration (ANH) for many patients has been life-saving. ANH can be provided via the enteral route with a naso-enteric tube or gastrostomy tube or via the parenteral route delivered though a central catheter. ANH has also become one of the most contentious of the life-prolonging treatments when deciding whether to initiate, withhold or withdraw treatment [1]. The controversy stems partially from disagreement about whether ANH is a medical treatment, and therefore similar to a mechanical ventilator or dialysis; or "basic care and comfort" to be provided to all patients, and therefore similar to turning a patient to prevent bed sores or keeping a patient clean. As basic care, ANH can prevent sensations of hunger and thirst, help to maintain a patient's life, and prevent death by malnutrition or dehydration. Additionally, because of the symbolic, cultural and even religious associations with eating and drinking [2], not providing "food and water," even when it is "artificial" or "medical," may be viewed by some as starvation, neglectful, and inhumane. These negatively critical views about forgoing ANH can be held not only by patients and families, but also by health care professionals who, in turn, might appeal to their personal consciences or to professional integrity as reasons not to participate in decisions to withhold or discontinue ANH. Further, prominent court cases such as Elizabeth Bouvia, Claire Conroy, Paul Brophy, Nancy Cruzan [3], and Terri Schiavo [4] have focused legal and ethical discussion and debate on troubling ethical dilemmas related to providing ANH for patients with significant debilities (although not necessarily resulting from stroke).

In the developing world of clinical ethics, a major foundational principle, especially when focused on adults, is respect for patient autonomy or self-determination. This core component and principle is fundamental for multiple ethics-related "standards of care" such as the process of informed consent and refusal, the recognition and honoring of an extensive list of patients' rights [5], the assessment of a patient's decision-making capacity (DMC) when there are concerns about a patient's cognitive abilities, the partnership model for decision-making between clinician and patient, the expectation that clinicians provide "patient-centered care" [6] and the promotion of advance care planning [7] often memorialized by patients completing advance directives such as Living Wills and Health Care Powers of Attorney.

However, the many ethical issues that can arise regarding clinical nutrition and stroke patients cannot and should not be reduced to issues related only to patient autonomy. As will be noted and discussed below, other ethical principles and considerations [8] have significance when making decisions with or on behalf of stroke patients. For example, ethical analyses and ethically supportable decisions are also dependent on appeals to beneficence (i.e., promoting a patient's benefit, health, and well-being), nonmaleficence (i.e., the do-no-harm principle), justice or fairness (i.e., treating similar cases similarly), patient best interests (i.e., maximizing the benefits and minimizing the burdens, risks and harms of treatment), and professional integrity (i.e., fidelity to one's professional commitments, values, and principles). Nevertheless, because stroke can directly impact patients' abilities to exercise their autonomy temporarily or permanently secondary to a diminution of orientation, consciousness, and cognition, ethical considerations related to patient autonomy are appropriate starting points for discussing ethical issues in stroke patients.

The aim of this chapter is to provide an ethical framework and a foundation for making ethically supportable decisions related to stroke patients and the provision of nutrition and hydration, especially when medically supplied. Due to space limitations, this chapter does not address every clinical scenario that raises ethical issues related to nutrition and stroke patients.

Decision-Making Capacity

Decision-making capacity (DMC) refers to a set of cognitive skills that a patient possesses and demonstrates, and that are used when a patient makes a specific health care decision. For various reasons (e.g., stroke, sedating medications, dementia, mental retardation, debilitating depression, head trauma, extreme fatigue), patients can experience temporary or permanent loss or diminution of these cognitive abilities. When concerns or doubts arise about a patient's cognition, the primary physician or attending neurologist has the responsibility to assess the patient's DMC. Seeking the assistance and input of others (e.g., bedside nurses; a psychiatrist, psychologist, or clinical social worker; a patient's family members and friends) can be helpful and appropriate.

A patient with doubtful DMC should be assessed for specific cognitive skills or abilities [9]. Four cognitive skills to be assessed are: (1) expression of a choice, (2) understanding information relevant to the specific decision at hand, (3) appreciation of the medical situation and its consequences, and (4) reasoning with relevant information. A DMC assessment should be focused on the specific decision to be made, and should occur after a process of information-disclosure about the specific decision. In other words, the question is not whether the patient has general cognitive abilities to manage all spheres of her life, but to make a specific medical decision after having received relevant and understandable information about the proposed therapeutic or diagnostic intervention and its goals.

A DMC assessment is not dependent on whether the patient is able to vocalize or orally communicate. For example, a patient immediately after a stroke who is in an intensive care unit (ICU) and is intubated and supported by mechanical ventilation could still retain DMC despite aphasia. Such patients might be able to participate in DMC assessments via alternate means of communication such as sign language, hand signals, writing, lip reading, computer keyboard use, eye blinking, or head nodding and shaking. Speech-language pathologists may be helpful in facilitating communication with such nonverbal patients.

Related to the four cognitive skills listed above, the clinician performing a DMC assessment should structure a set of questions around each skill being assessed [9]. For example, for the ability to *express a choice*, the patient could be asked: "Have you decided whether to go along with your doctor's suggestions for treatment? Can you tell me what your decision is?" For the ability to *understand relevant information*, the patient could be instructed to: "Tell me in your own words what your doctor told you about the nature of your condition, the recommended treatment, the possible benefits, risks or discomforts, and the risks and benefits of alternative treatments or of no treatment at all." For the ability to *appreciate the situation and its consequences*, the patient could be instructed: "Tell me what you believe is wrong with your health now?" and then asked: "Do you believe that you need some kind of treatment? What is the treatment likely to do for you? What do you think will happen if you are not treated?" Finally, pertaining to the ability to *reason with relevant information*, the physician or other professional performing the assessment might inquire: "Tell me how you reached the decision to accept [or reject] the recommended treatment? What were the factors that were important to you in reaching the decision?"

Despite the significance that DMC holds for an effective and interactive shared decision-making process and for actualizing a patient's autonomy, "there are currently no formal guidelines from professional societies for the assessment of a patient's capacity to consent to treatment" [10]. However, a variety of standardized instruments for assessing DMC have gained recognition in practice and in the published literature. One such tool is the Mini Mental State Examination (MMSE) [11] which is heavily weighted toward orientation, attention, and memory. However, the MMSE is not a substitute for a formal assessment of DMC for a specific clinical decision, as described above. No components of the MMSE are flexible enough to allow for an assessment of a patient's understanding and appreciation of particular clinical circumstances and the specific decisions to be made. Further, the MMSE relies significantly on verbal responses, reading, and writing. For patients with hearing or visual impairments, with marginal English language skills, or who are intubated, MMSE scores may falsely indicate that a patient has significant cognitive impairments whereas in reality the patient may have adequate cognitive skills to make a specific decision. The MMSE's usefulness, then, is as an initial screening tool that may then lead to a more formal assessment of DMC for a specific decision which the patient is being asked to make.

A second useful DMC assessment tool is the Aid to Capacity Evaluation (ACE) that appropriately uses the patient's own medical situation and diagnosis or treatment decision as the basis for the assessment [12]. The instrument consists of eight questions that assess the patient's understanding of the clinical problem, the treatment proposed, treatment alternatives, the option to refuse treatment, possible consequences of the decision, and the effect of any underlying cognitive problems or disorders on the decision to be made. The ACE can be performed in less than 30 minutes, is available free online [13] and includes training or instruction materials.

Even after the best efforts by members of the health care team to assess DMC, a reliable determination may be unachievable. In such situations, the patient should still have the opportunity to participate in conversations and the decision-making process to the extent that the patient is able and willing. This approach is analogous to decision making for some older pediatric or adolescent patients who should be included in their own health care decisions to the extent that they are able to participate, with their assent and cooperation with the treatment plan being sought [14].

Standards for Decision Making

The gold standard for clinical decision making involves a patient who currently has DMC and is able to engage presently in the process of informed consent. Most adult patients in the outpatient setting, and many hospitalized patients, meet this gold standard. When a patient's DMC is judged to be insufficient (as could be the case for many stroke patients, at least initially and depending on the location and severity of the stroke), a silver standard for decision making should be invoked and used. The silver standard entails turning to and using proxy or surrogate decision makers, when available. The ethical and legal expectation of a surrogate decision maker is to provide a substituted judgment, i.e., voicing the values, preferences, and wishes of the patient, and based on those, making decisions that the patient would have made. In the words of Beauchamp and Childress:

> Accordingly, if the surrogate can reliably answer the question, "What would *the patient* want in this circumstance?" substituted judgment is an appropriate standard. But if the

surrogate can only answer the question, "What do *you* want for the patient?" then this standard is inappropriate [8].

Occasionally patients express specific and concrete wishes or preferences in advance or proactively to their physicians, other health care professionals, or to family members and friends. When this has occurred, and especially when a patient's wishes and statements have been documented in the patient's medical record, such indicators of a patient's advance directives (whether given orally or in writing) can extend patient autonomy into the time period when the patient lacks DMC. When previously expressed wishes of the patient exist and have been well-documented, the silver standard of substituted judgment is more confidently actualized.

When proxy or surrogate decision makers are unable to formulate a substituted judgment because of a lack of knowledge about the patient, a third or bronze standard for decision making should be used, i.e., the standard of best interest. Strictly speaking, this standard is neither connected to nor an extension of patient autonomy and preferences. Rather, the best interest standard attempts objectively to weigh the benefits and burdens of the proposed treatment or diagnostic procedure, with the goal of maximizing benefit and minimizing risks and harms. This standard for decision making is useful not only when an available proxy or surrogate lacks specific knowledge about patient preferences, but also when the health care team must make decisions for a patient because no surrogate has been found, designated, or identified.

In the abstract, there might appear to be a relatively bright line between the silver (substituted judgment) and bronze (best interest) standards. In many clinical situations, this is not the case. Sulmasy and Snyder have noted that this hierarchical model of separate standards does not always reflect clinical reality or the interests of patients and families [15]. They propose an integrated model for surrogate decision making that they call "substituted interests and best judgments." Their proposal aims to reframe the silver and bronze standards as shared decision making that incorporates the patient's authentic values, wishes, and preferences, with clinician and physician recommendations for what is medically judged to be best for the patient. Sulmasy and Snyder write: "Under substituted interests' model, the clinician draws on expertise and clinical experience to help the surrogate define the patient's individualized interests, as a particular person in particular clinical circumstances." In their view, this model reframes surrogate decision making in a way that promotes the uniqueness of the patient in the context of a patient's relationships, and applies the patient's authentic values, wishes, and interests as best as these can be known.

Decisions to Forgo Life-Sustaining Treatments

Severe strokes with significant residual debilities routinely raise questions for patients (or more commonly, for their surrogates) about the patient's current and future quality of life. In general, clinical ethics has been cautious about someone making quality of life judgments for another person (in essence, making a determination whether life is worth living under specific circumstances of disability). With such quality of life judgments, subjective factors, potential biases, and conflicts of interests can too easily become entangled in the decision process. Nevertheless, when patients can no longer perform many or most activities of daily living, especially those that give meaning and enjoyment to their lives, and those same patients have become dependent on life-sustaining treatment (e.g., mechanical ventilator, dialysis, ANH), patients, surrogates, and even health care professionals can appropriately raise questions about the goals of treatment and whether the goals will likely be achieved. In this context, specific questions that can arise include: When is it time to discontinue the mechanical ventilator? Should a Do-Not-Resuscitate (DNR) order be written? Can we stop ANH?

Finding answers to these questions is often challenging. In best case scenarios, forthcoming answers result from consideration of diagnoses, co-morbidities and clinical complications, prognosis, the patient's values and wishes, along with a weighing of the benefits and burdens of current and projected treatments and interventions (e.g., rehabilitation). When challenging questions are raised and difficult decisions must be made, serious consideration should be given to convening an interdisciplinary family/patient conference [16]. In addition to the patient, surrogates and family members, attendance by clinical services directly involved in a patient's care is essential (e.g., neurology, nutrition, nursing). Such family conferences are likely to be enhanced if they include representation from rehabilitative medicine, palliative care, social work, and chaplaincy. An interdisciplinary conference can help to clarify relevant clinical information, including uncertainties related to clinical information and prognoses; the values and preferences of the patient as well as pre-stroke and base-line activities of daily living; and medical recommendations and goals of care. When interdisciplinary family conferences are conducted in a respectful and compassionate manner, with the health care professionals listening and not only speaking and disclosing clinical information, patients' and/or surrogates' trust of professionals can be enhanced. Ideally, an interdisciplinary conference can arrive at a consensus regarding a patient management plan that is consistent with evidence-based medical practice, clinical recommendations, and patient values and preferences.

Due to uncertainties about recoverability after stroke, especially during the immediate and acute phase, a time-limited trial (TLT) of life-sustaining treatment is often ethically justifiable. Quill and Holloway have written:

> A TLT is an agreement between clinicians and a patient/family to use certain medical therapies over a defined period to see if the patient improves or deteriorates according to agreed-on clinical outcomes. If the patient improves, disease directed therapy continues. If the patient deteriorates, the therapies involved in the trial are withdrawn, and goals frequently shift more purely to palliation. If significant clinical uncertainty remains, another TLT might be renegotiated [17].

A TLT may provide an opportunity for a stroke patient to recover sufficient DMC to make her own decisions if the silver (substituted judgment), bronze (best interest), or integrated (substituted interest or best judgment) standards have been used.

A TLT of ANH after stroke may provide an opportunity for a patient to recover from aphagia or dysphagia and regain an ability to swallow; or it could "buy some time" to see if the patient will recover sufficient cognitive and motor function to have a projected quality of life acceptable to the patient.

Limited time trials are an acceptable alternative when benefits of ANH are questionable and the trial nature of ANH is communicated and consented to by the patient and family prior to its initiation [18].

A TLT of mechanical ventilation after severe stroke could help determine whether the patient will regain brainstem responses. Most importantly, a TLT can create a middle ground between prematurely forgoing treatments that might help, and the risk of unwanted and indefinite exposure to burdensome treatment.

Discussing a stroke patient's desires regarding cardiopulmonary resuscitation (CPR) in the event of a cardiac or respiratory arrest can and should be a part of goal-setting conversations. Since the 1980s, discussions with patients about resuscitation status have become more commonplace. Most, if not all, hospitals have policies addressing CPR and "code status." Although most hospitals have chosen to designate decisions and corresponding medical orders to not provide CPR as DNR orders, there is not a uniform designation for such orders. For example, some hospitals and health care facilities have chosen instead to designate such orders as Do-Not-Attempt Resuscitation (DNAR) orders or Allow Natural Death (AND) orders [19]. When patients are in transit from one care setting to another (e.g., via ground or air ambulance) or are able to be cared for in a private home, many states have passed legislation allowing emergency medical personnel to honor out-of-hospital or portable DNR orders [20]. A growing number of states are now using the Physician or Medical Orders for Life-Sustaining Treatment (POLST or MOLST) paradigm to provide clear medical orders that are portable outside of the hospital setting [21].

Addressing resuscitation status in a proactive, timely way is crucial for many stroke patients, especially for those who have significant disabilities that are likely irreversible, or who have co-morbidities or major organ failures. Within a context of "hoping for the best, preparing for the worst" [22], clinicians should first help patients or their surrogates understand the realities of CPR and the resuscitative modalities that are entailed (i.e., chest compressions, electric shock, intubation, pharmacological agents). Further, clinicians should include in such conversations empirical data that demonstrate the relatively low rates of survival-to-discharge for all inpatient CPR attempts (approximately 16%) [23]. In general, the more preexisting and significant comorbidities patients have (including acute stroke, preexisting malignancy, and pre-arrest use of vasopressors or mechanical ventilation), the less likely they are to survive attempted CPR. Patients and their surrogates should also be informed that a DNR order does not mean that a patient will be abandoned by the physician or health care team (i.e., a DNR order is not equivalent to a Do-Not-Treat order), and that a DNR order can be compatible with continuing other aggressive treatments.

Discussions about CPR with patients or their surrogates can be excellent opportunities to review and revise explicitly the goals of treatment. Initially treatment goals may realistically include recovery of many physical and cognitive functions after stroke. Over time, depending on whether a patient responds to rehabilitation and the tincture of time, the goals may need to incorporate palliation or eventually shift to comfort care only. In addition to addressing and helping with symptom management, palliative care professionals can assist with other unmet patient needs such as independence and functional abilities, advance care planning, psychosocial distress, spiritual and existential issues, caregiver and family support, and prognostic understanding [24].

Although not always persuasive for patients, surrogates, and health care professionals who are reluctant or opposed to forgoing ANH, position statements by health care organizations have generally concluded that ANH is medical treatment that should be subject to the same principles of decision making as other treatments, and that patients or their surrogates are in the best position to weigh the harms and benefits of nutrition and hydration [25–28]. Health care institutions should have clear institutional policies about ANH so that personnel as well as patients and surrogates can know an institution's stance regarding ANH. Institutions and organizations should also have procedures that address "conscientious objection" for individual clinicians, and that support patient transfer if a patient's wishes or a surrogate's decision about ANH cannot be honored by particular clinicians or by the institution [29].

Forgoing ANH should not be cause for a patient to experience pain or discomfort. Consultation with professionals knowledgeable and expert regarding palliative care and symptom management should accompany decisions to forgo ANH. A commitment to patient comfort should be assured and communicated to patients and surrogates.

Conclusion: Ethics Consultation

Most hospitals in the United States have ethics committees [30] whose primary functions are to provide clinical ethics education, revise and recommend ethics-related policies, and facilitate ethics consultations for individual cases. Ethics consultation has been defined as: a set of services provided by an individual or group in response to questions from patients, families, surrogates, healthcare professionals, or other involved parties who seek to resolve uncertainty or conflict regarding value-laden concerns that emerge in health care [31].

Ethics consultation services (ECSs) usually have a policy or practice of open access, that is, anyone with a legitimate interest in a case can request assistance from the ECS. Assistance from an ECS is often sought when stakeholders in a case have exhausted their own resources and skills to resolve an ethics issue or dilemma, or when a case is especially complex, is not clearly or adequately addressed by hospital policy, or has institutional or organizational implications. The goals of ethics consultation are to: (1) promote an ethical resolution of the case at hand; (2) establish comfortable and respectful communication among the parties involved; (3) help those involved learn to work through ethical uncertainties and disagreements on their own; and (4) help the ethics committee recognize patterns within the organization and consider reviewing procedures or policies [32]. An active ECS can be a valuable resource for providing guidance and identifying ethically supportable options for stroke patients when ethical concerns and dilemmas arise.

Interpersonal skills and character traits that health care professionals may already possess can aid in the effective resolution of ethical challenges and dilemmas: attentive listening and communication; negotiation, mediation and conflict resolution; tolerance for ambiguity; cultural competence; awareness of one's own beliefs, values and biases; compassion, honesty, and humility; and practical wisdom acquired by reflection on past experience. Knowledge of core ethical principles and concepts as discussed in this chapter will also contribute to appropriately addressing ethical conflicts.

To assist stakeholders in a case to think ethically about the situation, arrive at an ethically supportable consensus, and use a somewhat standardized process from case to case, various frameworks and multi-step procedures have been proposed. Monod et al. [33] have proposed an eight-step process and guide for achieving these multiple aims:

1. Identify clinically relevant facts and clarify the ethical question(s).
2. Identify the patient's psychosocial–familial context and all stakeholders in the case.
3. Identify the care responsibilities of each stakeholder.
4. Identify the values considered by each stakeholder as essential to address the ethical question.
5. Analyze the ethical conflicts at stake in the clinical situation.
6. Identify all possible options to resolve the ethical conflicts.
7. Identify the option that best integrates the values of the patient and other stakeholders.
8. Discuss the moral and ethical justifications for the decision.

This process will not necessarily and always lead to consensus and agreement among stakeholders in a specific case, or arrive at a single best option for action. However, this process, coupled with a use of the ethics resources already noted (i.e., principles, concepts, skills, character traits), can increase the likelihood that a good and ethically supportable outcome can be achieved when difficult issues, conflicts, and dilemmas arise in the care of stroke patients.

References

1. Brody H, Hermer LD, Scott LD, Grumbles LL, Kutac JE, McCammon SD. Artificial nutrition and hydration: the evolution of ethics, evidence, and policy. J Gen Intern Med. 2011;26: 1053–8.
2. Slomka J. What do apple pie and motherhood have to do with feeding tubes and caring for the patient? Arch Intern Med. 1995;155:1258–63.

3. Poland SC. Landmark legal cases in bioethics. Kennedy Inst Ethics J. 1997;7:191–209.
4. Caplan AL, McCartney JJ, Sisti DA, editors. The case of Terri Schiavo: ethics at the end of life. Amherst, NY: Prometheus Books; 2006.
5. Smith ML, Eves M. Patient rights. In: Kattan M, editor. Encyclopedia of medical decision making. Thousand Oaks, CA: Sage Publications; 2009. p. 862–6.
6. Barry MJ, Edgman-Levitan S. Shared decision making—the pinnacle of patient-centered care. N Eng J Med. 2012;366:780–1.
7. Emanuel LL, Danis M, Pearlman RA, Singer PA. Advance care planning as a process: structuring the discussions in practice. J Am Geriatr Soc. 1995;43:440–6.
8. Beauchamp TL, Childress JF. Principles of biomedical ethics. 6th ed. New York: Oxford University Press; 2009.
9. Grisso T, Appelbaum PS. Assessing competence to consent to treatment, a guide for physicians and other health professionals. New York: Oxford University Press; 1998.
10. Appelbaum PS. Assessment of patients' competence to consent to treatment. N Engl J Med. 2007;357:1834–8.
11. Tombaugh TN, McIntyre NJ. The mini-mental state examination: a comprehensive review. J Am Geriatr Soc. 1992;40:922–35.
12. Sessums LL, Zembrzuska H, Jackson JL. Does this patient have medical decision-making capacity? JAMA. 2011;306:420–7.
13. Joint Centre for Bioethics, University of Toronto. Community tools: aid to capacity evaluation (Ace); 2008. http://www.jointcentreforbioethics.ca/tools/ace_download.shtml. Accessed 9 Jul 2012.
14. Committee on Bioethics. Informed consent, parental permission, and assent in pediatric practice. Pediatrics. 1995;95:314–7.
15. Sulmasy DP, Snyder L. Substituted interests and best judgments, an integrated model for surrogate decision making. JAMA. 2010;304:1946–7.
16. Curtis JR, Patrick DL, Shannon SE, Treece PD, Engelberg RA, Rubenfeld GD. The family conference as a focus to improve communication about end-of-life care in the intensive care unit: opportunities for improvement. Crit Care Med. 2001;29(Suppl):N26–33.
17. Quill TE, Holloway R. Time-limited trials near the end of life. JAMA. 2011;306:1483–4.
18. American Society for Parenteral & Enteral Nutrition (ASPEN). A.S.P.E.N. ethics position paper. Nutr Clin Pract. 2010;25:672–9.
19. Venneman SS, Narnor-Harris P, Perish M, Hamilton M. "Allow natural death" versus "do not resuscitate": Three words that can change a life. J Med Ethics. 2008;34:2–6.
20. Sabatino CP. Survey of state EMS-DNR laws and protocols. J Law Med Ethics. 1999;27:297–315.
21. Sabatino CP, Karp N. Improving advanced illness care: the evolution of state POLST programs. AARP Public Policy Institute; April 2011. http://www.aarp.org/ppi.
22. Back AL, Arnold RM, Quill TE. Hope for the best and prepare for the worst. Ann Intern Med. 2003;138:439–43.
23. Larkin GL, Copes WS, Nathanson BH, Kaye W. Pre-resuscitation factors associated with mortality in 49,130 cases of in-hospital cardiac arrest: a report from the National Registry for Cardiopulmonary Resuscitation. Resuscitation. 2010;81:302–11.
24. Swetz KM, Kamal AH. Palliative care. Ann Intern Med. 2012;ITC2:1–16.
25. American Medical Association (AMA). Withholding or withdrawing life-sustaining medical treatment (Policy E-2.20); 1996. www.ama-assn.org&uri=%2fresources%2fdoc%2fPolicyFinder%2fpolicyfiles%2fHnE%2fE-2.20.HTM. Accessed 18 Mar 2012.
26. American Dietetic Association (ADA). Position of the ADA: ethical and legal issues in nutrition, hydration, and feeding. J Am Diet Assoc. 2008;108(5):873–82.
27. American Nurses Association (ANA). Position statement: forgoing nutrition and hydration; 2011. www.nursingworld.org/positionstatements. Accessed 18 Mar 2012.
28. American College of Physicians (ACP). Ethics manual, 6th ed. Ann Intern Med. 2012;156:73–104.

29. Casarett D, Kapo J, Caplan A. Appropriate use of artificial nutrition and hydration—fundamental principles and recommendations. N Eng J Med. 2005;353:2607–12.
30. McGee G, Spanogle JP, Caplan AL, Asch DA. A national study of ethics committees. Am J Bioeth. 2001;1:60–4.
31. American Society for Bioethics and Humanities (ASBH). Core competencies for healthcare ethics consultation. 2nd ed. Glenview: American Society for Bioethics and Humanities; 2011.
32. Andre J. Goals of ethics consultation: toward clarity, utility and fidelity. J Clin Ethics. 1997; 8:193–8.
33. Monod S, Chiolero R, Bula C, Benaroyo L. Ethical issues in nutrition support of severely disabled elderly persons: a guide for health professionals. J Parenter Enteral Nutr. 2011;35: 295–302.

Chapter 19
Suggested Stroke Related Resources for the Practitioner and Patient

Arlene A. Escuro and Mandy L. Corrigan

Key Points

- There are a vast number of resources available for practitioners and patients on topics related to stroke.
- Medications such as propofol and phenytoin can affect the delivery of nutrients among critically ill stroke patients.
- Enteral nutrition is the mainstay of nutrition treatment for stroke patients and use of parenteral nutrition is rare. Calculations for both types of nutrition support are provided as a reference for the practitioner.

Keywords Dysphagia diet • Thickening agent • Propofol • Phenytoin • Enteral nutrition • Parenteral nutrition

Abbreviations

ASPEN   American Society For Parenteral And Enteral Nutrition
EN   Enteral Nutrition
LCT   Long Chain Triglycerides
mEq   Mili Equivalents

A.A. Escuro (✉)
Nutrition Therapy, Cleveland Clinic, 9500 Euclid Avenue/M17, Cleveland, OH 44195, USA
e-mail: escuroa@ccf.org

M.L. Corrigan
Nutrition Support Team, Center for Human Nutrition, Cleveland Clinic,
9500 Euclid Avenue/TT2, Cleveland, OH 44195, USA
e-mail: mandycorrigan1@gmail.com

M.L. Corrigan et al. (eds.), *Handbook of Clinical Nutrition and Stroke*,
Nutrition and Health, DOI 10.1007/978-1-62703-380-0_19,
© Springer Science+Business Media New York 2013

NDD   National Dysphagia Diet
PPN   Peripheral Parenteral Nutrition
PN   Parenteral Nutrition

Introduction

This chapter provides many up-to-date resources for individuals involved in the care of stroke patients. The first part covers information and websites of professional organizations. Clinicians are provided with guidelines on modifying enteral nutrition support for stroke patients on medications such as propofol and phenytoin. A comprehensive tutorial in calculating parenteral nutrition (PN) is included. The second part outlines resources for patients and their families on organizations involved in the care of stroke patients. A sample menu of National Dysphagia Diet (NDD) and a list of commercially available thickening agents is provided for patients with dysphagia.

Part 1: Resources for Practitioners

A. *Organizations and Professional Societies*

National Stroke Association
www.stroke.org

American Stroke Association
www.strokeassociation.org

Brain Aneurysm Foundation
www.bafound.org

Brain Attack Coalition
www.stroke-site.org

Hazel K. Goddess Fund for Stroke Research in Women
www.thegoddessfund.org

Childrens Hemiplegia and Stroke Association (CHASA)
www.chasa.org

Professional Societies

Academy of Nutrition and Dietetics
www.eatright.org

American Academy of Neurology
www.aan.com

American Association of Neuroscience Nurses
www.aann.org

American Association of Neurological Surgeons
www.aans.org

American Neurological Association
www.aneuroa.org

American Occupational Therapy Association
www.aota.org

American Occupational Therapy Foundation
www.aotf.org

American Speech-Language-Hearing Association (ASHA)
www.asha.org

Association of Rehabilitation Nurses
www.rehabnurse.org

European Federation of Neurological Societies
www.efns.org

International Stroke Society
www.world-stroke.org

National Aphasia Association
www.aphasia.org

Northern Ireland Multidisciplinary Association for Stroke Teams
www.nimast.org.uk

B. Sample Calculation for Modifying Nutrition Support with Propofol Administration

Propofol is a short acting anesthetic and sedative commonly used in neurocritical patients because it is easily titrated to desirable clinical effects, and its actions are rapidly terminated with drug discontinuation [1]. The oil source of propofol is soybean, composed of long-chain triglycerides (LCTs) and omega-6 fatty acid. This 10 % lipid vehicle provides 1.1 kcal/mL (0.1 mg/mL) calories in the form of fat, primarily linoleic acid. The extra calories provided are taken into consideration during assessment of a nutrition support regimen.

NOTE: Propofol = 1.1 kcal/mL (0.1 g/mL) fat, 10 mg = 1 mL, 1 mg = 1,000 mcg
If the propofol order is 25 mcg/kg/min, how much fat kcal will a 70-kg patient receive?

1. 25 mcg × 70 kg = 1,750 mcg
2. 1,750 mcg × 60 min/h = 105,000 mcg/h
3. 105,000 mcg/h ÷ 1,000 mcg/mg = 105 mg/h
4. 105 mg/h ÷ 10 mg/mL = 10.5 mL/h
5. 10.5 mL/h × 24 h/day = 252 mL/day
6. 252 mL/day × 1.1 fat kcal/mL = 277 fat kcal/day

C. Sample Calculation for Modifying Enteral Nutrition (EN) Formulation with Oral/Enteral Phenytoin Administration

Phenytoin is an anticonvulsant often used for the prevention and treatment of post-traumatic seizures. Holding EN for 1 h before and after each dose of the acid suspension appears to be feasible and effective option for circumventing the impaired absorption of phenytoin with patients on enteral feeding [2].

A patient is receiving a 1.5 kcal/mL EN formula infusing at goal rate of 50 mL/h and started on phenytoin twice daily via feeding tube. Hold EN infusion for 4 h total per day (1 h before and 1 h after each phenytoin dose).

1. 1.5 kcal/mL EN solution × 50 mL/h × 24 h/day = 1,800 kcal/day
2. 1,800 kcal/day ÷ 20 h- infusion using a 1.5 kcal/mL EN solution = Increase TF rate to 60 mL/h × 20 h

D. Calculating Peripheral Parenteral Nutrition

Peripheral Parenteral Nutrition (PPN) can be infused thru a peripheral vein while keeping the osmolarity of the solution less than 900 mOsm/L.

Step 1: Determine the patient's fluid requirements.

A non-fluid restricted, euvolemic patient usually requires 2,000–2,400 mL of fluid daily (a general rule of thumb is 1,000–1,500 mL for urine, 500 mL for insensible losses). When using PPN, the patient's nutritional needs are likely to not be fully met. If the patient can tolerate increased amount of fluid (provided the patient will be closely monitored), the clinician can consider giving a large volume of fluid (not to exceed 3,000 mL) to therefore provide larger quantities of the macronutrients to better meet the patient's nutritional requirements. PPN shouldn't be used in fluid restricted patients.

In the following example, we will use 2,400 mL of fluid.

Sample patient data: 70 kg, 69″, BMI 23, 55-year-old male

Estimated Needs:

1,600–2,100 cal
105–140 g protein
2,400 mL fluid

Step 2: Determine the amount of calories, protein, dextrose, and fat
A general rule of thumb for calculating PPN:

~700 cal/L	4 cal/g of protein
~30–35 g protein/L	3.4 cal/g of dextrose
	10 cal/g of fat

(a) Determine the amount of protein that will fit in the volume of fluid:
2.4 L×30 g protein/L=72 g of protein

72 g of protein×4 kcal/g of protein=288 protein kcal

(b) Determine the total amount of calories that will fit in the volume of fluid:

2.4 L×700 cal/L=1,680 cal

(c) Subtract the protein calories from the total amount of calories

1,680 total calories—288 protein calories=1,392 nonprotein calories

(d) Determine the amount of dextrose and fat calories
    A general rule of thumb is that 40 % of the nonprotein calories will come from dextrose and 60 % of the nonprotein calories will come from fat. The distribution is higher in fat since fat contributes the least amount to the osmolarity of the solution. Using a higher amount of fat also helps provide the patient with more calories (fat is the most calorically dense macronutrient source). Since PPN is only used for a maximum of 1–2 weeks, more fat is commonly provided (above the 1 g/kg as recommended by A.S.P.E.N.) to provide the patient with calories. The commercially available intravenous fat emulsions come in either a 20 or 30 % concentration.

1,392 nonprotein calories×40 %=556 cal as dextrose
1,392 nonprotein calories×60 %=835 cal as fat

Convert the dextrose calories to grams:
        556 dextrose calories/3.4 cal per gram=164 g dextrose

Convert the fat calories to grams:
        835 fat calories/10 cal/g=~83 g fat

(e) Final macronutrient prescription:

72 g of protein
164 g of dextrose
83 g of fat
in 2.4 L of Fluid

Note: the format for ordering of PPN solutions varies by institution—check with your pharmacy for specific order forms and format. Some institutions order PPN by grams, calories, or as percentages of the volume.

(f) Determine the patient's electrolyte additives based on laboratory studies and add mEq of the following electrolytes:

Calcium gluconate
Magnesium sulfate
Sodium or potassium phosphates
Potassium chloride or acetate
Sodium chloride or acetate

Step 3: Determine the osmolarity of the PPN solution

Use this simple formula to calculate osmolarity and ensure it is 900 mOsm or less.

(a) Estimation of Osmolarity

10 mOsm × 72 g of protein ÷ PN volume in L = 720/2.4 L = 300 mOsm
5 mOsm × 164 g of dextrose ÷ PN volume in L = 164/2.4 L = 341 mOsm
0.67 × 83 g lipid ÷ PN volume in L = 55.6/2.4 L = *23 mOsm*
Approximate Osmolarity from Macronutrients: 664 mOsm

(b) Determine the amount of mOsm contributed by electrolytes
(Electrolytes in mEq)
Example:

10 mEq Calcium gluconate
8 mEq Magnesium sulfate
60 mEq Potassium Acetate
100 mEq Sodium Chloride
in 2.4 L of fluid

Add total the amount of mEq provided by Calcium, Magnesium, Potassium and Sodium then multiply by 2 and divide by the total volume of PN in liters.

2 × (mEq of electrolytes) ÷ PN volume in L
2 × (178 mEq. ÷ 2.4 L = 148 mOsm from electrolytes

(c) Determine the total osmolarity (macronutrients + electrolytes) and ensure it is below the 900 mOsm limit

300 mOsm from protein
341 mOsm from dextrose
23 mOsm from fat
148 mOsm from electrolytes
Total Osmolarity of the PPN solution = 812 mOsm

Step 4: Determine compatibility of the PPN solution

Since all the macronutrients are in one PN solution (fat, dextrose, and protein) this is commonly referred to as a 3-in-1 solution. When using a 3-in-1 solution,

Table 19.1
Compatibility chart for 3-in-1 PN solutions used by Cleveland clinic
nutrition support team

Additive	Acceptable stability range
Protein	20–60 g/L
Dextrose	40–250 g/L
Lipid	20–60 g/L
Divalent Cations (mEq Magnesium + mEq Calcium)	≤20 mEq/L
Calcium Phosphorus Product (Calcium mEq/L) × (Phosphorus mEq/L)	<200

compatibility becomes an issue since the intravenous fat solutions are sensitive and easily can crack or destabilize rendering the solution unsafe for delivery. Using Table 19.1 below, ensure the PPN solution meets the pharmacy compounding guidelines for stability. Compounding guidelines for compatibility vary by institution and clinicians should seek this information from their institution's pharmacy department.

Example PPN solution (from earlier)

72 g of protein
164 g of dextrose
83 g of fat
10 mEq Calcium gluconate
8 mEq Magnesium sulfate
60 mEq Potassium Acetate
100 mEq Sodium Chloride
2.4 L of fluid

(a) Determine macronutrient stability (see Table 19.1)

Grams of protein ÷ PN volume in L (acceptable range 20–60 g/L)
Grams of dextrose ÷ PN volume in L (acceptable range 40–250 g/L)
Grams of fat ÷ PN volume in L (acceptable range 20–60 g/L)
72 g of protein ÷ 2.4 L = 30 g/L = within acceptable range
164 g of dextrose ÷ 2.4 L = 68 g/L = within acceptable range
83 g of fat ÷ 2.4 L = 34 g/L = within acceptable range

(b) Determine divalent cation stability

mEq of Magnesium + mEq of Calcium must be ≤ 20 mEq/L
With our example from above:
8 mEq of Magnesium sulfate + 10 mEq of Calcium Gluconate = 18 mEq
Total mEq ÷ PN volume in L = 18 mEq ÷ 2.4 L = *7.5 mEq/l*
     = acceptable (range ≤ 20 mEq/L)

(c) Determine the calcium phosphorus product

Example:
10 mEq Calcium gluconate
30 mEq of Sodium phosphate
$= (10 \text{ mEq Calcium} \div 2.4 \text{ L}) \times (30 \text{ mEq Phosphorus} \div 2.4 \text{ L})$
$= \mathbf{53}$
$=$ acceptable (range <200/L)

E. Calculating Parenteral Nutrition (3-in-1 PN)

Requires central Vascular Access Device
Step 1: Determine the patient's fluid requirements.

Sample patient data: 70 kg, 69″, BMI 23, 55-year-old male

Estimated Needs:

> 1,600–2,100 cal
> 105–140 g protein
> 2,400 mL fluid

A non-fluid restricted, euvolemic patient usually requires 2,000–2,400 mL of fluid daily (a general rule of thumb is 1,000–1,500 mL for urine, 500 mL for insensible losses). PN can be concentrated if the patient is fluid restricted.
In the following example, we will use 2,400 mL of fluid.

Step 2: Determine the amount of calories, protein, dextrose, and fat

Sample patient data: 70 kg, 69″, BMI 23, 55-year-old male

Estimated Needs:

> 1,600–2,100 cal
> 1,600–2,100 cal
> 105–140 g protein
> 2,400 mL fluid

On the first day PN is initiated, provide only part of the total nutritional needs to avoid refeeding syndrome (in malnourished patients) and glucose abnormalities. A general rule of thumb is to provide half the patients calories on the first day initiating PN and provide the full amount of protein. Gradually increasing from half to full calories can be done over 1–3 days by increasing the dextrose load by ~150–200 g/day pending the laboratory studies (especially electrolytes and blood sugars) and patient status. The example on calculating 3-in-1 PN solutions will be the solution that provides goal calories.

(a) Provide the patients full protein needs.

> 140 g protein = goal
> 140 g of protein × 4 cal/g = 560 protein calories

(b) Subtract the protein calories from the total amount of calories

2,100 total calories—560 protein calories = 1,540 nonprotein calories

(c) Determine the amount of dextrose and fat calories

A general rule of thumb is that 60 % of the nonprotein calories will come from dextrose and 40 % of the nonprotein calories will come from fat when there is a central line available to utilize a 3-in-1 PN solution. Since the patient has a central line, there is no need to restrict the osmolarity of the solution, and more dextrose can be provided and fat limited. The American Society for Parenteral and Enteral Nutrition (A.S.P.E.N), fat should be limited to no more than 1 g of fat per kilogram.

1,540 nonprotein calories × 60 % = 924 cal as dextrose
1,540 nonprotein calories × 40 % = 616 cal as fat
Convert the dextrose calories to grams:
924 dextrose calories/3.4 cal/g = 271 g dextrose
Convert the fat calories to grams:
616 fat calories/10 cal/g = ~62 g fat

(d) Final macronutrient prescription (at goal calories):

140 g of protein
271 g of dextrose
62 g of fat

in 2.4 L of Fluid

Step 3: Determine compatibility of the 3-in-1 PN solution

Since all the macronutrients are in one PN solution (fat, dextrose, and protein) this is commonly referred to as a 3-in-1 solution. When using a 3-in-1 solution, compatibility becomes an issue since the intravenous fat solutions are sensitive and easily can crack or destabilize rendering the solution unsafe for delivery. Using Table 19.1 below, ensure the 3-in-1 PN solution meets the pharmacy compounding guidelines for stability. Compounding guidelines for compatibility vary by institution and clinicians should seek this information from their institution's pharmacy department.

Example 3-in-1 PN solution (from earlier)

140 g of protein
271 g of dextrose
62 g of fat

in 2.4 L of Fluid

(a) Determine macronutrient stability (see Table 19.1)

Grams of protein ÷ PN volume in L (acceptable range 20–60 g/L)
Grams of dextrose ÷ PN volume in L (acceptable range 40–250 g/L)
Grams of fat ÷ PN volume in L (acceptable range 20–60 g/L)
140 g of protein ÷ 2.4 L = 58 g/L = within acceptable range
271 g of dextrose ÷ 2.4 L = 112 g/L = within acceptable range
62 g of fat ÷ 2.4 L = 26 g/L = within acceptable range

(b) Also check divalent cations and calcium phosphorus product.
   See example under section B (calculating PPN) & follow same steps

F. Calculating Parenteral Nutrition (2-in-1 PN)

Requires Central Vascular Access Device
Step 1: Determine the patient's fluid requirements.

Sample patient data: 70 kg, 69″, BMI 23, 55-year-old male

Estimated Needs:

   1,600–2,100 cal
   1,600–2,100 cal
   105–140 g protein
   2,400 mL fluid

A non-fluid restricted, euvolemic patient usually requires 2,000–2,400 mL of fluid daily (a general rule of thumb is 1,000–1,500 mL for urine, 500 mL for insensible losses). PN can be concentrated if the patient is fluid restricted.
   In the following example, we will use 2,400 mL of fluid.

Step 2: Determine the amount of calories, protein, dextrose, and fat

Sample patient data: 70 kg, 69″, BMI 23, 55-year-old male

Estimated Needs:
1,600–2,100 cal
105–140 g protein
2,400 mL fluid

On the first day PN is initiated only providing part of the nutritional needs is wise to avoid refeeding syndrome (in malnourished patients) and glucose abnormalities. A general rule of thumb is to provide half the patients calories on the first day initiating PN and provide the full amount of protein. Gradually increasing from half to full calories can be done over 1–3 days by increasing the dextrose load by ~150–200 g/day pending the laboratory studies (especially electrolytes and blood sugars) and patient status. The example on calculating 2-in-1 PN solutions will be the solution that provides goal calories.

(a) Provide the patients full protein needs.

   140 g protein=goal
   140 g of protein×4 cal/g=560 protein calories

(b) Subtract the protein calories from the total amount of calories

   2,100 total calories − 560 protein calories = 1,540 nonprotein calories

Table 19.2
Examples of PN solutions for a 70 kg, 69″, BMI 23, 55-year-old male

	Peripheral PN	2-in-1 Central PN	3-in-1 Central PN
Volume	2.4 L	2.4 L	2.4 L
Amino acids	72 g	140 g	140 g
Dextrose	164 g	390 g	271 g
Lipid	83 g	0	62 g
IV Piggyback Lipid, 20 % Lipid	0	250 mL, three times weekly	0
Total Calories/kilogram	24 kcal/kg	30 kcal/kg/day	30 kcal/kg/day
Macronutrient Distribution	17 % Calories as Protein	27 % Calories as Protein	27 % Calories as Protein
	33 % Calories as Dextrose	63 % Calories as Dextrose	44 % Calories as Dextrose
	50 % Calories as Lipid	10 % Calories as Lipid[a]	29 % Calories as Lipid
Approximate Osmolarity (excluding electrolytes)	812	1,395	1,164

Estimated Needs:
2,100 cal/day
105–140 g protein/day
[a]Given as IV Piggyback, 250 mL, three times weekly

(c) Determine the amount of dextrose and fat calories

Since the patient has a central line, there is no need to restrict the osmolarity of the solution.

Note: Since a 2-in-1 PN solution is being utilized, the only two components in the PN bag are dextrose and protein. Intravenous fat solutions are then "piggybacked" or delivered from a separate bag.

For this example: 250 mL of 20 % Lipid emulsion will be given three times weekly (Equivalent to 1,500 fat calories per week, or an average of 214 fat calories daily)

Subtract the calories provided from fat out of the nonprotein calories and this will be the goal dextrose load.

1,540 nonprotein calories – 214 cal from fat = 1,326 dextrose calories

Convert dextrose calories to grams of dextrose:
1,326 dextrose calories ÷ 3.4 cal/g = 390 g dextrose

(d) Final macronutrient prescription (at goal calories)

140 g of protein
390 g of dextrose
in 2.4 L of Fluid

with 250 mL of 20 % Intravenous fat emulsion three times weekly piggybacked

Step 3: Calculate the calcium phosphorus product

Calculate the calcium phosphorus product (see equation in Table 19.1)

2-in-1 PN solutions do not require calculations for stability or have limits on the divalent cations delivered since there is no lipid added to the solution.

See Table 19.2 for a comparison of the different PN solutions given in the examples above.

Part 2. Resources for Patients and Families

A. *Organizations*

NINDS Information—NINDS Disorders Index: Stroke http://www.aan.com/apps/disorders/index.cfm?event=database:disorder.view&disorder_id=1072http://www.ninds.nih.gov/disorders/stroke/stroke_needtoknow.htm

Medline Plus
http://www.nlm.nih.gov/medlineplus/stroke.html

Medscape
www.medscape.com/resource/stroke

Professional and Patient/Family Publication

American Academy of Neurology—Neurology Now
http://journals.lww.com/neurologynow/pages/default.aspx

Research and Clinical Trials

NINDS—Stroke Clinical Trials
http://www.ninds.nih.gov/disorders/clinical_trials/index_all.htm#Stroke

Research Center for Stroke and Heart Disease—Jacobs Neurological Institute
www.strokeheart.org/

NINDS—Patient Recruitment for Clinical Trials
http://patientinfo.ninds.nih.gov/Disorders.aspx?did=139

Locating a Primary Stroke Center

Joint Commission
http://www.jointcommission.org/certification/primary_stroke_centers.aspx

B. National Dysphagia Diet Sample Menu [3]

Level 1 (Dysphagia Pureed)

Meal	Menu
Breakfast	½ cup fruit juice without pulp*
	½ cup thinned oatmeal with no lumps or ½ cup Cream of Wheat®
	1 pureed bread or pancakes with butter or margarine
	1 pureed scrambled egg
	1 cup coffee, tea, or milk*
Lunch	½ cup strained creamed soup; no lumps or grainy texture
	½ cup pureed chicken with gravy
	½ cup mashed potatoes with gravy
	½ cup pureed carrots
	½ cup pureed applesauce
	6 ounces plain or flavored smooth yogurt without fruit pieces
	1 cup beverage*
Evening Meal	½ cup pureed tomato soup made with milk
	½ cup pureed beef with gravy
	½ cup pureed green beans
	½ cup pureed pasta or noodles
	½ cup vanilla pudding
	½ cup pureed peaches
	1 cup beverage*

*Prepared to the prescribed liquid consistency

Level 2 (Dysphagia Mechanically Altered)

Meal	Menu
Breakfast	½ cup fruit juice*
	½ cup oatmeal with no lumps or ½ cup dry cereals with little texture such as corn flakes, Rice Krispies®
	1 soft scrambled egg with melted cheese
	Pancakes moistened with syrup or muffin with butter or margarine
	1 cup coffee, tea, or milk*
Lunch	½ cup tomato soup
	½ cup soft macaroni and cheese
	3 ounces moist meatloaf
	½ cup well-cooked green beans
	½ cup diced peaches
	½ cup custard
	1 cup beverage*
Evening Meal	½ cup potato soup
	1 cup moist tuna noodle casserole
	½ cup well-cooked carrots
	½ cup canned fruit
	½ cup ice cream
	1 cup beverage*

*Prepared to the prescribed liquid consistency

Level 3 (Dysphagia Advanced)

Meal	Menu
Breakfast	½ cup fruit juice* ½ cup dry cereal with milk or ½ cup oatmeal 1 scrambled egg with melted cheese on toast with soft crust 1 cup coffee, tea, or milk*
Lunch	lasagna with finely minced onions and ground meats or ravioli with smooth marinara sauce 1 slice soft bread with butter or margarine ½ cup well-cooked carrots 1 small banana ½ cup pudding 1 cup beverage*
Evening Meal	½ cup soup without tough meats or large chunks 3 ounces moist meatloaf or 3 ounces moist chicken ½ cup mashed potatoes with gravy or ½ cup soft-cooked rice ½ cup well-cooked broccoli 1 slice pie with pudding-like filling such as pumpkin, lemon, or chocolate 1 cup beverage*

*Prepared to the prescribed liquid consistency

C. Liquid Thickening Agents

Note: Many drug store pharmacies and medical supply store can order these products for you if they do not have them on hand.

Product	Where to buy	How to use	Types of liquids for use
Resource Thicken Up®	nestlenutritionstore. com 1.888.240.2713 gfsmarketplace.com 1.800.968.6525 walgreens.com 1.877.250.5823	Measure recommended amount using measuring spoon to achieve desired consistency. Slowly add Thicken up® to beverage while stirring briskly for 15 s using utensil or blender on low speed. When thickening larger amounts, stir for 30 s	All hot and cold beverages
Simply Thick®	simplythick.com 1.800.205.7115 gfsmarketplace.com 1.800.968.6525	Use 1 packet for each 4 ounces of liquid, shake for 5–10 s in a closed container, or mix vigorously with a *fork* for 20–30 s. Do not shake hot or carbonated beverages	Gel-type thickener for hot and cold beverages
Thick & Easy®	homecarenutrition. com 1.888.617.3482	Add recommended amount to beverage and stir	All hot and cold beverages
Thick-it®	walgreens.com 1.877.250.5823 cvs.com 1.888.607.4287 thickitdelivered.com 1.800.778.5704	Measure recommended amount using measuring spoon. Add Thick-it® slowly and blend for 5–10 s using utensil or blender at low speed. Do not overmix	All hot and cold beverages

D. Household Thickeners

Note: To use, follow instructions for thickening on the package. If there are no directions, start by adding a teaspoon of thickener to the beverage and stir. Continue to add additional teaspoons until desired thickness is achieved

- Food starches: corn, potato, tapioca, rice
- Xanthan gum
- Arrowroot
- Pectin
- Custard powder

Conclusion

The aforementioned resources are important for practitioners and family members alike. Frequently family members would like additional information and these components will assist the clinician in providing them with a quick yet comprehensive resource list. Health care providers caring for stroke patients should be familiar with the National Dysphagia Diet, thickening agents, and the necessary adjustments to avoid drug-nutrient interactions.

References

1. de Leon-Knapp I. The effects of propofol on nutrition support. Support Line. 2009;31(6): 12–9.
2. Cook AM, Peppard A, Magnuson B. Nutrition considerations in traumatic brain injury. Nutr Clin Pract. 2008;23:608–20.
3. National Dysphagia Diet Task Force. National dysphagia diet: standardization for optimal care. Chicago, IL: American Dietetic Association; 2002. p. 10–25.

Index

M.L. Corrigan et al. (eds.), *Handbook of Clinical Nutrition and Stroke*, Nutrition and Health, DOI 10.1007/978-1-62703-380-0, © Springer Science+Business Media New York 2013

Printed by Printforce, the Netherlands